AF846815

Bullying and Victimization Across the Lifespan

Paul R. Smokowski • Caroline B. R. Evans

Bullying and Victimization Across the Lifespan

Playground Politics and Power

Springer

Paul R. Smokowski, MSW, Ph.D.
School of Social Welfare
University of Kansas
Lawrence, KS, USA

Caroline B. R. Evans
Rhode Island College
Providence, RI, USA

ISBN 978-3-030-20292-7 ISBN 978-3-030-20293-4 (eBook)
https://doi.org/10.1007/978-3-030-20293-4

© Springer Nature Switzerland AG 2019
This work is subject to copyright. All rights are reserved by the Publisher, whether the whole or part of the material is concerned, specifically the rights of translation, reprinting, reuse of illustrations, recitation, broadcasting, reproduction on microfilms or in any other physical way, and transmission or information storage and retrieval, electronic adaptation, computer software, or by similar or dissimilar methodology now known or hereafter developed.
The use of general descriptive names, registered names, trademarks, service marks, etc. in this publication does not imply, even in the absence of a specific statement, that such names are exempt from the relevant protective laws and regulations and therefore free for general use.
The publisher, the authors, and the editors are safe to assume that the advice and information in this book are believed to be true and accurate at the date of publication. Neither the publisher nor the authors or the editors give a warranty, express or implied, with respect to the material contained herein or for any errors or omissions that may have been made. The publisher remains neutral with regard to jurisdictional claims in published maps and institutional affiliations.

This Springer imprint is published by the registered company Springer Nature Switzerland AG
The registered company address is: Gewerbestrasse 11, 6330 Cham, Switzerland

This book is dedicated to our families, who provided us with invaluable inspiration and support.

Paul R. Smokowski, Ph.D.: For my belated father, Richard T. Smokowski, who was my unwavering advocate and taught me how to guide my sons, Jose and Cesar. And for my wife, Martica Bacallao, as we journey through life together.

Caroline Evans, Ph.D.: For my husband and best friend Louis, who always provides unwavering support and wise council. And for our two wonderful daughters Alia and Alena—the next generation of strong upstanders.

This book is also dedicated to:

All the people who have been bullied, you did not deserve such disrespect.

All the people who bullied others, you can break the cycle of violence and aggression.

All the people who stood by as frightened witnesses, may you find the courage to intervene.

All the people who stood up for a victim, you are everyday heroes. Some day, we will all be upstanders rather than bystanders.

Contents

About the Authors

Paul R. Smokowski, Ph.D., M.S.W., C.P. is a Professor in the University of Kansas's School of Education. He has an interdisciplinary background in social welfare, child development, and public health. Before joining KU, Dr. Smokowski was a faculty member at the University of North Carolina-Chapel Hill for 16 years. His past 15 years of work in youth violence prevention culminated in the North Carolina Youth Violence Prevention Center (NC-YVPC), a nonprofit agency specializing in helping rural communities promote healthy youth development that Dr. Smokowski directs. Dr. Smokowski's research teams have procured more than $15 million worth of federal funding from the Centers for Disease Control, the National Institute of Justice, and the National Institutes of Health. As a prolific author, he has published more than 100 articles and book chapters on issues related to risk, resilience, acculturation, adolescent mental health, family stress, and youth violence prevention. Dr. Smokowski has received national awards for his youth violence prevention research, such as the 2010 Collaborator's Award from the American Society of Group Psychotherapy and Psychodrama and the best article of the year award from the Society for Social Work Research. He served on the National Institutes of Health's Youth Violence Consortium and was a member of the inaugural class of Health Protection Research Awardees funded by the Center for Disease Control's Office of the Director. Dr. Smokowski directed the Latino Acculturation and Health Project, a multisite longitudinal study examining youth violence risk and protective factors in Latino youth, and the Entre Dos Mundos/Between Two Worlds program for helping Latino immigrant families cope with acculturation stressors. This research program culminated in Dr. Smokowski's previous book published by New York University Press titled *Becoming Bicultural: Risk and Resilience in Latino Youth.* In his current work, Dr. Smokowski is guiding the implementation and evaluation of a multilevel youth violence prevention initiative in one of the most ethnically diverse rural counties in the United States.

Caroline B. R. Evans, Ph.D. is adjunct faculty at Rhode Island College and works on a community violence prevention grant based in Tucson, AZ. Prior to this work Dr. Evans was a research associate for the North Carolina Youth Violence Prevention

Center (NC-YVPC). In this role, she helped run a youth violence prevention program funded by the National Institute of Justice and worked to disseminate research findings through conference presentations and publications. Dr. Evans graduated from the University of North Carolina at Chapel Hill in 2015 with her doctorate in social work, and during her academic tenure worked for the NC-YVPC on a youth violence prevention grant funded by the Centers for Disease Control. Dr. Evans's research focuses on youth violence, specifically childhood and adolescent bullying victimization and perpetration, bystander behavior, and aggression. She is particularly interested in youth violence prevention through evidence-based programs.

Chapter 1
Playground Politics: How the Bullying Framework Can Be Applied to Multiple Forms of Violence

1.1 Introduction

Bullying. A single word that conjures up many strong images. What comes to your mind? The traditional image of the biggest kid in the classroom stealing lunch money? Or the geeky looking boy in glasses getting stuffed into a locker? Perhaps a group of popular girls whispering and snickering around an exclusive lunch table while a left-out onlooker sits alone? Or maybe a string of mean and hurtful text messages sent day after day? Bullying comes in many shapes and sizes, and for the last two decades or so, the national spotlight on bullying has intensified. Increased media attention to bullying, frantic parents, worried school personnel, and the multiple suicides of bullied youth have spurred bullying researchers to investigate the devastating consequences of bullying and to create and test bullying intervention programs. As a result, bullying research now has a unique niche under the umbrella of violence research.

Despite the publicity and integration into our cultural consciousness, bullying often remains a "know it when you see it" phenomenon for many people. What is bullying? How is it different from aggression and violence? Where and when does it happen? Who gets victimized? Bullying is all around us and always has been. The vignettes below provide some examples of bullying at different life stages and across multiple venues.

> Jose and Ernie were at the top of the slide during playtime at preschool. Jose was a big, sturdy boy who had trouble waiting his turn. Ernie fidgeted anxiously at the top of the slide as he looked down, taking his time. Jose pushed him so that he would go faster. Ernie flew off the slide and broke his arm when he hit the ground.
>
> "Drink bleach and die." "Why don't you go kill yourself?" "You're ugly." "You should die." These are a few of the phrases 12-year-old Rebecca Sedwick heard every day for a year from at least 15 of her classmates. When the harassment moved from in person to online, there was no escape and Sedwick could not take the abuse any longer. In 2014, she jumped from a silo tower to her death.

© Springer Nature Switzerland AG 2019

P. R. Smokowski, C. B. R. Evans, *Bullying and Victimization Across the Lifespan*, https://doi.org/10.1007/978-3-030-20293-4_1

At age 10, Daniel W. Smith was routinely beaten up by his older brother. Put in a headlock or stranglehold, Smith's brother would punch him repeatedly. Fighting back made it worse, so Smith just took the beatings and waited for them to end.

Fifteen-year-old Audrie Pott hung herself in 2012 one week after being sexually assaulted by three teenage boys at a party. Instead of receiving support after the trauma of sexual assault, pictures of the assault were posted online and spread like wild fire throughout the school.

The five Ferguson siblings endured years of child abuse. Hit with baseball bats, burned with irons, starved, and forced to drink urine, the children never told the family "secret" and it took years for them to be rescued. Now, both of their parents are serving 65-year prison terms.

Eighth grader Marcus McTear started out as a loving and sweet boyfriend. But as time went on, he began to control Rae Anne Spence's every move. He dictated what she wore, forbid her to wear makeup, and punched or slapped her if she disrespected him. Spence attempted to end the relationship on multiple occasions, but McTear threatened suicide and would write loving apology notes. Almost two years later, Spence finally changed schools in order to extricate herself from this harmful relationship and McTear set his sights on 16-year-old Ortralla Mosely. In 2003, McTear stabbed Mosely to death in the hallway of their high school when Mosely tried to end their relationship.

In July 2014, 17-year-old Michelle Carter convinced her boyfriend Conrad Roy III to commit suicide via carbon monoxide poisoning. As Roy sat in his truck breathing in carbon monoxide texting Carter that he was having doubts, Carter texted, "When are you going to do it? Stop ignoring the question."

In 2011, drum major Robert Champion died after participating in a ritual called "Crossing Bus C." As Champion made his way to the back of the bus, his bandmates from the Florida A&M University marching band punched him and beat him with mallets and drumsticks. Minutes later, Champion lost his eyesight, went into cardiac arrest, and died.

Football player Tim Piazza just wanted to be accepted by the Beta Theta Pi brothers and earn a spot in the Pennsylvania State University fraternity. Surely his future brothers would look out for him and keep him safe. After drinking copious amounts of alcohol while engaging in an obstacle course called "The Gauntlet," Piazza fell down the basement stairs and lost consciousness. After being hauled to a couch, the fraternity "brothers" poured beer on Piazza and slapped him in the face to help him regain consciousness. No one called for help until 12 hours after the fall. Piazza died the next day with an estimated blood alcohol content of 0.40.

Katie fell in love with her husband quickly; they were engaged and married within 3 months. He gradually cut her off from her family and friends, and took over all of their finances, leaving Katie with little access to money and forcing her to put all big purchases on her credit card. Katie's husband had guns in the house and would constantly clean them in front of her as if to remind her of their presence and that he could use one any time he pleased. Sometimes he would slap Katie in the face or shove her around. Then one night, he beat her so badly she ended up in the ICU and he was sent to prison for 7 years.

Forty-seven-year-old Eric Donovan died of a heart attack deemed to be directly related to harassment by his supervisor, Nadine Hendricken. Hendricken constantly made hostile personal comments and was rude and demeaning towards Donovan in the presence of coworkers. Dealing with this day after day caused Donovan extreme stress, anxiety, and panic attacks that ultimately led to his death.

At 83, Barbara Jean had no children of her own and her nieces and nephews lived a few hours away, which meant she had no one to take care of her. When the caretaker of her home and lawn, Mike, offered to move in to help take care of her, Barbara Jean was elated. However, Mike gradually took over Barbara Jean's finances and stopped sending the checks she wrote to pay for her home's utility bills. When overdue notices arrived, Mike berated

Barbara Jean for forgetting to send in the money. He started stealing money from her and had her rewrite her will and became her power of attorney.

An African American girl walking in an all-white neighborhood was chased by a white man wielding a stick shouting, "Go back home!" A black man out for a run in the early morning was stopped by a policeman and held at gun point because he "looked suspicious." A group of Latino teenagers were followed closely by a store clerk as they perused the merchandise at a store, while their white counterparts browsed the aisles unencumbered. These types of events happen to people of color all the time.

In 2017, US President Donald Trump was strolling with other world leaders at the NATO conference when he shoved Dusko Markovic, the president of Montenegro, out of his way. Trump was apparently trying to reach the front row for a photograph. However, as Trump pushed Markovic aside, he uttered no apology or a polite "excuse-me," Trump did not even acknowledge Markovic's existence, it was almost as if Markovic was invisible. The leader of the most powerful country in the world rode roughshod over the president of a small country of 600,000. Trump then straightened his tie and was in the center of the picture.

What themes do you see across these examples—aggression, violence, domination, harassment, callous disrespect? Traditionally, different forms of violence have been studied in isolation. Researchers studying bullying, sibling violence, child maltreatment, teen dating violence, domestic violence, college hazing, workplace bullying, elder maltreatment, discrimination, and violence within and between larger social units (e.g., communities, countries) work in isolated silos with minimal communication (Hamby & Grych, 2013; Wilkins, Tsao, Hertz, Davis, & Klevens, 2014). These researchers all study forms of violence, however, each form of violence is viewed as a distinct entity, when in fact they are all related and interconnected (Wilkins et al., 2014). In an attempt to unite violence researches and break down the barriers between research on various forms of violence, the Centers for Disease Control and Prevention's (CDC) Division of Violence Prevention (DVP; 2016) has recently embarked on a 5-year mission to understand the interconnections between these multiple forms of violence.

The CDC's mission is rooted in the fact that different forms of violence often co-occur, indicating that all forms of violence must be understood and studied together. Violent victimization can be cumulative and youth who are victimized by one form of violence are likely to experience other forms of violence (Finkelhor, Turner, Hamby, & Ormrod, 2011; Hamby & Grych, 2013). For example, the National Survey of Children's Exposure to Violence found that 64.5% of surveyed youth reported more than one type of direct victimization and 10.9% reported five or more types of direct victimization (Finkelhor et al., 2011). Further, youth who were physically assaulted in the past year were five times as likely to have also been sexually victimized and more than four times as likely to have also been maltreated compared to non-victimized youth (Finkelhor, Turner, Ormrod, Hamby, & Kracke, 2009). The same is true of violent perpetration; individuals who have behaved violently in one context are more likely to behave violently in other contexts (Foshee et al., 2015; Herrenkohl, Sousa, Tajima, Herrnkohl, & Moylan, 2008; Klevens, Simon, & Chen, 2012); indeed, engaging in one type of aggression increases the odds of engaging in additional types of aggression from 1.5 to 4 times (Klevens et al., 2012). For example, youth who engaged in peer violence were more likely to also be violent towards their dating partners (Foshee et al., 2015) and adults who domestically abused their partners were more likely to abuse their children (See Herrenkohl et al., 2008 for a review). This means that youth who are bullied at school could be victims of other forms of violence such as child maltreatment, dating violence, or sibling violence. Likewise, youth who bully others might also be engaging in violence against their siblings or dating partners. Clearly, there are groups of perpetrators who manipulate, harass, and abuse others across multiple social contexts. There are also victims who are often abused at different times over the human life span. And even more people witness this perpetration and victimization from different distances, reacting or withdrawing—we all play a role in the bullying dynamic.

Further connecting the various forms of violence is the fact that different forms of violence have similar risk factors for perpetrators and similar consequences for victims. Perpetrator risk factors for violence span the entire ecology and include individual, family, peer, school, community, and cultural factors. For example, individual temperament (e.g., anger, poor impulse control, substance use, viewing the world as hostile), family relationships (e.g., high levels of conflict, poor parent-child relationships, economic stress), deviant peer behavior, community characteristics (e.g., disadvantaged neighborhood, neighborhood violence, low neighborhood cohesion), and societal stressors (e.g., income inequality, high rates of poverty; Foshee et al., 2015; Sumner et al., 2015) are all risk factors for violence. In terms of consequences, violent victimization, regardless of the form, can result in multiple negative outcomes including injury, sexually transmitted diseases and infections, mental health disorders (e.g., depression, anxiety, post-traumatic stress disorder, conduct disorder), eating disorders, substance use, suicidality, and death (Division of violence Prevention, 2016; See Sumner et al., 2015 for a review).

Given the multiple connections between various forms of violence, it is vital that researchers begin collaborating. Collaboration will increase researchers' ability to create wide ranging and functional intervention programs. One possible means to increase collaboration is to create a common framework through which researchers, practitioners, policy makers, and all concerned citizens can view and understand violence. We will use the bullying dynamic as a framework through which to view and understand multiple forms of violence at different ages and stages and within diverse contexts. Applying the bullying dynamic to multiple forms of violence provides a nuanced understanding of the power relationships inherent in violent behavior, providing a new and innovative way of viewing violence across the life span.

1.2 The Definition of Bullying

"I know it when I see it." These words were uttered by Supreme Court Justice Potter Stewart in 1964 in the case Jacobellis v. Ohio. This phrase has become somewhat of a colloquial expression that attempts to define something subjective that lacks a clear definition. Many school personnel, parents, and youth take this approach when it comes to identifying bullying and as a result, behaviors are often mislabeled as bullying. A certain amount of aggression and conflict is normative. This is not to say that such behavior should be tolerated or condoned, but children and adolescents have conflicts and arguments and are sometimes mean to one another. Being left out or pushed on the playground once or twice, while not pleasant, does not constitute bullying. However, these isolated behaviors are often erroneously labeled as bullying, especially by adults (e.g., parents, school personnel) who themselves were bullied as children. The example of Jose and Ernie on the preschool slide ended very badly, with Ernie's arm broken and Jose expelled from preschool. The event, and the intense arguments among the adults involved, would define much of their childhood experiences. But it was not bullying. It was a poor decision made by a preschooler paired with physical force that was not adequately controlled.

Being bullied often leaves permanent scars and results in a hypersensitivity or a bullying radar of sorts. Adults who were bullied as children might be overly sensitive to bullying and therefore overreact to any form of interpersonal conflict they witness. This inclination to label minor aggressive interactions as bullying might be especially strong for parents who witness or hear about their own child being hassled at school, especially if the parent was bullied. Thus, when a child comes home saying he/she was pushed on the playground or excluded from a particular lunch table, parents often storm into school, demand a meeting with the principal, and report that their child is being bullied. In reality, their child has experienced one of the painful and unpleasant realities of growing up. If, however, the pushing or exclusion continues day after day, labeling the behavior as bullying and demanding school intervention are certainly warranted.

Conversely, depending upon how parents and school personnel envision and define bullying, they might neglect to intervene in behaviors that actually are bullying, especially with more covert forms of bullying such as rumor spreading or cyberbullying. If adults are desensitized to bullying or believe that bullying is a rite of passage or a normal part of growing up, they can easily fail to recognize when bullying is right in front of them or they could recognize it but not intervene. Perhaps some adults who were bullied as children, rather than becoming hypersensitive to bullying, believe that bullying is a normal part of life and helps toughen kids up. Adults might also believe that kids should work through conflicts on their own and therefore refrain from intervening. Covert forms of bullying like nasty looks, whispered rumors, or mean text messages are easy to slip past adults and a lack of adult response could simply be due to ignorance that the bullying is even occurring. Further, bullying can be difficult to define and identify because it depends upon the victim's reactions and interpretations. Bottom line: relying on "I know it when I see" to define bullying situations is much too subjective and leads to people incorrectly identifying or ignoring bullying situations or failing to intervene when intervention is necessary and warranted. It follows that there is a need for a standardized and widely accepted definition of bullying.

However, difficulty arises because researchers, practitioners, and policy makers often define bullying differently. In fact, the three national surveys on bullying all provide slightly different definitions of bullying (see below in Sect. 1.4 on prevalence rates). Because researchers use inconsistent definitions of bullying, prevalence rates of bullying differ across studies, making comparisons difficult (Gladden, Vivolo-Kantor, Hamburger, & Lumpkin, 2014). While there is no standardized definition of bullying, bullying researchers generally rely on three, distinct, defining features of bullying established by international bullying researcher Dan Olweus (1993):

1. *repetition*—bullying occurs repeatedly over time;
2. *power imbalance*—the perpetrator has more social and/or physical power than the victim; and
3. *intent to harm*—the perpetrator engages in aggression that is intended to physically and/or emotionally harm the victim (Olweus, 1993).

These definitional criteria were recently expanded by the CDC to include three additional key elements: bullying is unwanted, occurs between youth who are not siblings or dating partners, and likely causes the victim distress or harm (Gladden et al., 2014).

Although the above definition is helpful in terms of identifying bullying, it is important to discuss the ambiguity imbedded within the definition. First, the criteria of repetition should be addressed. In general, bullying is repeated over time, however, certain one-time aggressive acts are so egregious they could and should be defined as bullying; however, under the current definition a singular event would not be defined as bullying (Evans & Smokowski, 2016; Finkelhor, Turner, & Hamby, 2012). For example, during the 2012 US presidential race, it came to light that when Republican candidate Mitt Romney was a senior in high school, he incited a group of five friends to forcibly hold down underclassman John Lauber. While Lauber struggled and yelled for help, Romney cut off his ponytail. Lauber reported being haunted by this traumatic incident decades later (Horowitz, 2012), while Romney claimed to have no memory of the event (Bazelon, 2012). Although this was a seemingly single event, the intensity and cruelty surpassed an act of aggression and should be labeled as bullying (Evans & Smokowski, 2016). The term bullying denotes severe and intense aggression and to avoid labeling horrendous one-time events as bullying fails to impart to the perpetrator, victim, and bystanders the seriousness of the event. In the proceeding chapters, we will include intense one-time events that are intended to cause physical or psychological harm to the victim, such as the hazing that killed Robert Champion in the example at the beginning of this chapter, as bullying.

However, the difficulty with expanding the definition of bullying to include single events, is that identifying what single events are horrendous enough to be labeled as bullying is subjective. Given the above discussion about the difficulty adults have in correctly identifying and labeling bullying, disagreement could also arise about whether a specific one-time act of interpersonal aggression constitutes bullying. There is no easy way to solve this conundrum except to say that certain single acts of aggression, like forcibly cutting off someone's ponytail, cross a line from routine aggression to bullying. Being shoved on the playground once should not be considered bullying, but being tied up to a tree with a jump rope at recess and left is a different story. Below, we have amended the definition of bullying to say that it "usually" occurs repeatedly over time; this subtle change in wording gives youth, parents, school personnel, practitioners, and researchers the leeway to identify particularly horrible one-time events as bullying.

Power imbalance is the second part of the definition of bullying that requires additional explanation as this concept is quite complex and difficult to define. For example, sources of power might not align: "If a stronger but less popular girl repeatedly intimidates a weaker but popular boy, is the controlling dimension popularity, gender, or physical strength?" (Finkelhor et al., 2012, p. 272). To further complicate issues, if the girl is from a high socioeconomic status (SES) family and is dressed in trendy and desirable clothing and the boy comes from a low SES family and is wearing worn out hand-me-down clothing, income becomes another dimension of power. The difficulty with the concept of power imbalance is that the significance depends upon the victim's perceptions (Evans & Smokowski, 2016). If the girl's physical strength and high SES status cause the boy to feel powerless and afraid, then he might perceive the girl to have more power and could view her repeated harassment as bullying. However, if the boy is sufficiently popular among his classmates and is supported by a group of friends and/or feels more powerful than the girl due to being a male, than he might not be intimidated by the girl's physical strength and flashy clothing; in this case, the boy would perceive his social power and gender to be more salient than the girl's physical strength and SES and he might view her taunting as harmless and not define it as bullying. Further, once an act of aggression has begun, the act itself can create a power differential where the perpetrator has more power than the victim. However, the aggressive act could have created this power differential or exacerbated an existing power differential (Finkelhor et al., 2012). There is not an easy solution for the complexities inherent in defining and recognizing a power differential. We highlight these intricacies because it is important for adults witnessing bullying to be aware of and attend to dynamics of power. School personnel should try to understand how students involved in bullying dynamics view the distribution of power; talking with students about power imbalance is a vital step that adults should take to help better understand the bullying dynamic. Power differentials are central to the other forms of violence that we will discuss throughout this book and are actually often more clear cut than the power differential in a bullying dynamic (e.g., the power differential between a parent and child is very clear cut).

In terms of the three additional definitional components added by the CDC, we argue that violence between siblings and dating partners can and should be defined as bullying (to be discussed later). The CDC also added in the definitional component that bullying likely causes harm to the victim. The only foreseeable way bullying would not harm the victim is if the victim had a developmental disability that prevented him/her from understanding the content of the bullying. However, even if this was the case, the presence of the bullying would harm bystanders by potentially making them feel scared and unsafe and would also contribute to a negative school culture and climate. Therefore, it is more accurate to define bullying by saying that bullying causes harm to one or all of the following: victim; bystanders; and the culture and climate of the environment in which the bullying takes place. However, we agree with the CDC that bullying is always unwanted and that this should become part of the formal definition of bullying.

For the purpose of this book, we will rely on a combination of Olweus's and the CDC's definition of bullying. Bullying is: ***Unwanted behavior* that occurs between a more *powerful* perpetrator(s) and weaker victim and *usually* occurs *repeatedly* over time; the behavior is *intended to harm* the victim and does *cause harm* to the victim, bystanders, and/or culture and climate within the environment where the bullying occurs**. We will often refer to the "bullying dynamic" because of the public nature of bullying events that often include witnesses and bystanders. Bullying is not usually a discreet phenomenon between a perpetrator and victim; it has large group effects on the social networks within the environment where it occurs.

Throughout this book, we will apply this definition of bullying to various forms of interpersonal violence across the life span including violence at home (i.e., sibling violence, child maltreatment), violence in intimate partner relationships (i.e., teen dating violence, domestic violence), college hazing, work place bullying, elder maltreatment, discrimination (i.e., minority-majority group level bullying), and higher level bullying (e.g., conflict between communities and countries). Each of these forms of violence display the majority of the above defining characteristics of bullying (i.e., unwanted, power differential, repeated over time, intended to harm, causes harm), however, they are not generally understood or examined in light of the bullying dynamic.

Before addressing each of these forms of violence, it is important to fully understand the bullying dynamic. In the remainder of this chapter, we will discuss forms of bullying and the scope of the problem in the USA and worldwide; explain the economic cost of bullying; and provide some recommendations for practitioners and school personnel. Chapter 2 discusses the roles in the bullying dynamic and provides a theoretical explanation for why bullying occurs. Chapter 3 addresses the short- and long-term consequences of bullying victimization with special attention to mental and behavioral health, neuroscience, peer relationships, cumulative victimization, longitudinal studies, and trauma. Chapter 4 focuses on bystanders in the bullying dynamic with a discussion of prosocial and antisocial bystanders, and Chap. 5 discusses cyberbullying. Each of the remaining chapters of the book focuses on a specific form of violence and applies the aforementioned bullying definition in order to understand the violent dynamics in a new and innovative way. Chapter 6 discusses bullying in childhood at home and includes an overview of child maltreatment as well as sibling violence; Chap. 7 looks at hazing in college and applies the bullying framework to this form of interpersonal violence; Chap. 8 delves into violence in intimate partner relationships and discusses teen dating violence as well as intimate partner violence; Chap. 9 reviews bullying in adulthood and discusses workplace harassment and bullying; Chap. 10 focuses on elder maltreatment and defines this problem as one of bullying; Chap. 11 examines bullying at a higher level between groups, corporations, communities, and countries with attention on how racial discrimination and hatred can actually be considered a form of bullying; and Chap. 12 provides an overarching concluding summary, focusing on bullying prevention and intervention strategies.

1.3 Forms of Bullying

Bullying includes direct aggressive behaviors that occur in the presence of the victim and indirect aggressive behaviors that occur when the victim is not present but are still intended to cause harm. Direct and indirect bullying behaviors are classified into four types:

1. Physical bullying is physical force intended to harm the victim such as hitting, kicking, or pushing.
2. Verbal bullying is oral or written communication like name calling, teasing, or threatening.
3. Relational bullying is any action intended to harm the victim's reputation and social relationships such as spreading rumors, excluding, or making embarrassing images of the victim public through the internet, cellphones, or other means.
4. Bullying by property damage includes stealing and/or destroying the victim's property (Gladden et al., 2014).

The Centers for Disease Control and Prevention (CDC; Gladden et al., 2014) consider electronic bullying to be a form of verbal and relational bullying executed using electronic means (e.g., e-mail, instant messaging, chat rooms, websites [e.g., Facebook, Twitter], gaming sites, cell phones [e.g., applications such as Instagram, Snapchat, text messages]) to harass, insult, exclude, and/or ostracize victims. Electronic bullying includes behaviors ranging from harassing text messages or pictures sent via cellphone to creating defamatory websites intended to embarrass or humiliate the victim (Kowalski, Limber, & Agatston, 2012; Raskaukas & Stoltz, 2007).

These forms of bullying behavior occur everywhere, regardless of social class, geography, age, or gender. National assessments throughout the USA, and some across the globe, unfortunately reveal that over one fifth of middle and high school-aged youth are victims of bullying. The prevalence climbs dramatically when perpetrators, bully/victims, and bystanders are added up to capture the full bullying dynamic. Consequently, we use the phrase "playground politics" to describe the bullying dynamic because this behavior often has its roots in jockeying for social status in early to middle childhood. Yet the aggressive, hierarchical politics we often learn on the school playground commonly extend to adverse interactions across the life span.

1.4 Prevalence of Bullying Nationally and Internationally

National prevalence rates of bullying in the USA come from three major sources: the Health Behavior of School-Aged Children Survey (HBSC), the School Crime Supplement (SCS), and the Youth Risk Behavior Surveillance System (YRBSS). Each source provides a different definition of bullying, measures bullying differently (i.e., yes/no response versus multiple response options), and assesses bullying across different age ranges (i.e., middle school only, middle and high school, high school only) resulting in slightly different prevalence rates. Further, only one study (HBSC) assesses bullying perpetration as well as victimization (See Table 1.1 for a summary of the three survey results).

The HBSC is a cross-national survey that began in 1983/1984 with five participating countries. The next year (1985/1986), participation increased to 13 countries. Following 1986, the HBSC was administered every 3 years and in the ensuing decades participation gradually increased until the most recent HBSC (2013/2014), which included 42 countries. The USA began participating and providing national data in 1997/1998 and provided data in 2001/2002, 2005/2006, and 2009/2010, but did not participate in the most recent HBSC survey (2013/2014; WHO, 2016). However, the USA did participate in the 2009/2010 HBSC survey which defined bullying as,

> We say a student is being bullied when another student, or a group of students, say or do nasty and unpleasant things to him or her. It is also bullying when a student is teased repeatedly in a way he or she does not like or when he or she is deliberately left out of things. But it is not bullying when two students of about the same strength or power argue or fight. It is also not bullying when a student is teased in a friendly and playful way (World Health Organization, 2012).

This definition touches on repetition, power imbalance, and negative behaviors but in a very cursory manner. First, this definition states that teasing is done repeatedly but does not state that other negative behaviors (e.g., hitting, rumor spreading) must be repeated for a behavior to be defined as bullying. Second, power is not defined and power imbalance is not mentioned; it is not clear that the perpetrator has more power than the victim. Third, very limited examples of bullying behaviors are provided and no examples of cyberbullying or physical bullying are provided. In addition, harm to the victim is not mentioned. Further, who determines if the teasing is being done in a friendly and playful way? If the perpetrator intends the teasing to be a joke, but the victim takes offense, would the HBSC definition consider the behavior to be bullying? The limitations of this definition could impact how youth answer the survey questions and could account for the relatively low rates of bullying victimization that the HBSC found.

HBSC respondents were limited to youth ages 11, 13, and 15. Participants were asked if they had been bullied at least twice in the past couple of months and response options ranged from zero to several times per week. In addition, the HBSC asked if youth had bullied others. In the USA, 13% of 11-year-old girls and 15% of 11-year-old boys reported being bullied; these rates dropped to 12% of 13-year-old girls and 13% of 13-year-old boys and 7% of 15-year-old girls and 6% of 15-year-old boys. In terms of bullying others 3% of 11-year old girls and 8% of boys reported bullying others at least twice in the past couple of months. These rates increased to 8% of 13-year-old girls and 10% of 13-year-old boys and 6% of 15-year-old girls and 9% of 15-year-old boys (World Health Organization, 2012).

Table 1.1 Rates of victimization across national studies

	Health behavior of school-aged children survey (HBSC)	School crime supplement (SCS)	High school youth risk behavior surveillance system (YRBSS)	Middle school youth risk behavior surveillance system (YRBSS)
N	6274	2317	15,448	67,825
Sample age	11-, 13-, 15-years	6th–12th Grade	9th–12th Grade	6th–8th Grade
Overall % victimized	N/A	20.8%	20.2%	Lowest-Rhode Island: 38.0% Highest-West Virginia: 53.4%
Female	N/A	22.8%	24.8%	Lowest-Rhode Island: 44.6% Highest-West Virginia: 60.9%
Male	N/A	18.8%	15.8%	Lowest-Rhode Island: 31.9% Highest-West Virginia: 44.4%
6th Grade	Female: 13% Male: 15%	31.0%	N/A	Lowest-Rhode Island: 38.1% Highest-West Virginia: 50.7%
7th Grade	N/A	25.5%	N/A	Lowest-Rhode Island: 38.1% Highest-West Virginia: 50.7%
8th Grade	Female: 12% Male: 13%	22.2%	N/A	Lowest-Rhode Island: 35.4% Highest-West Virginia: 53.5%
9th Grade	N/A	19.0%	23.4%	N/A
10th Grade	Female: 7% Male: 6%	21.2%	20.8%	N/A
11th Grade	N/A	15.8%	20.3%	N/A
12th Grade	N/A	14.9%	15.9%	N/A
African American	N/A	24.7%	13.2%	Lowest-Maine: 28.7% Highest-Virginia: 43.0%
Asian	N/A	15.6%	14.8%	Lowest-Vermont: 31.1% Highest-Hawaii: 43.5%
Caucasian	N/A	21.6%	23.5%	Lowest-Rhode Island: 39.6% Highest-New Mexico: 53.4%

(continued)

Table 1.1 (continued)

	Health behavior of school-aged children survey (HBSC)	School crime supplement (SCS)	High school youth risk behavior surveillance system (YRBSS)	Middle school youth risk behavior surveillance system (YRBSS)
Hispanic/ Latino	N/A	17.2%	16.5%	Lowest-Delaware: 32.9% Highest-Hawaii: 50.9%
Multiple Races	N/A	N/A	25.8%	Lowest-Hawaii: 45.1% Highest-Maine: 61.4%

The 2015 SCS provided a slightly more comprehensive definition of bullying that more accurately highlights the three definitional components established by Olweus (1993):

> Bullying happens when one or more students tease, threaten, spread rumors about, hit, shove or hurt another student. It is not bullying when students of about the same strength or power argue or fight or tease each other in a friendly way. Bullies are usually stronger, or have more friends or more money, or some other power over the student being bullied. Usually, bullying happens over and over, or the student being bullied thinks it might happen over and over (National Center for Education Statistics, 2015).

This definition provides examples of power imbalance and explains that power imbalance is present in a bullying dynamic. A diverse array of bullying behaviors are presented, which gives respondents a comprehensive template of how to define bullying in their own lives. However, this definition does not mention intent to harm and does not state that the victim is harmed.

Participants were asked a series of yes or no questions about whether they were bullied in the current school year and if it was verbal, physical, or social bullying. Youth were then asked how often they were bullied and where the bullying occurred, if they told an adult, how much the bullying impacted various aspects of their life (e.g., work, health), and why they were bullied (e.g., race, religion; National Center for Education Statistics, 2015). The SCS survey was administered to 2317 students in grades 6 through 12 and findings indicated that 20.8% of the sample reported being bullied in the 2014–2015 school year. A slightly higher percentage of females (22.8%) reported being bullied compared to males (18.8%) and in general, rates decreased from sixth grade through middle school and high school. In terms of race, 21.6% of White youth reported being bullied, compared to 24.7% of black youth, 17.2% of Hispanic/Latino youth, and 15.6% of Asian youth (U.S. Department of Education, 2016).

Finally, the most recent YRBSS (CDC, 2015a, 2015b) provided a more cursory definition of bullying:

> Bullying is when 1 or more students tease, threaten, spread rumors about, hit, shove, or hurt another student over and over again. It is not bullying when 2 students of about the same strength or power argue or fight or tease each other in a friendly way.

This definition does provide a comprehensive array of examples of bullying behavior but, similar to the HBSC definition, fails to fully explain the concept of power imbalance and does not discuss the harm caused to the victim. Two questions asked youth if they had been bullied or electronically bullied on school property in the year preceding the survey with a yes/no response option. About 15,448 US high school students were surveyed and 20.2% reported being bullied in the year before the survey; a significantly higher percentage of females (24.8%) endorsed being bullied compared to males (15.8%). Bullying decreased across high school from 23.4% in ninth grade to 15.9% in 12th grade (CDC, 2015a).

The YRBSS also collected data from 67,825 middle school youth from 11 states; due to the small state response rate, no national middle school prevalence rate is available. State rates of bullying victimization ranged from 52.4% in West Virginia to 38.0% in Rhode Island. Across all 11 states females were significantly more likely to report being bullied compared to males. Nine states collected data from all three middle school grades and in one (Vermont) a significantly higher percentage of seventh graders reported being bullied compared to sixth graders (sixth grade 45.8% versus seventh grade 48.1%) and eighth graders (seventh grade 48.1% versus eighth grade 44.8%), but in the other eight states there were no significant differences between sixth and seventh graders, between sixth and eighth grade, or seventh and eighth graders in terms of victimization rates (CDC, 2015b. See Table 1.1 for states with the highest and lowest percentages).

In summary, the USA national prevalence rates for bullying vary slightly across the three aforementioned studies. According to the SCS and YRBSS rates of bullying victimization for high school alone and middle and high school combined are about 20%. Rates for middle school youth from the HBSC survey are slightly lower and range from 6% to 15%. However, these rates might be conservative and, as discussed above, could also be impacted by the limitations in the definitions of bullying that were provided. Other studies, including meta-analyses, have found higher rates of bullying. For example, a meta-analysis of 80 studies of traditional and cyberbullying in middle and high school found a prevalence rate of 35% for traditional bullying and 15% for cyberbullying (Modecki, Minchin, Harbaugh, Guerra, & Runions, 2014). Further, when specific forms of bullying are assessed, prevalence rates are higher. For example, the 2005/2006 version of the HBSC assessed specific forms of bullying and found that in a sample of 7182 youth in Grades 6 through 10, 41% reported being the victim of relational bullying, 37% were verbal victims, 13% were physical victims, and 10% were electronic victims (overall prevalence adds to 70%, but some victims experience multiple forms of bullying; Wang, Iannotti, & Nansel, 2009). In a study of 1874 youth across 14 middle- and high-schools in North Carolina, 50% reported being verbally bullied, 29% were physically bullied, and 13% reported cyberbullying (Turner, Exum, Brame, & Holt, 2013). It is possible that assessing specific forms of bullying is more straightforward for youth because they are being asked about a specific behavior as opposed to bullying in general, which is very broad. Taken together, findings indicate that at least one fifth of US middle and high school students have been bullied and as many as two fifths to half have been relational and/or verbal victims, but rates could be higher in certain geographic regions (e.g., study conducted in North Carolina; Turner et al., 2013). The middle school YRBSS rates shown in Table 1.1 underscore bullying victimization as nothing less than a public health epidemic, with a low of 38% of youth in Rhode Island and 54% of middle schoolers in West Virginia reporting victimization. Figure 1.1 displays rates of high school bullying victimization by state. These high school rates are lower than the middle school rates. Further, these rates are only reports from victims, adding bullies and bystanders would substantially increase these rates. There is one inescapable conclusion from examining the map; bullying is everywhere. We cannot consider this as an urban crises or one happening in some states but not others. Moving the family to Alaska is not likely to help. Combined with the negative long-term consequences of victimization that we discuss in Chap. 3, these rates should alarm all parents, educators, psychologists, social workers, public policymakers, and anyone who cares about America's children.

The variation in victimization rates across age groups found in the three national studies is worth mentioning. According to the SCS, high school YRBSS, and the HBSC, rates of bullying decrease across middle and high school. Perhaps as youth mature and gain more sophisticated social skills they are able to relay on these skills as opposed to bullying to navigate complex social situations. It is also possible that when youth transition to middle school (in sixth or seventh grade depending upon the school system) that rates of bullying are high as they jockey for social standing. Perhaps early on in middle school, bullying is used as a means of establishing a social pecking order and as social positions solidify across middle and high school, bullying becomes less necessary as a means of establishing dominance because the pecking order is established. In this explanation, the damage is already done in middle school and high school roles are largely set. It is also possible that bullying changes forms as youth age. Perhaps traditional bullying between peers (e.g., physi-

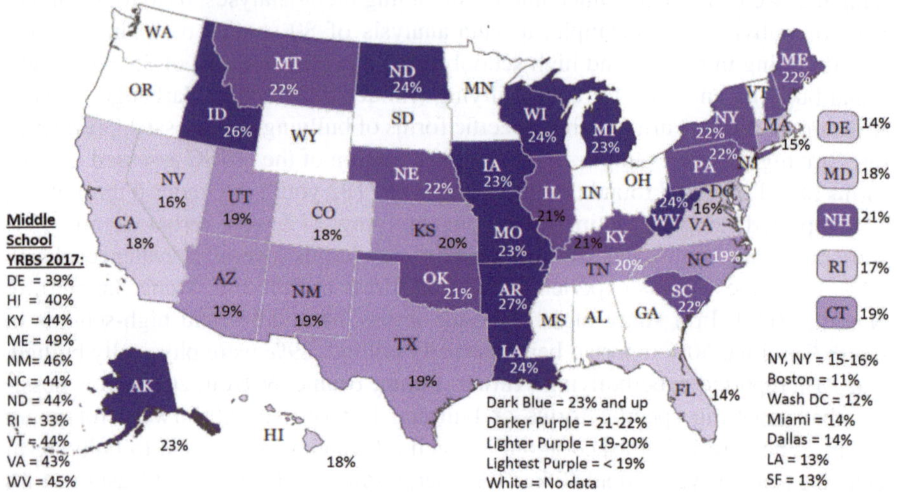

Fig. 1.1 Percent Reporting Being Bullied on School Property in last 12 Months. High School YRBS 2017, CDC data

cal pushing and hitting, rumor spreading) decreases and other forms of bullying like dating violence increase and in a sense replace traditional bullying. Rather than taking their aggression out on their peers, youth who bully might set their sights on dating partners. Indeed, according to the YRBSS, rates of dating violence increased across high school with 8.1% of ninth graders, 9.6% of tenth graders, 10.1% of 11th graders, and 10.5% of 12th graders reporting physical dating violence (CDC, 2015a). Youth might not consider or label dating violence as bullying and therefore do not endorse bullying victimization when they are victimized by dating partners. Thus, it appears that rates of bullying decrease as youth age, but it could just be that the bullying takes a different form (e.g., dating violence) that youth fail to recognize and label as bullying.

It is also interesting to examine bullying internationally as rates of bullying victimization and perpetration vary across countries. The 2013/2014 HBSC found that rates of bullying victimization were highest in Lithuania where 29% of 11-year-old girls and 35% of 11-year-old boys; 29% of 13-year-old girls and 31% of 13-year-old boys; and 22% of 15-year-old girls and 29% of 15-year-old boys reported being bullied at school at least two or three times per month in the past couple of months. Rates for 11-year-olds (3% of girls, 4% of boys), and 13-year-olds (1% of girls, 4% of boys) were lowest in Armenia and for 15-year-olds were lowest in Iceland (1% of girls, 2% of boys; World Health Organization, 2016). For bullying perpetration, rates were highest for 11-year-old girls in Latvia (14%) and highest for 11-year-old boys in Greenland (26%); rates for 13-year-old girls and boys was highest in Latvia (20% girls and 33% boys); and for 15-year-old girls rates were highest in Latvia (19%) and for 15-year-old boys were highest in Lithuania (34%). For 11-year-old girls rates were lowest in Sweden and Iceland (0%) and lowest for 11-year-old boys in Sweden, Iceland, and Malta (2%); rates for 13-year-old girls and boys were lowest in Iceland (0% of girls, 1% of boys); rates were lowest for 15-year-old girls in Sweden, England, Italy, Ireland, and Norway (1%) and lowest for boys in Ireland and Sweden (3%). See Table 1.2 for rates of 13-year-old bullying victimization and perpetration across countries.

It is interesting to consider what factors contribute to the different rates of bullying victimization and perpetration across the world. Perhaps countries with an inherent power imbalance imbedded within their society (i.e., social inequality) are more prone to bullying; that is, countries with a very unequal distribution of resources and power where there is a large gap between the "haves" and the "have nots" might foster a culture of bullying. Or perhaps overall levels of life satisfaction and happiness impact bullying. For example, Lithuania has the highest suicide rates in Europe (Tamosiunas, Reklaitiene, Virvicute, & Sopagiene, 2006) and also the highest rate of bullying victimization and one of the highest rates of bullying perpetration (World Health Organization, 2016). Lithuania has a long and traumatic history of subjugation and only obtained independence from the Soviet Union in 1990. This history of historical trauma no doubt lingers and perhaps plays a role in the high rates of bullying victimization and perpetration.

It is interesting to note that for 13-year-old youth (Table 1.2), for all countries listed, bullying perpetration rates were higher for boys than for girls and in 30 coun-

Table 1.2 Rates of bullying victimization and perpetration for 13-year-old youth by Country

	Bullying victimization age 13	Bullying perpetration age 13
Lithuania	Girls: 29% Boys: 31%	Girls: 18% Boys: 31%
Latvia	Girls: 24% Boys: 26%	Girls: 20% Boys: 33%
Belgium (French)	Girls: 16% Boys: 26%	Girls: 9% Boys: 12%
Austria	Girls: 17% Boys: 21%	Girls: 10% Boys: 26%
Russian Federation	Girls: 15% Boys: 21%	Girls: 14% Boys: 24%
Estonia	Girls: 13% Boys: 19%	Girls: 7% Boys: 16%
Bulgaria	Girls: 15% Boys: 17%	Girls: 11% Boys: 17%
Scotland	Girls: 18% Boys: 13%	Girls: 2% Boys: 3%
Wales	Girls: 15% Boys: 16%	Girls: 2% Boys: 4%
Ukraine	Girls: 15% Boys: 15%	Girls: 10% Boys: 17%
Portugal	Girls: 14% Boys: 16%	Girls: 7% Boys: 12%
Canada	Girls: 17% Boys: 13%	Girls: 3% Boys: 5%
Romania	Girls: 12% Boys: 16%	Girls: 14% Boys: 23%
Greenland	Girls: 13% Boys: 15%	Girls: 15% Boys: 18%
Republic of Moldova	Girls: 12% Boys: 14%	Girls: 10% Boys: 16%
Poland	Girls: 10% Boys: 15%	Girls: 7% Boys: 15%
France	Girls: 12% Boys: 13%	Girls: 8% Boys: 12%
USA[a]	Girls: 12% Boys: 13%	Girls: 8% Boys: 10%
Luxembourg	Girls: 12% Boys: 11%	Girls: 10% Boys: 14%
England	Girls: 12% Boys: 11%	Girls: 2% Boys: 4%
Germany	Girls: 12% Boys: 10%	Girls: 6% Boys: 13%
Switzerland	Girls: 11% Boys: 11%	Girls: 5% Boys: 13%

(continued)

Table 1.2 (continued)

	Bullying victimization age 13	Bullying perpetration age 13
Finland	Girls: 11% Boys: 11%	Girls: 1% Boys: 6%
Former Yugoslav Republic of Macedonia	Girls: 10% Boys: 12%	Girls: 5% Boys: 13%
Israel	Girls: 5% Boys: 16%	Girls: 4% Boys: 13%
Hungary	Girls: 10% Boys: 11%	Girls: 2% Boys: 6%
Slovakia	Girls: 9% Boys: 12%	Girls: 13% Boys: 15%
Malta	Girls: 8% Boys: 12%	Girls: 1% Boys: 6%
Croatia	Girls: 8% Boys: 11%	Girls: 5% Boys: 12%
Belgium (Flemish)	Girls: 7% Boys: 11%	Girls: 3% Boys: 6%
Slovenia	Girls: 8% Boys: 10%	Girls: 6% Boys: 13%
Albania	Girls: 8% Boys: 10%	Girls: 11% Boys: 14%
Netherlands	Girls: 8% Boys: 9%	Girls: 4% Boys: 6%
Ireland	Girls: 7% Boys: 8%	Girls: 1% Boys: 2%
Greece	Girls: 9% Boys: 6%	Girls: 6% Boys: 13%
Norway	Girls: 6% Boys: 7%	Girls: 0% Boys: 3%
Czech Republic	Girls: 5% Boys: 7%	Girls: 2% Boys: 4%
Denmark	Girls: 7% Boys: 5%	Girls: 3% Boys: 6%
Spain	Girls: 5% Boys: 7%	Girls: 4% Boys: 8%
Iceland	Girls: 6% Boys: 5%	Girls: 1% Boys: 2%
Italy	Girls: 6% Boys: 5%	Girls: 3% Boys: 5%
Sweden	Girls: 6% Boys: 4%	Girls: 2% Boys: 3%
Armenia	Girls: 1% Boys: 4%	Girls: 2% Boys: 6%

Order of countries goes from the highest to the lowest rates of bullying victimization
[a]Rate from 2009/2010 HBSC

tries boys reported higher rates of victimization compared to girls, whereas in ten countries girls had higher rates (rates of victimization between boys and girls were equal in three countries). This suggests that worldwide, boys are more prone to involvement in the bullying dynamic than girls. However, the HBSC survey did not assess for specific forms of bullying, which would have changed the results as girls are often more involved in verbal and relational bullying while boys tend be more physically oriented. Table 1.2 illustrates the bullying victimization and bullying perpetration rates across countries; although data are available for ages 11, 13, and 15, we have opted to include only age 13 for simplicity. Although rates of bullying vary across countries, states, and age groups, it is easy to see that the bullying dynamic is a universal phenomenon across the globe with more severe manifestations in some places over others.

1.5 The Economic Impact of Bullying

The negative impact of bullying on victims, perpetrators, and the overall school climate and culture is widely discussed in the research literature (and will be discussed in Chap. 3). However, an often overlooked impact of bullying is the enormous economic toll it takes on schools and society as a whole. In 2010, an estimated 160,000 students missed school each day due to bullying (Bully Statistics, 2010). Given that the federal government reimburses schools based on average daily attendance (Phillips, 2011), the decreased attendance due to bullying translates into decreased federal funding for schools. Thus, the suspensions, expulsions, truancy, and dropping out of school related to bullying result in thousands of lost dollars for schools. For example, in a fictional school with 1000 students, a 12% dropout rate would translate into $2,160,000 in lost federal funding (Kemp-Graham & Hendricks, 2015; Phillips, 2011). Considering the high percentage of youth both in the USA and worldwide who are involved in the bullying dynamic, it follows that many of these youth miss school. Victims are often fearful and skip school to avoid further harassment, and perpetrators are suspended or expelled for their harmful behavior, which translates into hundreds of thousands of lost federal funding dollars for schools.

In addition to the loss of school funding, bullying causes increased medical costs. It is well documented that victimized youth suffer from poor mental health in the short and long term (Aluede, Adeleke, Omoike, & Afen-Akpaida, 2008; Nazir & Piskin, 2015; Ttofi, Farrington, & Losel, 2012; Ttofi, Farrington, Losel, & Loeber, 2011) and thus might require additional mental health care services with extreme societal cost. In 2015, mental health services cost an average of $3384 per person under age 18 (Center for Financing, Access and Cost Trends, Agency for Healthcare Research and Quality, Medical Expenditure Panel Survey, 2015). The high percentage of youth victimized by bullying who suffer from the ensuing poor mental health, likely require additional mental health services, resulting in increased cost to society. In 2016, there were 49.7 million youth in the USA between the ages of 6 and 17. If 20% of this group was victimized, then 9.94 million youth required mental health service at an average cost of $3384 per child. That represents a potential cost of $33,636,960,000 for society each year due to bullying victimization just for mental health services.

Overall, the societal cost of bullying is exorbitant. A cost–benefit model examining a cohort of high schools students 25 years after graduation compared the societal cost for those who were not bullied with those who were bullied or bullied others in high school. The model considered employment, justice system involvement, and reliance on public assistance. Findings indicated that per year, an individual who bullied others cost society an additional $951,327 compared to someone not engaged in bullying and an individual who was bullied cost an additional $461,668 per year (Highmark Foundation, n.d.). Once again, with 49.7 million youth in the USA in 2016, we can estimate 20% were victimized (9,940,000 victims) and 15% were bullies (7,455,000 perpetrators). Thus, there is an estimated annual perpetration cost of $7 trillion (7,455,000 × 951,327 = 7, 092,142,785,000). The estimated annual victimization cost is $4.5 trillion (9,94 0,000 × 461,668 = 4,588,979,920,000). Consequently, it is reasonable to estimate that society spends approximately $11.5 trillion on the bullying dynamic each year.

1.6 Practitioner and School Recommendations

If a practitioners and/or schools wish to assess the issue of bullying in a clinical or school setting, we have specific recommendations based on past research and our discussion of the definition of bullying. Using a survey (as opposed to individual interviews or focus groups) is the most expeditious manner in which to collect large amounts data and information on bullying related behaviors. It is vital to ensure that participants filling out the survey have a clear understanding of the definition of bullying. We therefore suggest providing participants with the definition of bullying we include in this chapter as well as providing some examples of bullying. Following the definition provided in this chapter we suggest stating that bullying includes actions like physical violence (hitting, kicking, pushing), threatening, teasing, name-calling, ignoring, rumor spreading, sending hurtful e-mails or text messages, and/or leaving someone out on purpose (Evans & Smokowski, 2016). We suggest then providing participants with a list of possible ways in which they might have been victimized and then a separate list of ways in which they might have bullied others. Items assessing each type of bullying (physical, verbal [including electronic bullying], relational, and property damage) should be included. Items should be rated on a Likert scale that includes response options of Never, 1–2 times, 3–10 times, and more than ten times.

Victimization items should include the following:

1. Someone at school harmed me physically, for example, by pushing, shoving, or hitting me.
2. Someone at school told lies or spread rumors about me.
3. Someone at school made fun of or picked on me.
4. Someone at school called me mean names.
5. Someone at school excluded me or made me feel left out.
6. Someone at school stole my money or possessions or damaged something I own.
7. Someone at school sent me mean messages (text message or e-mail) or pictures on my cell phone or over the Internet.
8. Someone spread rumors about me or sent a hurtful picture of me to other people over the Internet or cell phone.

Bullying items should include the following:

1. I harmed someone at school physically by pushing, hitting, or kicking them.
2. I told lies or spread rumors about someone at school.
3. I made fun of or picked on someone at school.
4. I called someone at school mean names.
5. I excluded someone at school or made them feel left out.
6. I stole someone's money or possessions or damaged something that belongs to someone else at school.
7. I sent someone mean messages (text message or e-mail) or pictures to their cell phone or over the internet.
8. I spread rumors about someone or sent a hurtful picture of them to other people over the internet or cell phone.

In addition to assessing the ways in which youth are bullied or bully others, it is also important to gather information on why youth perceive they were bullied or why they decided to bully others.

Reasons why youth perceived they were bullied:

1. I was bullied because of my race/ethnicity.
2. I was bullied because of my religion.
3. I was bullied because people think I'm gay/lesbian/bisexual/queer/questioning/transgender or I am gay/lesbian/bisexual/queer/questioning/transgender.
4. I was bullied because I have a disability.
5. I was bullied because I am overweight.
6. I was bullied because of something else about my body or my physical appearance.
7. I was bullied because of the way I dress.
8. I was bullied because I do well in school.
9. I was bullied because I do not do well in school.
10. I was bullied for some other reason. Explain ________________

Reasons why youth bullied others:

1. I bullied someone because of their race/ethnicity.
2. I bullied someone because of their religion.
3. I bullied someone because I think they are gay/lesbian/bisexual/queer/questioning/transgender.
4. I bullied someone because they have a disability.
5. I bullied someone because they are overweight.
6. I bullied someone because of something else about their body or physical appearance.
7. I bullied someone because of the way they dress.
8. I bullied someone because they do well in school.
9. I bullied someone because they do not do well in school.
10. I bullied someone for some other reason. Explain ______________

Following these suggested guidelines will provide a comprehensive picture of the bullying dynamic in a clinical or school setting. Ensuring that all participants fully understand the definition of bullying prior to filling out the survey is key. If possible, we suggest having an open dialogue with participants to discuss the nuances of the provided definition of bullying thus ensuring that all participants are on the same page when it comes to defining bullying.

1.7 Conclusion

Various forms of violence are often studied in isolation. The purpose of this book is to use the bullying dynamic as a universal framework to understand violence across the life span. In order to accomplish this goal, bullying will be defined as *unwanted behavior* that occurs between a more *powerful* perpetrator(s) and weaker victim and *usually* occurs *repeatedly* over time; the behavior is *intended to harm* the victim and does *cause harm* to the victim, bystanders, and/or culture and climate within the environment where the bullying occurs. It is clear that bullying is a serious problem in the USA and directly impacts 20–50% of youth; in fact, almost every student in a school worldwide is negatively impacted by the presence of bullying. Although the power imbalance in the bullying dynamic is fundamental to the definition of bullying, it can be ambiguous and difficult to identify. The concept of power imbalance is central to other forms of violence discussed throughout this book and will be addressed in later chapters. We have provided practitioners, school personnel, or anyone else who wants to assess bullying with some important guidelines for a comprehensive assessment. We now turn our attention to theoretical explanations of bullying by examining the roles in the bullying dynamic and why youth are bullied and bully others.

References

Aluede, O., Adeleke, F., Omoike, D., & Afen-Akpaida, J. (2008). A review of the extent, nature, characteristics, and effects of bullying behaviour in schools. *Journal of Instructional Psychology, 35*, 151–158.

Bazelon, E. (May 10, 2012). How bad was Mitt Romney's prep school bullying? *Slate*. Retrieved from http://www.slate.com/articles/news_and_politics/bulle/2012/05/romney_s_bullying_how_bad_was_the_vicious_incident_reported_by_the_washington_post_html

Bully Statistics. (2010). *Bullying statistics 2010*. Retrieved from www.bullyingstatistics.org

Center for Financing, Access and Cost Trends, Agency for Healthcare Research and Quality, Medical Expenditure Panel Survey. (2015). *Medical expenditure panel survey (MEPS) summary data tables – Household component*. Rockville, MD: Agency for Healthcare Research and Quality. Retrieved from https://meps.ahrq.gov/mepstrends/hc_cond/

Centers for Disease Control and Prevention. (2015a). *Youth risk behavior surveillance system: High school YRBSS*. Atlanta, GA: Author. Retrieved from https://nccd.cdc.gov/youthonline/

Centers for Disease Control and Prevention. (2015b). *Youth risk behavior surveillance system: Middle school YRBSS*. Atlanta, GA: Author. Retrieved from https://nccd.cdc.gov/youthonline/

Division of Violence Prevention. (2016). *Preventing multiple forms of violence: A strategic vision for connecting the dots*. Atlanta, GA: Division of Violence Prevention, National Center for Injury Prevention and Control, Centers for Disease Control and Prevention.

Evans, C. B. R., & Smokowski, P. R. (2016). Understanding weaknesses in bullying research: How school personnel can help strengthen bullying research and practice. *Children and Youth Services Review, 69*, 143–150.

Finkelhor, D., Turner, H., Hamby, S., & Ormrod, R. (2011). *Polyvictimization: Children's exposure to multiple types of violence, crime, and abuse*. Washington, DC: U.S. Department of Justice, Office of Justice Programs, Office of Juvenile Justice and Delinquency Prevention.

Finkelhor, D., Turner, H. A., & Hamby, S. (2012). Let's prevent peer victimization, not just bullying. *Child Abuse & Neglect, 36*, 271–274.

Finkelhor, D., Turner, H. A., Ormrod, R., Hamby, S. L., & Kracke, K. (2009). *Children's exposure to violence: A comprehensive national survey*. Washington, DC: U.S. Department of Justice, Office of Justice Programs, Office of Juvenile Justice and Delinquency Prevention.

Foshee, V. A., Reyes, L. M., Tharp, A. T., Chang, L., Ennett, S. T., Simon, S. T., … Suchindran, C. (2015). Shared longitudinal predictors of physical peer and dating violence. *Journal of Adolescent Health, 56*(1), 106–112.

Gladden, R. M., Vivolo-Kantor, A. M., Hamburger, M. E., & Lumpkin, C. D. (2014). *Bullying surveillance among youths: Uniform definitions for public health and recommended data elements, Version 1.0*. Atlanta, GA: National Center for Injury Prevention and Control, Centers for Disease Control and Prevention and U.S. Department of Education.

Hamby, S., & Grych, J. (2013). *The web of violence: Exploring connections among different forms of interpersonal violence and abuse*. New York, NY: Springer Briefs in Sociology.

Herrenkohl, T. I., Sousa, C., Tajima, E. A., Herrnkohl, R. C., & Moylan, C. A. (2008). Intersection of child abuse and children's exposure to domestic violence. *Trauma, Violence, & Abuse, 9*(2), 84–99.

Highmark Foundation. (n.d.). *The cost benefit of bullying prevention: A first-time analysis of savings*. Pittsburgh, PA: Author. Retrieved from https://www.highmarkfoundation.org/pdf/publications/HMK_Bullying%20Report_final.pdf

Horowitz, J. (May 10, 2012). Mitt Romney's prep school classmates recall pranks, but also troubling incidents. *Washington Post*. Retrieved from http://www.washingtonpost.com/politics/mitt-romneys-prep-school-classmates-recall-pranks-but-alsotroubling-incidents/2012/05/10/gIQA3WOKFU_story.html

Kemp-Graham, K. Y., & Hendricks, L. (2015). The socio-emotional and financial costs of bullying. *Journal of Bullying and Social Aggression, 1*(1). Online.

Klevens, J., Simon, T. R., & Chen, J. (2012). Are the perpetrators of violence one and the same? Exploring the co-occurrence of physical aggression in the United States. *Journal of Interpersonal Violence, 27*(10), 1987–2002.

Kowalski, R. M., Limber, S. P., & Agatston, P. W. (2012). *Cyberbullying: Bullying in the digital age*. Malden, MA: Wiley-Blackwell.

Modecki, K. L., Minchin, J., Harbaugh, A. G., Guerra, N. G., & Runions, K. C. (2014). Bullying prevalence across contexts: A meta-analysis measuring cyber and traditional bullying. *Journal of Adolescent Health, 55*, 602–611.

National Center for Education Statistics. (2015). *School crime supplement to the national crime victimization survey 2015 questionnaire*. Washington, DC: U.S. Department of Commerce Economics and Statistics Administration. Retrieved from https://nces.ed.gov/programs/crime/student_questionnaires.aspcrime/pdf/student/SCS2015.pdf

Nazir, T., & Piskin, M. (2015). School bullying: Effecting child's mental health. *The International Journal of Indian Psychology, 2*(4), 130–135.

Olweus, D. (1993). *Bullying at school: What we know and what we can do*. Malden, MA: Blackwell.

Phillips, R. (2011). *The financial costs of bullying, violence, and vandalism*. Reston, VA: National Association of Secondary Principals: Leading Schools. Retrieved from http://community-matters.org/downloads/SLATE%20magazine.%20Financial%20Cost%20of%20Bullying,%20Violence%20and%20Vandalism%20Feb%202011.pdf

Raskaukas, J., & Stoltz, A. D. (2007). Involvement in traditional and electronic bullying among adolescents. *Developmental Psychology, 43*(3), 564–575.

Sumner, S. A., Mercy, J. A., Dahlberg, L. L., Hillis, S. D., Klevens, J., & Houry, D. (2015). Violence in the United States: Status, challenges, and opportunities. *Journal of American Medical Association, 314*(5), 478–488.

Tamosiunas, A., Reklaitiene, R., Virvicute, D., & Sopagiene, D. (2006). Trends in suicide in Lithuanian urban population over the period 1984-2003. *BMC Public Health, 6*, 184–190.

Ttofi, M., Farrington, D. P., & Losel, F. (2012). School bullying as predictor of violence later in life: A systematic review and meta-analysis of prospective longitudinal studies. *Aggression and Violent Behavior, 17*, 405–418.

Ttofi, M. M., Farrington, D. P., Losel, F., & Loeber, R. (2011). Do victims of school bullies tend to become depressed later in life? A systematic review and meta-analysis of longitudinal studies. *Journal of Aggression, Conflict, and Peace Research, 3*(11), 63–73.

Turner, M. B., Exum, M. L., Brame, R., & Holt, T. J. (2013). Bullying victimization and adolescent mental health: General and typological effects across sex. *Journal of Criminal Justice, 41*(1), 53–59.

U.S. Department of Education. (2016). *Student reports of bullying: Results from the 2015 School Crime Supplement to the National Crime Victimization Survey*. Washington, DC: National Center for Education Statistics. Retrieved from https://nces.ed.gov/pubs2017/2017015.pdf

Wang, J., Iannotti, R. J., & Nansel, T. R. (2009). School bullying among adolescents in the United States: Physical, verbal, relational, and cyber. *Journal of Adolescent Health, 45*(4), 368–375.

Wilkins, N., Tsao, B., Hertz, M., Davis, R., & Klevens, J. (2014). *Connecting the dots: An overview of the links among multiple forms of violence*. Atlanta, GA; Oakland, CA: National Center for Injury Prevention and Control, Centers for Disease Control and Prevention; Prevention Institute.

World Health Organization. (2012). *Social determinants of health and well-being among young people-Health behavior in school-aged children (HBSC) study: International report from the 2009/2010 survey*. Geneva: Author. Retrieved from http://www.euro.who.int/__data/assets/pdf_file/0003/163857/Social-determinants-of-health-and-well-being-among-young-people.pdf

World Health Organization. (2016). *Growing up unequal-Gender and socioeconomic differences in young people's health and well-being: Health Behavior in school-aged children (HBSC) Study: International Report from the 2013/2014 survey*. Geneva: Author. Retrieved from http://www.euro.who.int/__data/assets/pdf_file/0003/303438/HSBC-No.7-Growing-up-unequal-Full-Report.pdf?ua=1

Chapter 2
Roles Youth Play in the Bullying Dynamic and Theoretical Explanations for Why Bullying Happens

2.1 Introduction

Bullying is a complex dynamic with multiple participants. Figure 2.1 is a drawing made by a sixth grade boy about his experience being bullied. The drawing expertly captures the multiple roles inherent in the bullying dynamic. The victim is clearly in a powerless position, on the floor, begging for his book bag to be returned. He is experiencing public humiliation, pleading for the bully to stop. What are the psychological consequences of this type of interpersonal traumatic event? The abuse is carried out in front of the victims' peers who cheer the bully on, except for one potential friend willing to help him up. Will his social relationships ever heal? Will his sense of self-esteem and personal efficacy to impact his environment develop? The victim cannot even trust the adult in the room, the teacher on the right-hand side, who is saying, "Oh Lord!" and not intervening in any effective way. It is likely that the emotional impact of this event will linger in the victim's mind for months, years, or possibly decades.

The perpetrator in the drawing is central, powerful, and not just standing, but with arms wide and savoring his plundered backpack. He has a helper and a cheering section of peers, an audience watching his dominating performance. What are the consequences for this bully perpetrator? He does not fear the teacher who wants to avoid dealing with this behavior. The harsher he becomes, the more power he reaps from the event. This is a drama where he is the star.

The crowd of bystanders provides an electric energy for the bullying event; it is a social event with winners and losers, which raises the stakes dramatically for both bullies and victims. This is a social process; one that can hardly be avoided if you are a student in that classroom or that school. A small minority of one student offers to help the victim as a prosocial bystander. The main negative bystander contributes to the bully perpetrator's power in tormenting the victim (e.g., "Crybaby! Stop crying, little girl!"). The rest of the class laughs or cheers, embracing the experience or, embodied by the teacher, trying to avoid the scene. All of these actors experience

© Springer Nature Switzerland AG 2019

P. R. Smokowski, C. B. R. Evans, *Bullying and Victimization Across the Lifespan*, https://doi.org/10.1007/978-3-030-20293-4_2

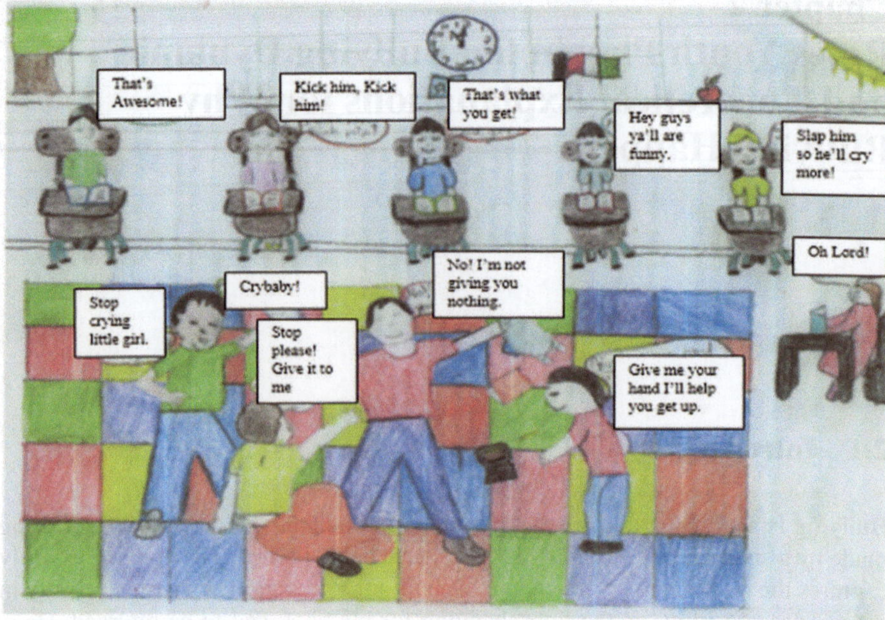
That's Awesome!
Kick him, Kick him!
That's what you get!
Hey guys ya'll are funny.
Slap him so he'll cry more!
Oh Lord!
Crybaby!
No! I'm not giving you nothing.
Stop crying little girl.
Stop please! Give it to me
Give me your hand I'll help you get up.

Fig. 2.1 Victimization portrait by sixth grade male

consequences that impact their personal psychology, their social processes, and the shared context. In this chapter, we explore these roles within the bullying dynamic and theories to help explain why bullying occurs and is so hard to eradicate. In Chap. 3, we explore the diverse bioecological consequences of the bullying dynamic.

2.2 Roles in the Bullying Dynamic

The roles in the bullying dynamic are consistent across place and time. Youth can be actively involved in the bullying dynamic as a perpetrator (i.e., bullying others), a victim (i.e., bullied by others), or a bully-victim (i.e., alternates between bullying others and being a victim) or more passively involved as a bystander who offers varying degrees of support to the perpetrator or victim (Salmivalli, 2010). Regardless of a child's role in the bullying dynamic, the presence of bullying in a school has a negative impact on the entire student body, with the most pernicious impact being on those students who are most directly involved in the bullying. Each of the roles in the bullying dynamic is discussed below.

Youth who bully others are typically aggressive. However, it is important to remember that this does not just refer to physical aggression but also includes verbal and relational aggression as well. Relationally aggressive children and adolescents who bully others might never physically harm a peer, but their malicious rumors, spiteful looks, and pernicious whispers can do just as much harm as a slap in the face. As noted in Chap. 1, youth who bully are also often powerful; this power is social and comes from relegating the victim to a lower social standing but also comes from other sources as well. For example, physically larger youth often bully others, thus physical size provides a source of power. Having a lot of money, which provides access to the best clothing and technology, is also a source of power that might give youth the confidence to bully others.

It is interesting to consider what motivates youth to bully others. Bullying others is often a means to an end, with the desired goal being social power or status. Indeed, research suggests that while kids do not always like their peers who bully, they view them as popular (Cillessen & Mayeux, 2004; Prinstein & Cillessen, 2003). Liking a peer and viewing him/her as popular do not always go hand in hand. Popularity refers to social power and youth who have social power and are seen as popular are not always liked. This makes sense in light of the fact that bullying tactics might be used to gain popularity; the peer group dislikes these aggressive perpetrators but also views them as powerful and popular. Bullying others could also be a way to prevent one's own bullying; bullies are viewed as tough and strong, and classmates might be hesitant to mess with someone who is physically or verbally aggressive. It is also possible that if youth feel that their social position is at risk or that they might become a victim, they lash out and proactively bully others to establish dominance and prevent themselves from being bullied. Finally, it is possible that some youth like causing others pain and that bullying others actually gives them pleasure. Between 2% and 6% of youth under 18 are thought to be "fledgling psychopaths," that is they lack empathy, guilt, and remorse (Fersch, 2006) and might find it easy and/or enjoyable to cause others harm. Indeed, bullying is an early warning sign of psychopathic tendencies (Fersch, 2006). According to his journal writings, Eric Harris, one of the Columbine shooters, fell into this category and seemed to enjoy hurting others (Langman, 2009a) and prior to the shooting at Columbine, bullied and harassed some of his classmates (Langman, 2009b).

Victims are typically insecure and anxious and often have something about their physical body, clothing, speech, or behavior that makes them easy targets. The North Carolina Youth Violence Prevention Center (NC-YVPC) collected data from over 5000 middle- and high-school students from two counties in North Carolina on bullying related experiences. Table 2.1 illustrates the most common reasons youth were bullied and bullied others. The highest percentage of youth were bullied due to their race/ethnicity (17.3%), something about their body (16.4%), being overweight (13.9%), and their clothing (13.0%). Similarly, in the School Crime Supplement (SCS) sample (discussed in Chap. 1), the highest percentage of youth were bullied due to their appearance (26.9%) and race (10.1%).

Indeed, youth who do not fit in with the rest of their peers are easy targets. Other research confirms that overweight youth are often victimized. In one study of 1555 high school students, 84% witnessed overweight students being teased and 65–77% observed overweight peers being ignored, avoided, excluded, or having rumors spread about them (Puhl, Luedicke, & Heuer, 2011). Sexual orientation is also a common reason youth are bullied. The 2013 National School Climate Survey found

Table 2.1 Percentage of NC-YVPC and SCS participants who reported being victimized or bullying others for specific reasons

	SCS victimized[a]	NC-YVPC victimized[b]	NC-YVPC bullied others[b]
Race/(Ethnicity; NC-YVPC)	10.1%	17.3%	3.8%
Ethnic origin	6.9%	N/A	N/A
Religion	3.7%	8.6%	3.1%
Sexual orientation	3.4%	9.8%	6.0%
Disability	4.4%	5.9%	3.5%
Gender	6.7%	N/A	N/A
Appearance	26.9%	N/A	N/A
Overweight	N/A	13.9%	6.3%
Something else about body	N/A	16.4%	4.9%
Clothing	N/A	13.0%	6.2%
Do well in school	N/A	10.8%	3.5%
Do poorly in school	N/A	7.4%	4.4%

[a]Items were dichotomous yes/no and percentages refer to the percentage of the 2317 participants who endorsed yes (National Center for Education Statistics, 2015)
[b]Percentages refer to once, sometimes, or often being victimized or bullying others for a specific reason; data comes from year 7 of the NC-YVPC study $N = 3363$

that 74.1% of LGBT students were verbally bullied (e.g., called names, threatened), 16.5% were physically bullied (e.g., punched, kicked), and 49.0% were electronically bullied (e.g., via text messages or Facebook) in the past year due to their sexual orientation (Kosciw, Greytak, Palmer, & Boesen, 2014). Race/ethnicity is also a contributing factor to bullying victimization and more African American youth (25%) were bullied compared to Caucasian youth (22%; U.S. Department of Education, 2016). North America has a long history of racial tension dating back at least to 1619 when the first 20 African slaves were brought over by a Dutch ship to the British colony of Jamestown, Virginia. Throughout the last 400 years, racism has been a pressing issue ripe with complex power dynamics that might get played out in bullying dynamics. Discrimination against immigrant groups is strongly integrated in this dynamic (Smokowski & Bacallao, 2010; this will be discussed further in Chap. 10). Youth who look different from their peers might already feel powerless and being bullied further strips them of power and confidence. Victims of bullying respond in various ways to being bullied. Some become depressed, anxious, and isolated, while others bully weaker classmates in an attempt to regain social power; these youth are referred to as bully-victims.

Bully-victims, also referred to as reactive bullies or proactive victims (Smokowski & Kopasz, 2005), are youth who bully others but are also bullied themselves. The difficulty with the concept of a bully-victim is that there are nuances to this category that have not yet been researched. For example, there are likely subsets of bully-victims: there are bully-victims who are bullied and victimized equally (balanced bully-victim), there are those who are predominately victimized but bully others occasionally (predominately victimized bully-victim), and then there are those who predominantly bully others but are occasionally victimized (predominately bullying bully-victims). These three distinct groups are all bully-victims but might vary widely in their developmental outcomes and reasons for bullying others/being bullied, yet research on bully-victims looks at all bully-victims as one group regardless of the amount of time spent bullying or being victimized. Further, youth can be mislabeled as bully-victims, when in reality they are victims simply trying to protect themselves via self-defense. For example, a victim who responds to being bullied with aggressive self-defense (e.g., hits or kicks their bully) might erroneously be labeled as a bully-victim. This child could be a bully-victim or he/she could be reactively aggressive (i.e., an aggressive response to provocation) or could be at his/her wits end and feels that lashing out aggressively is the only way to end his/her bullying. Further research is needed to more clearly delineate the different subtypes of bully-victims and to further distinguish reactively aggressive victims from victims responding with self-defense from true bully-victims.

The final role in the bullying dynamic encompasses bystanders. The importance of bystanders captured the nation's attention following the brutal 1964 murder of Catherine Susan (Kitty) Genovese, which was supposedly witnessed by 38 of her neighbors who took no action to help her. Although the details of the story have been disputed (maybe far fewer than 38 witnesses were present, two neighbors reported that they called the police although there is no record of the calls, and one neighbor supposedly ran to comfort the dying Genovese), the lessons of the story live on even decades later. Shortly after this horrific incident, social psychologists began studying the bystander effect: the social phenomenon that witnesses to an event requiring intervention are less likely to provide assistance if other actual or perceived people are present (Howard, Landau, & Pryor, 2013). Bullying almost always occurs when others are present; in fact, bystanders are present for almost 90% of bullying episodes, making bystanders of central importance to the bullying dynamic (Atlas & Pepler, 1998; Hawkins, Pepler, & Craig, 2001). There are three basic roles bystanders can play: (1) prosocial bystanders intervene to support the victim; (2) negative bystanders perpetuate the bullying by joining in or verbally supporting the perpetrator; and (3) inactive bystanders passively observe the bullying without taking any action. Although there is limited research on bystander behavior, findings indicate that 17–20% of middle school bystanders behave in a positive way and support the victim (Salmivalli, Lappalainen, & Lagerspetz, 1998). This means that the vast majority of bystanders support the bully or stand idly by. What might impact a bystander's proclivity to support the victim versus jumping on the bully's bandwagon? The social psychology of this bullying dynamic remains largely unanswered, but below we will offer theories to help explain bullying behavior.

Youth who feel supported by a loyal cadre of friends might have the confidence and courage to confront the bully. Part of the danger of confronting the bully is becoming the next victim, but if youth are confident that their friends will stand by them no matter what, then even if the bully lashes out at them, their friends will have their back and they will not become a social pariah. Youth who have been bullied in the past and remember how painful it is or youth who have high levels of empathy and can easily imagine how horrible it must be to be bullied might be likely to jump in and support the victim. Conversely, youth who have been bullied before might want to avoid being bullied again and could therefore decide to support the bully in an effort to garner his/her respect and avoid becoming victimized again. Or these youth could quietly witness the bullying, the fear of becoming victimized again keeping them quiet. Improving bystanders' self-efficacy is one key step to increasing prosocial bystander intervention. If youth are taught how to intervene and stop bullying this might increase their self-efficacy and make them more likely to step in and support the victim (Thornberg et al., 2012). Bystanders are discussed in more depth in Chap. 4.

2.3 Group Sociometry and the Bullying Dynamic: The Playground Politics of Forming Social Hierarchies

There is a strong consensus among developmental psychologists that peer groups have a significant, pervasive impact on individual social, emotional, and behavioral functioning and adjustment, especially in larger social settings (i.e., in schools, neighborhoods, youth groups; Rubin, Chen, Coplan, & Buskirk, 2005). Researchers have studied childhood peer group formation for more than 70 years. According to Fine (1987), peer groups teach children about cooperative activity, how to pursue collective goals, social skills for leading and following other children, how to control hostility towards other group members, and how to mobilize aggression towards others outside the group in order to promote the group the child belongs to. With such key social learning happening in childhood peer groups, it is important to understand how peer groups function and how children relate to peers in different ascribed roles.

Urie Bronfenbrenner (1943) defined sociometry as "a method for discovering, describing, and evaluating social status, structure, and development through measuring the extent of acceptance or rejection between individuals in groups" (p. 364). Sociometric testing is widely used by developmental psychologists as a measure of childhood adjustment because the testing methods are clear-cut, easy to administer, reliable, can be predictive of adaptive and maladaptive outcomes in both social (Parker, Rubin, Erath, Wojslawwowicz, & Buskirk, 2006) and academic domains (Poulin & Dishion, 2008; Véronneau & Vitaro, 2007; Williams & Gilmour, 1994). Most sociometric studies have been conducted in schools because schools are not only the environment in which children spend substantial time but also the context in which children are exposed to a stable peer group.

Sociometric popularity, also referred to as acceptance, is the extent to which an individual is liked or disliked by his or her peer group (Asher & Coie, 1990). One method of assessing sociometric popularity uses *peer nominations* rating that ask youth to nominate or choose the three peers they like most and three peers they like least (e.g., Bell-Dolan, Foster, & Sikora, 1989). The next step in the sociometric testing is to tally the peer nominations to form groups of students based on the number of "like most" and "like least" nominations. These aggregate scores can be used to create sociometric categories (e.g., rejected, popular, controversial, neglected, and average) or a continuous index of peer status (e.g., acceptance, rejection, social preference). For example, a student with many "like least" nominations would be rejected, a student with many "like most" nominations would be popular, a student with a mixture of both nominations would be controversial, a student with no nominations would be neglected, and a student with a few nominations of either type would be average.

Along with sociometric popularity, researchers have defined the concept of perceived popularity. Perceived popularity is based on reputation rather than children choosing each other as in sociometric popularity and is measured by asking youth to nominate the peers they perceive as being the most popular and least popular (Cillessen & Rose, 2006). Perceived popularity is important. A youth can be perceived as being popular by the peer group; however, the youth does not get chosen by others on sociometric criteria and may even be disliked. This is the case for some antisocial teenagers who are perceived as popular due to their dominance and visibility but could be disliked by classmates. Yet popular-antisocial youth mainly socialize with other antisocial youths (Rubin et al., 2005).

A second sociometric measurement strategy of *peer rating* is similar to peer nomination but is more comprehensive. Whereas peer nomination considers only the three most preferred and the three least preferred classmates, other researchers have used Likert scales, ranging from 3-point to 7-point scales, that ask participants to rate how much they like each of their classmates (e.g., Parker & Asher, 1993). In this strategy, students can also use a Likert scale to give their responses to other specific criteria such as how much they like to "spend time with" or "work with" each child in the class. Categorization is based on two dimensions: social preference and social impact. Preference ratings are determined by the extent to which the child was liked or disliked by peers, and impact ratings describe the child's social salience or visibility (Coie, Dodge, & Coppotelli, 1982). Preference and impact scores can be calculated using the nomination totals, and children are categorized into a sociometric status group based on those scores.

Many studies have documented the relationships between sociometric status and adolescents' antisocial behavior and academic achievement (Cillessen & Mayeux, 2004; Véronneau & Vitaro, 2007). One commonly accepted classification system assigns a child to one of six sociometric status groups: popular, rejected, neglected, controversial, average, and other (Coie et al., 1982). We use this classification system as a guide to review existing knowledge on sociometric status and bullying. As shown in Table 2.2, we have defined these groups and delineated risk and protective factors inherent in each classification.

Table 2.2 Sociometric classifications and bullying

Sociometric category	Definition	Risk factors	Protective factors	Relationship to bullying
Popular	Many peers like and few dislike the child; the child displays high visibility and preference in the group. Two subgroups: popular-prosocial and popular-antisocial.	These children may feel the need to protect their high status. Popular-antisocial children seek dominance and status. May use status in negative ways (e.g., to exclude others).	Popular-prosocial behavior, respect for authority and rules, helpfulness, engagement in interactions with peers, intelligence, adult protection. High levels of social skills.	Popular-prosocial children may be positive bystanders helping victims or just witness bullying. Under stress, popular-antisocial children may engage in relational aggression. May bully others if their popularity is threatened. Bully others for dominance.
Average	Some peers like and some dislike the child; the child displays mid-range visibility and preference in the group.	These children may feel the need to protect the relationships they have. They may seek more popularity and fear becoming controversial, neglected, or rejected.	Peer support from the friends they have, moderate level of social skills.	Witnesses to bullying. These children may not intervene because they fear becoming the next victim.
Controversial	Many peers both like and dislike the child; High visibility; mid-range preference. Child may take risks or speak out in unconventional ways.	Disruptive, aggressive behavior, the child's friends may also be controversial.	Possess leadership skills, may have friends. May have resilience and rebellious spirit.	May become bully-victims. When victimized by bullies, the child may seek other children to bully. May engage in relational aggression. May stir controversy by spreading rumors, starting conflicts.

(continued)

Table 2.2 (continued)

Sociometric category	Definition	Risk factors	Protective factors	Relationship to bullying
Neglected	Few peers like or dislike the child; low visibility. Child may withdraw or hide during group interactions. He or she may want to interact but does not know how.	Unsociable, prefer solitary play, engage in fewer verbal interactions with peers, ignored by peers. Low levels of social support.	May or may not be lonely, may have one or two reliable friends. Child may be sensitive, creative, and unconventional. May have a dynamic inner life to compensate for interpersonal difficulties.	At high risk for becoming victims. Easy targets with little capacity for retaliation. Low social support to protect from victimization.
Rejected	Few children like and many dislike the child; high visibility and low preference in the group; lack popularity but may not be entirely friendless or isolated. Two subgroups identified—rejected-withdrawn and rejected-aggressive.	Lack of social skills, inappropriate behavior, anxiety, aggression, immaturity, hyperactivity, impulsivity, having a disability, less intelligent, underlying disturbance.	Rejected-withdrawn children may cope by hiding, may have a dynamic inner life. Rejected-aggressive children may have some friends. These friends may be older and engaged in delinquent or deviant behavior.	Rejected-withdrawn—Worry about being victimized and/or humiliated, are easy targets, are often victims Rejected-aggressive—Tend to be bullies.

2.3.1 *Popular Status*

Children classified as popular received many positive nominations and received few, if any, negative nominations. Children considered to be popular are skilled in initiating and maintaining positive relationships. They are able to adopt the frame of reference of groups they are joining, do not draw negative attention to themselves or talk exclusively about themselves (Putallaz & Wasserman, 1990). Popular children tended to demonstrate prosocial behavior, were helpful and considerate, respected authority and rules, and actively engaged in interactions with their peers without disrupting ongoing group activities (Coie, Dodge, & Kupersmidt, 1990; Coie & Kupersmidt, 1983). These children prefer cooperative strategies, negotiation, and compromise during conflict (Rubin et al., 2005). Further, the popularity of some students appears to be based on their athletic or academic competence (Dunn, Dunn, & Bayduza, 2007; Newcomb, Bukowski, & Pattee, 1993). Researchers have found a positive relationship between a child's intelligence and popularity among peers (Czeschlik & Rost, 1995). Popular status children tended to have adult support from both teachers and parents, indicating that they were socially competent in building diverse relationships.

Researchers found two subgroups of children considered popular. Along with the socially competent, prosocial group described above, there emerged a second group of popular antisocial children who were dominant, aggressive, stuck-up, manipulative, unkind, and not trustworthy. These popular antisocial children were focused on social prestige and influence, material possessions, personal attainment, glamour, and appearance (Adler, Kless, & Adler, 1992; Parkhurst & Hopmeyer, 1998). Popular-antisocial boys were defiant of authority, challenged rules, and received more discipline while popular-antisocial girls used exclusionary tactics to limit access to their social circles and bullied others through relational aggression (Adler et al., 1992; LaFontana & Cillessen, 2002; Rodkin, Farmer, Pearl, & Van Acker, 2000; Rubin, 2002).

2.3.2 Rejected Status

Children classified as rejected status received few, if any, positive nominations and many negative nominations. These children are distinguished from those in the neglected group in that rejected children are actively disliked by their peers. However, despite rejected children's lack of popularity and general acceptance, researchers have indicated that these children are seldom entirely friendless or completely isolated (Cadwallader, 2000/2001). Further, the rejected category typically contains two subgroups: children who are rejected for being overly aggressive and children who are rejected for being withdrawn or immature. However, most peers express a dislike for both subgroups. In addition, researchers have suggested that peer rejection was negatively related to intelligence and that rejected children are likely to be at risk for later adjustment difficulties (Asher & Coie, 1990; Asher & Parker, 1989; Czeschlik & Rost, 1995; Kupersmidt, Coie, & Dodge, 1990; Putallaz, 1983).

Withdrawn-rejected children, who are disliked by peers, were found to be at risk for becoming victims of bullying. However, rejected children also tended to become bullies if they were physically larger than other children and relied on aggressive behavior to respond to social situations (i.e., rejected-aggressive children). Rejected status children seemed to be a heterogeneous group usually divided into rejected-aggressive and rejected-withdrawn subgroups. Nearly half of rejected children (40–50%) were perceived by their peers as aggressive, whereas 10–20% of rejected children were perceived by their peers as socially withdrawn (Cillessen, van IJzendoorn, van Lieshout, & Hartup, 1992). The rejected-aggressive group was described as "impulsive, disruptive, dishonest, hypersensitive, and non-cooperative" (Cillessen et al., 1992, p. 902). In contrast, children in the rejected-withdrawn group were active-isolates, rather immature and socially unskilled children who wanted to play with others but were usually unable to find willing partners (Harrist, Zaia,

Bates, Dodge, & Petit, 1997). These children often became withdrawn as a result of their rejection. Rejected-withdrawn children tend to think poorly of their own social skills and have negative cognitions that hamper them in social situations (e.g., "I can't join the group. Other kids will not like me."). In contrast rejected aggressive children tend to overestimate their social competence and peer acceptance (Rubin et al., 2005). Further, rejected-withdrawn children reported loneliness in childhood and adolescence, whereas rejected-aggressive youth did not report loneliness. Indeed, rejected-aggressive youth tend to form friendships with other aggressive children and instead of feeling lonely and internalizing social difficulties like the rejected withdrawn kids, the aggressive youth often subgroup into an antisocial peer hierarchy (Cairns & Cairns, 1994).

In the research conducted to date, these two rejected subtypes have applied more to rejected boys than to rejected girls. Moreover, in examining peer-rejected girls, French (1990) found that two further subgroups emerged based on deviant behavior. The more deviant group was characterized by withdrawal, anxiety, and low academic functioning whereas the less deviant group was distinguished by behavior disorders, aggression, and self-control deficits relative to popular girls (French, 1990). Therefore, although aggression appeared to be the most common reason for rejection among boys, withdrawal distinguished rejected girls. In addition, the presence of aggression differentiated the subgroups of rejected boys, whereas the presence of internalizing disorders seemed to differentiate the subgroups of rejected girls (French, 1990).

On the whole, however, rejected children tended to be less sociable than average children (Newcomb et al., 1993). In addition, those in the rejected status tended to be perceived by peers as lacking positive qualities to balance unfavorable reputations and were viewed as lacking friendships (Newcomb et al., 1993). Compared to popular children, rejected children reported significantly higher feelings of loneliness and lower levels of athletic ability (Dunn et al., 2007). Despite this characterization, rejected children were not entirely alone (Cairns, Cairns, Neckerman, Gest, & Gariepy, 1988). Some research has suggested that although rejected children have a social network, they engaged in lower levels of social participation as compared with average children (Newcomb et al., 1993). Other researchers have offered an alternate scenario in which rejected children commonly formed subgroups, banding together in a counterculture with the covert message, "If I'm not 'good enough,' then I can be 'bad enough.'" In terms of family, rejected children, similar to neglected children, tend to have parents who rely on authoritarian parenting styles (Franz & Gross, 2001).

A growing body of research has established a link between childhood aggression and peer rejection (Cillessen & Mayeux, 2004; Véronneau & Vitaro, 2007). Children who were rejected by their peers, were also more likely than other children to use aggression to achieve social goals (Bierman, Smoot, & Aumiller, 1993; Miller-Johnson, Coie, Maumary-Gremaud, Bierman, and The Conduct Problems Prevention Research Group, 2002). Moreover, rejected children were more likely to escalate their aggressive behavior if they were the targets of harassing acts such as teasing or taunting. Rejected children were quick to fight and slow to employ negotiation, bargaining, and other forms of problem-solving. Although fighting back may be perceived as self-defense in some circumstances, the result was often increased rejection and marginalization by other children (Hanish & Guerra, 2002). One rare longitudinal study conducted by Nelson and Dishion (2004) has demonstrated the relation of childhood sociometric status of 200 fourth-grade boys to their outcomes as young adults. Nelson and Dishion found that when young men were compared on measures of antisocial behavior and work/school engagement as young adults (ages 23–24 years), those who had been rejected and isolated boys differed from those who had been amiable and popular boys, even when these behaviors were accounted for at earlier time points.

Similar to Nelson and Dishion, a substantial body of evidence has shown that childhood sociometric status has implications that persist beyond the classroom. Neglected and rejected children are at increased risk of problems in their schools and communities because they lack connections with prosocial peer groups (Coie, Lochman, Terry, & Hyman, 1992; Hawkins & Weis, 1985; Kaplow, Curran, Dodge, and The Conduct Problems Prevention Research Group, 2002; Kupersmidt et al., 1990; Rieffe, Villanueva, & Meerum Terwogt, 2005). Rejection by prosocial peers heightened the probability of a rejected child associating with delinquent peers, which is an important risk factor for subsequent crime, delinquency, conduct disorder, emotional difficulties, and substance use (Cairns & Cairns, 1994; Fergusson, Swain-Campbell, & Horwood, 2002; Hanish & Guerra, 2002; Kupersmidt & Coie, 1990). Researchers have indicated that the rejected status group may be more stable than the other status groups. However, some investigators have argued that—even though some movement between groups may occur over time—within a consistent social environment, children tend to remain perceived in broadly the same terms by their peers (Williams & Gilmour, 1994). Consequently, rejection by peers is one of the most commonly cited factors in a risk sequence associated with poor developmental outcomes (see Cillessen & Mayeux, 2004; Fraser, Kirby, & Smokowski, 2004; Hanish & Guerra, 2002; Kaplow et al., 2002; Lonczak et al., 2001; Miller-Johnson et al., 2002; Miller-Johnson, Coie, Maumary-Gremaud, Lochman, & Terry, 1999; Véronneau & Vitaro, 2007).

2.3.3 *Neglected Status*

In contrast to the other classifications, neglected children are categorized as such because they receive few nominations at all. Peers tend to label these children as shy, and some research has shown that they often preferred to play by themselves (Coie et al., 1982). Although neglected children may have a few friends (French & Waas, 1985), overall this group was generally ignored by peers rather than actively liked or disliked. Neglected status children tend to play alone and were often characterized as withdrawn (Bergin, 1986; Williams & Gilmour, 1994). This group of children seemed to be low in approach motivation yet did not seem to be necessarily low in avoidance motivation (Asendorpf, 1990; Harrist et al., 1997). Thus, even though these children had the social competence to interact with other children, they often preferred to play alone (Harrist et al., 1997). This dynamic may be due to the neglected child's inability to initiate interactions with other children or a lack of confidence regarding their ability to engage with their peers. Once the difficulties of engagement were surmounted, neglected children interacted appropriately with others. However, some research has indicated that deficits in social competence (rather than lack of confidence) were the cause of neglected girls being ignored by peers (Feldman & Dodge, 1987). The parents of neglected status children tended to engage in fewer overall interactions with their children than did parents of other children (Franz & Gross, 2001). In addition, parents of neglected status children were inclined to use an authoritarian parenting style, which was characterized by criticism, excessive disciplinary control, and little praise or affection (Franz & Gross, 2001). Overall, neglected children tended to be less socially active and less aggressive, disruptive, and negative than other children when they interacted with their peers (Bergin, 1986; Coie et al., 1990; Rubin et al., 2005). Therefore, it appears that what distinguished neglected children from average children was that neglected children were not well known by their peers and lacked visibility within the peer group (Newcomb & Bukowski, 1983). This makes them vulnerable targets for bullies with no strong friends to back them up. Neglected status is unstable, meaning these children may go unnoticed by one group, but emerge in a different group with an average status.

2.3.4 *Controversial Status*

Children classified as controversial received both positive and negative nominations from peers but may also be aggressive or disruptive in the classroom. Despite this behavior, controversial children seem to possess social and leadership skills, which gain them popularity with some children. For example, the "class clown" who is disruptive but funny may engender positive and negative feelings from his classmates. In a study that investigated the sociometric status of adopted children in the Netherlands, Juffer, Stams, and van IJzendoorn (2004) reported that adopted children identified by peer reports as controversial or rejected had significantly higher scores on externalizing problems than did adopted children whose peer reports classified them as popular, average, or neglected.

2.3.5 *Average Status*

Children with average status generally received some positive and negative nominations and tended to be viewed as neither highly popular nor unpopular. Average-status children often served as the reference point for other groups (Williams & Gilmour, 1994). These average-status children commonly witness bullying as bystanders and have to decide whether or not to respond by supporting the victim or the bully. This is a fraught decision because average-status children have friends but lack the power of the popular group. They also may fear becoming members of the neglected or rejected groups if they intervene in the bullying. The final classification of children as "other status" comprises those who receive a mix of nomination types that do not fit clearly into any of these other five categories.

Although sociometry can be used to measure a child's relationships within his or her peer group, researchers caution that a child's status within a particular group is not necessarily reflective of their overall status (Cadwallader, 2000/2001; Williams & Gilmour, 1994). For example, a child may have been popular among his or her neighborhood friends and family members but neglected by peer groups at school. As adolescents move between social contexts their sociometric status might change. However, group dynamics are so powerful that being rejected or neglected in one important peer group may lead children and adolescents to form cognitions about themselves that they carry with them from one social context to another (i.e., "People don't like me," "No one cares about me," "I don't fit in").

One final note centers on friendship. Friendship is different from sociometric status in that it has to be reciprocal (i.e., there is a mutual choice of two children choosing each other). Given that reciprocity is the hallmark of friendship (Krappmann, 1996), friendship is assessed by providing youth with a class roster and asking them to circle the names of their three best friends; classmates who mutually nominate each other are deemed friends (e.g., Rose, 2002). Having at least one mutual friend is one of the most powerful protective factors in child development, especially for sociometrically neglected and rejected youth (Rubin et al., 2005) and can buffer some of the stress of bullying victimization.

2.4 Theories Explaining the Bullying Dynamic

Beginning in toddlerhood, around ages 2–3, children are more likely to socially imitate peers than adults (Ryalls, Gull, & Ryalls, 2000). Why would peer social relationships be so important to development? Why would sociometric hierarchies and roles in the bullying dynamic have such strong connections to childhood well-being? We will address these questions using social science theories. Theories are used to explain, understand, or predict phenomena (Dubin, 1978). The use of theory is particularly important to illuminate social processes, such as school bullying. Given the complexity of bullying behavior, multiple theories are needed to fully explicate this social dynamic and understand what motivates bullying behavior. Further, theory can also help elucidate the negative victim outcomes associated with bullying and explain how the organizational culture and climate of schools is associated with the prevalence of bullying behavior. Following Evans and Smokowski (2015), we will analyze the bullying dynamic using interpretative concepts from social capital theory, dominance theory, the theory of humiliation, and organizational culture theory. All of these theories link to evolutionary psychology through an emphasis on acquisition of power and control of resources, attention, and status within peer hierarchies.

2.4.1 *Evolutionary Psychology*

An emerging discussion amongst evolutionary psychologists suggests that bullying is a goal-driven behavior that is underpinned by the struggle for control of resources, sexual access, and social dominance or status (Ellis, Volk, Gonzalez, & Embry, 2016; Volk, Camilleri, Dane, & Marini, 2012a, 2012b; Volk, Dane, & Marini, 2014). From the perpetrator's perspective, repeated displays of power over others is considered the result of a positive cost–benefit ratio where the personal success advanced by bullying behavior (i.e., reputation, status, power, wealth, sexual access, privilege) outweighs the potential costs (i.e., disciplinary action from authorities that is often absent or inconsistent). Over time, the intensity of bullying often leads to gains in dominance for perpetrators (Reijntjes et al., 2013), reinforcing the effectiveness of this aggressive behavior. While bullying perpetrators can be disliked, they are usually feared, which is much more powerful in opening opportunities for resources, access, and status. These benefits outweigh the contextual costs or sanctions against this behavior, leading to one explanation for the ineffective nature of current anti-bullying strategies (Ellis et al., 2016).

Applying an evolutionary perspective, bullying perpetrators may see their pursuit of access, status, dominance, power, sex, wealth, and privilege as effective but also as alienating them from others (e.g., others may be "losers" with less power and privilege). Being mean and aggressive towards others over time could result in a worldview that is relentlessly competitive and threatened by rivals (Anderson & Graham, 2007). If youth engage in bullying over time, they may begin to view the world as aggressive and hostile, which would make it difficult to feel optimistic about the future, at least in the conventional prosocial sense. Bullying perpetration over an extended period may lead to a general cognitive model of the world as a coercive place filled with conflict where one's status is largely determined by power and control of others. This cognitive template may connect to a bleak view of the future as an ongoing struggle for dominance within a system where others dislike you. Popularity centers on power, not working relationships. Children who chronically bully others may create a worldview for themselves where they must constantly show their strength by humiliating others, a dystopian cycle that makes thoughts of the future unpleasant. According to Resource Control Theory (Hawley, 2003), these perpetrators have a coercive style for obtaining goals (e.g., they force or bully others to do what they want). Coercive perpetrators have low levels of self-reported agreeableness, attention to social cues, and conscientiousness and high levels of aggression, hostility, and cheating relative to youth who engage in prosocial behavior to obtain goals (Hawley, 2003).

The evolutionary perspective helps to interpret bullying perpetration yet warrants more discussion when applied to victims, negative bystanders, and prosocial bystanders. Victims are often singled out by perpetrators because they are low in status or on the periphery of the social hierarchy (Bacallao & Smokowski, 2010), leaving these vulnerable children with little power or support to defend themselves. There is little social cost for perpetrators in exerting power over the least powerful members of the social group. Victimization often results in further disempowering victims and increasing the perpetrator's reputation for dominance. Bullying is commonly a public event, quickly disseminating the perpetrators reputation for dominance and the victim's humiliation. As victimization experiences accumulate over time, victims appear to be at risk for displaying aggression (Evans, Smokowski, Rose, Mercado, & Marshall, 2018). Past research suggests that victims most commonly display reactive aggression (Camodeca & Goossens, 2005; Camodeca, Goossens, Terwogt, & Schuengel, 2002). If victims engage in reactive aggression in response to being bullied, this could anger the bully, ultimately increasing and perpetuating their victimization. However, adopting aggressive behaviors may be seen by victims as an adaptive response to the toxic stress of victimization and a reasonable accommodation to an adverse environmental context (Ellis, Bianchi, Griskevicius, & Frankenhuis, 2017). Bully-victims in particular may see aggression as a necessary defense mechanism or a way to retaliate in the context of cumulative victimization experiences. An evolutionary psychology interpretation of the positive relationship between cumulative victimization and aggression may be that adolescents who were victimized begin to use aggressive behavior as the characteristic way to compete for status and resources within their environmental context. Child and adolescent bullying victims consistently display poor adult mental health (Copeland, Wolke, Angold, & Costello, 2013) and physical health (Copeland et al., 2014). Evolutionary psychologists would also suggest that this pattern of effects makes sense for youth relegated to the bottom of the social dominance hierarchy. The deleterious results of victimization form a potential vicious cycle where insecure, pessimistic, anxious, and depressed youth are easy targets for bullying perpetrators to continue to dominate in different social contexts across the lifespan.

Negative bystanders may align with the bully to further their own social reputations and solidify their relationship to a powerful leader. Engagement in negative bystander behavior is one step removed from bullying others; rather than initiating bullying, negative bystanders support the actions of perpetrators. As youth increasingly engage in negative bystander behavior year after year, they could become enmeshed in an aggressive peer group that causes their overall level of aggression to increase. Negative bystanders resemble children who bully others in their aggression and low future optimism; however, their adjustment is even poorer in manifesting low academic achievement and internalizing symptoms (Evans et al., 2018). From an evolutionary perspective, this pattern brings up interesting speculation. Given that bullying perpetrators have been characterized as achieving status and power with their behavior, negative bystanders may be less dominant youth trying to affiliate with a powerful, albeit negative, leader. Negative bystanders may be struggling with prosocial pathways, such as academics and future optimism, and instead may seek the aggressive status and power that perpetrators have. This negative bystander behavior may be the gateway to becoming a full-fledged perpetrator or it may be an affiliation process for youth trying to find their place in the antisocial peer hierarchy.

Engaging in a positive behavior that helps others could cause prosocial bystanders to feel good about themselves, thus increasing future optimism, self-esteem, and academic achievement. Prosocial bystanders are defenders of the oppressed who display courage and conviction under stressful circumstances. However, they also pay the price of experiencing increases in internalizing symptoms (Evans et al., 2018). From the evolutionary perspective, this profile of effects for prosocial bystanders shows them to be high functioning youth who pursue their goals by conventional, positive means (i.e., academic achievement, future optimism, self-esteem). Because they are invested in these positive pathways to success, intervening in bullying by telling a teacher or helping the victim may enhance their reputations and lead to movement towards their goals. The prosocial bystander behavior can enhance their reputations in an analogous way to the perpetrator's negative power accumulation. Prosocial bystanders may also become closer to authorities (e.g., teachers, principals) from their actions to break up bullying situations. They may also be admired by grateful victims and, outside of the cost–benefit calculation, may feel empowered by their altruism and advocacy. Prosocial bystanders may intervene to promote their positive reputations with authority figures (e.g., talking with a teacher) or may be prompted by more complex higher-order impulses, such as altruism. It is also important to consider that these prosocial bystanders could also be victimized and that their internalizing symptoms may be a result of their own personal victimization and that their inclination to engage in prosocial bystander behavior arises out of high levels of empathy.

These evolutionary explanations are further illuminated using social science research from social capital, dominance, and humiliation, theories.

2.4.2 *Social Capital Theory*

Social capital refers to the benefits gained from social relationships (Putnam, 2000). Specifically, individuals form and invest in social relationships with the expectation of fulfilling goals and profiting from their interactions with others (Coleman, 1988; Lin, 2001). Putnam described the mutual benefit of social capital as the force that drives people to maintain social networks: "Social capital refers to features of social organization such as networks, norms, and social trust that facilitate coordination and cooperation for mutual benefit" (Putnam, 1995, p. 67). Social capital can be categorized as either bonding social capital or bridging social capital. Bonding social capital consists of social ties (i.e., interpersonal relationships) between similar individuals who belong to a homogenous group that creates a feeling of cohesion and shared belonging, whereas bridging social capital consists of social ties with people outside the homogenous group that creates a wider social network (Beugelsdijk & Smulders, 2003; Putnam, 2000).

According to social capital theory, individuals invest in social relationships to access the resources embedded within these relationships. Social capital theorists argue that social ties offer four beneficial resources (Lin, 2001; Lin, Cook, & Burt, 2001). First, social ties provide access to information about opportunities and choices that might not be available to those outside of the relationship. As applied to adolescent social networks, youth with social ties to the popular crowd likely have access to information about after school social events where they might interact with and form strong bonds with high-status peers. Bonding with high-status peers is a form of social capital that increases social standing and decreases the chances of being bullied and/or socially ostracized. Second, social ties with individuals connected to people with power are beneficial because these individuals might be able to influence the person in power. For example, having a social tie with the "queen bee's" best friend might provide protection from being the target of relational bullying. Similarly, being friends with a member of a bully's entourage could increase the chances of being protected from becoming a victim. Third, social ties provide individuals with social credentials; specifically, being socially connected to certain individuals indicates access to resources. For example, if a moderately popular girl starts dating the football star, this social tie increases her social capital. This dating relationship would potentially connect her to all of the resources or social credentials the football star possesses (e.g., respect, popularity, social engagements, social ties to other football players) and might subsequently increase her chances of being incorporated into the popular group of girls and gaining social status. Amassing social credentials can also provide protection against being bullied because adolescents are more likely to befriend someone with many social credentials as a way of gaining access to the other person's social resources. Fourth, social relationships reinforce an individual's identity and sense of self-worth. Being a member of a social group with others who share similar interests and values is a way of obtaining emotional support and affirmation. Thus, having a group of friends at school provides validation of an individual's self-worth and is a potential source of support (Lin, 2001; Lin et al., 2001).

The theory of social capital is often applied to business and economics (Beugelsdijk & Smulders, 2003); however, this theory is also pertinent to the school setting. Social capital in the school setting is best represented by friends and social status. Friendships provide youth with support and often buffer against social stressors such as peer rejection (Bagwell & Schmidt, 2011), whereas social status indicates popularity and power. Friendships and social status do not necessarily go together; that is, youth might have social capital in the form of a few or many friends but might not be viewed as popular or vice versa.

Youth victimized by bullying have few friends, and in turn, have low social status (Bagwell & Schmidt, 2011; Scholte et al., 2008) resulting in minimal social capital. Even when bullied youth have friends, these friendships do not provide social capital because victims' friends are often rejected by the larger peer group outside the friendship (Scholte et al., 2008). Although having one or a few friends could serve to reinforce a victim's self-worth, victims' friendships likely do not increase their access to valuable social information, improve their social credentials, or provide avenues to influence powerful social figures in the school. Further, victims' limited social capital likely precludes them from being invited to social gatherings where they would have the opportunity to interact and perhaps bond with peers who could provide social capital. Victims' lack of social capital intensifies and prolongs their victimization experiences and many victims lack friends or acquaintances who can protect them from being bullied. For example, victims are unlikely to receive help from bystanders given that research has shown only 10–20% of bystanders intervened to protect victims of bullying (Atlas & Pepler, 1998; Evans & Smokowski, 2015; Hawkins et al., 2001; Salmivalli et al., 1998). Thus, bullying behavior often continues uninterrupted. Acquiring additional social capital in the form of one supportive friend or a small group of friends willing to support the victim could help a victim escape further bullying. However, victims are often seen as undesirable friends because of their low social status and social awkwardness, making it difficult for victims to acquire either friends or additional social capital.

On the other hand, bullies often have an easier time acquiring social capital and use bullying tactics as a means of amassing social capital in the form of social status (Pellegrini, 2002). Bullies exert power over weaker peers, relegating those peers to a low position in the social hierarchy. Although bullies are usually disliked (Rodkin & Berger, 2008) they are often perceived as popular by their peer group (de Bruyn, Cillessen, & Wissink, 2010; Prinstein & Cillessen, 2003; Vaillancourt, Hymel, & McDougall, 2003). Perceived popularity indicates social status and is a form of social capital because it indicates that peers think of bullies as having power and social prestige. This power protects bullies from becoming victims and increases the likelihood of their peers rallying behind them.

Indeed, bullies who are able to effectively use intimidation and humiliation tactics often become the leaders of their cliques (Pellegrini, Bartini, & Brooks, 1999). Having a group of devoted followers reinforces an individual's self-worth, which is one of the benefits of social capital. Further, being a group leader provides opportunities for making social connections with leaders of other groups, and thus expanding the individual's social credentials through bridging social capital. Once a group amasses social power, group members benefit from that social power and strive to maintain it, oftentimes using bullying tactics as means to stay on top.

Bully-victims might also turn to bullying perpetration as a means of acquiring social capital, improving their social status in the classroom, and ending their victimization. For example, as classmates scramble for social capital, bully-victims are likely victimized, resulting in a low social status and a lack of social capital. However, rather than withdrawing like most victims, bully-victims might search out weaker classmates to bully in an effort to obtain social capital and improve their social status. In this regard bully-victims mimic the behavior of the bullies and bully weaker classmates in an effort to obtain social capital.

In summary, social capital refers to the resources embedded in social relationships. Both individuals and groups benefit from the resources of information, social influence, social credentials, and reinforcement of self-worth that social ties provide. Victims of bullying have few friends or social ties, and thus, have minimal social capital, which prevents them from exiting their role as a victim. Conversely, bullies use bullying tactics as a means of acquiring social capital in the form of perceived popularity. Youth often perceive bullies as powerful and popular, which serves as a form of social capital that protects bullies' social status. Finally, bully-victims attempt to end their victimization and gain social capital by bullying weaker peers.

2.4.3 Dominance Theory: Motivation for Bullying Behavior

The desire for power and dominance is a central motivating factor that fuels bullying behavior and bullies use intimidation and humiliation as a means of obtaining power. Social dominance theory (SDT; Sidanius & Pratto, 1999) and dominance theory (Long & Pellegrini, 2003) provide insight into the bullying dynamic. Both theories indicate that youth bully one another in their attempts to gain group and individual levels of social dominance and then maintain their social status through ongoing bullying. In other words, bullying perpetration is used as means of establishing and maintaining dominance. Bullying is a group process and the peer group dictates whether a bully can establish dominance (Salmivalli, 2010). For example, if classmates respect and support the bully, the bully gains dominance and social power within the classroom. Further, if the bully becomes the leader of a clique of admiring followers, the clique members might experience heightened power within the classroom based on their membership in a group led by a powerful, respected individual. To maintain social dominance, this group would use ongoing bullying as a means of oppressing less powerful members of the class. Indeed, youth who desire dominance act aggressively and bully others to gain social status (Long & Pellegrini, 2003).

In contrast to group-based social hierarchies, individual based social hierarchies are formed when an individual gains social status and power using personal characteristics such as a charismatic leadership style or intelligence (Sidanius & Pratto, 1999). For example, in the bullying dynamic, "ringleader" bullies can usually be identified (Salmivalli, 2010, p. 113) and these youth might use their charisma and skill for humiliating less powerful classmates as a means of gaining social prestige and establishing dominance. Indeed, research has suggested that bullying is a successful method of obtaining dominance; as compared with nonaggressive boys in sixth grade, aggressive boys had more access to girls (i.e., dated more; Pellegrini & Bartini, 2001) and bullies were often viewed as popular by their classmates (Cillessen & Mayeux, 2004; de Bruyn et al., 2010; Prinstein & Cillessen, 2003; Vaillancourt et al., 2003). However, bullies are not always successful in their quest for dominance and some do not obtain popularity. Certain characteristics such as physical attractiveness, athleticism, and stylish clothing increase the likelihood that bullies will obtain dominance and be viewed as powerful and popular by their classmates (Vaillancourt et al., 2003).

Both group- and individual-based social hierarchies are relevant in the bullying dynamic. The bully's goal of gaining power and status is an individual objective that requires the ability to establish an individual-based social hierarchy. However, the realization of this goal depends upon the peer group accepting and valuing the bullying behavior (Salmivalli, 2010) as well as forming a group that creates a group-based social hierarchy. These hierarchies are then maintained through ongoing bullying and humiliation of victims.

The highest levels of aggression are often exhibited during group formation when a social hierarchy is forming, with aggression decreasing after the hierarchy has been formed (Long & Pellegrini, 2003). During the formation process, when social dominance is not yet established, it is likely that youth might use bullying as a way of jockeying for a dominant social position. Indeed, bullying peaks in sixth grade and then decreases throughout middle and high school (Guerin & Hennessy, 2002; National Center for Educational Statistics, 2011; Peskin, Tortolero, & Markham, 2006). The higher rates of bullying during the outset of middle school might serve to establish a social pecking order as youth transition to a new school setting and social context. Although rates decrease thereafter, bullying continues at lower levels to maintain the social hierarchy.

An example of the way bullying can be used to establish social dominance can be found in relational bullying among girls. Relational bullying and relational aggression are closely related but distinct constructs, primarily distinguished by whether the behavior is repeated. Relational bullying is repetitive and ongoing, whereas relational aggression is limited to a few isolated acts. Relational bullying and aggression are intended to harm the victims' reputation and social relationships, and include actions such as rumor spreading, excluding, ignoring, and posting embarrassing images of the victim via physical or electronic means (Gladden, Vivolo-Kantor, Hamburger, & Lumpkin, 2014). These forms of relational aggression are less obvious and obtrusive than physical aggression, which makes them effective because incidents often go undetected by adults (Mishna, 2012). Further, the lack of overt aggression makes relational aggression especially appealing to girls; some studies have found that girls are more likely than boys to be relationally aggression (Crick & Grotpeter, 1995).

During adolescence, relationships are the focal point of many girls' lives (Simmons, 2002). Because these social relationships are in constant flux (Simmons, 2002), girls experience continuous competition to obtain social dominance, which is measured by popularity and social status. Social dominance is often established through relational bullying used to create alliances among some girls while turning girls against each other. "Indeed, popularity itself is in large part defined by the ability of one girl to turn her friends against someone else … Alliance building is a sign of peer affirmation, an unspoken contract that means … a girl will not be abandoned" (Simmons, 2002, p. 82). The desire for dominance is a catalyst for bullying behavior. Strategies used by girl bullies to obtain dominance and relegate others to a lower social status include rumor spreading, gossiping, excluding, and ignoring. These tactics are often successful. Research with seventh and ninth grade girls showed relational aggression was associated with increased perceived popularity over time (Rose, Swenson, & Waller, 2004). That is, the more a girl engaged in relational aggression, the more likely her classmates were to perceive her as having power. An increased perception or "reputation" of power among the group can lead to greater popularity for the bully.

Both individual- and group-based social hierarchies form because of relational aggression. Charismatic girls who are adept at manipulating others are more likely to successfully use strategies of relational aggression to garner respect, popularity, and social status for themselves. If other girls follow the perpetrator and form a group or clique, a group-based social hierarchy forms because the group shares social dominance and the members of this group would be accorded social power. If individuals join a group to affiliate with the group's social status, they are often pressured to take on characteristics of that group, promoting homogeneity. If bullying or relational aggression is a tool of that group, new members would likely become quickly socialized to the use of bullying tactics. Indeed, after this socialization process, a group member may be reluctant to leave the group because leaving may dramatically heighten the risk of becoming the group's next victim.

2.4.4 The Theory of Humiliation: Why Being Dominated Is Painful and Leads to Negative Victim Outcomes

Humiliation is "excessive overt derogation" that occurs when a more powerful individual publically reveals the inadequacies of a weaker victim, who feels the treatment is unjustified (Jackson, 1999, p. 2). The concept of humiliation is distinct from shame. An individual can shame him or herself, whereas humiliation requires action from an outside agent who engenders feelings of powerlessness in the victim (Hartling & Luchetta, 1999; Klein, 1991). Further, shame results in an internal feeling of inadequacy and embarrassment, whereas humiliation often causes anger towards the perpetrator and the desire for retaliation (Jackson, 1999). Conversely, the rage generated by humiliation can also be turned inwards in the form of depression (Lindner, 2007). These emotional reactions are quite common for victims after bullying incidents.

The effects of humiliation are far reaching and impact the humiliated individual as well as the surrounding community or society, and therefore, humiliation is considered a significant impediment to positive human development. From harmony on preschool playgrounds to global peace, experiences of humiliation disrupt social cohesion (Lindner, 2003). Bullying victimization is a form of humiliation (Meltzer, Vostanis, Ford, Bebbington, & Dennis, 2011; Simmons, 2002) given that bullying usually occurs in public, involves the subjugation of a less powerful victim, and effects the entire school community by limiting social cohesion.

Lindner's (2001a, 2006) theory of humiliation addresses humiliation on a global scale (e.g., feelings of humiliation among the German people after World War I set the stage for Hitler's rise to power). However, this theory can also be applied to school bullying to illuminate the role humiliation plays in the outcomes of victims and bully-victims, as well as to illustrate how bullying prevents the formation of a peaceful and cohesive school environment. The interpersonal nature of humiliation is vital to understanding and applying Lindner's theory. Klein (1991) coined the term humiliation dynamic to highlight the fact that although humiliation is an intensely personal feeling, humiliation is generated from social interactions and relationship dynamics such as bullying.

Humiliation involves “putting down and holding down” (Lindner, 2006, p. xi) and has such intense power that it is considered “the nuclear bomb of the emotions” (Lindner, 2006, p. 3). With the emergence of human rights and the recognition that all persons are deserving of dignity, humiliating another person became morally and ethically wrong (Lindner, 2001b). The basis for Lindner’s theory is the notion that all humans desire and deserve recognition and respect and humiliation violates this fundamental human right, resulting in eroded interpersonal relationships and disrupted social cohesion (Lindner, 2007).

The humiliation dynamic involves three roles: the humiliator (i.e., the person who inflicts humiliation), the victim (i.e., the person who experiences humiliation), and the witness (i.e., the person who observes and verifies that humiliation is occurring; Klein, 1991). Bullies physically, verbally, or relationally humiliate their victims, relegating their victims to a lower social status in an effort to establish power. Building on the work of Smith (2001), Lindner (2003, 2006) posited humiliation had four forms:

1. *Conquest humiliation*—an individual uses conquest humiliation to force a former equal into a subordinate position. Conquest humiliation is a precursor to bullying because this form of humiliation establishes the power differential inherent in the bullying dynamic. For example, if two adolescent girls of equal status are vying for the position of “queen bee” of a desired social group, one girl could use relational aggression (e.g., rumor spreading, exclusion) to humiliate her rival and turn other girls against the rival, thus relegating her rival to a lower social position and creating a power differential.
2. *Reinforcement humiliation* is used to maintain the social hierarchy established by conquest humiliation. Following from the above example, the new queen bee would continue to spread rumors about and exclude her rival as a means of ongoing humiliation to maintain her rival’s subjugation.
3. *Relegation humiliation* is used as a means of creating a larger power differential between the humiliator and the victim. If the new queen bee wanted to ensure the complete social demise of her rival, she could use relegation humiliation to sabotage her rival’s new friendships by increasing the intensity and frequency of bullying, thus making her rival appear socially undesirable and relegating her to an even lower social position.
4. *Exclusion humiliation* is the most stringent form of humiliation and involves banishing victims altogether by exiling or killing them. In the realm of bullying, this form of humiliation would occur if the queen bee ensured that everyone in the class completely ignored and avoided her rival, perhaps until the rival left school or, in extreme situations, committed suicide.

The humiliation of being bullied violates the individual’s fundamental need for respect and recognition. Humiliation also undermines social standing, engendering the psychological pain of ostracism. Being bullied results in anger; this anger can be externalized as retaliation or internalized as depression. The outward expression of anger as retaliation can take the form of bullying, which fits with the description of the bully-victim as a person who is a victim of bullying but also bullies others. In contrast, other victims internalize the humiliation and feel deep despair, which manifests as depression; this reaction to humiliation explains why victims often have higher rates of depression compared with non-victimized youth (Juvonen, Graham, & Schuster, 2003; Menesini et al., 2009). Further, the humiliation experience may cause victims to be excluded from social groups, which generates loneliness. In turn, loneliness is a significant risk factor eroding positive development and adjustment (Asher & Paquette, 2003).

Research has indicated that humiliation exacerbates interpersonal conflicts (Fitness, 2001) and results in strong, negative emotions. For example, individuals who reported they had been humiliated by their partner also reported feeling hatred towards their partner and tended to withdraw (Fitness & Fletcher, 1993). Qualitative interviews with ten students and ten teachers revealed that experiences of humiliation such as bullying resulted in substance use, attendance problems, dropping out of school, and suicidal thoughts (Frey & Fisher, 2008).

Given these strong reactions to humiliation, intense ongoing humiliation can be considered as a form of trauma (Lindner, 2001a). Recently, bullying victimization has been studied as a form of interpersonal trauma (D'Andrea, Ford, Stolbach, Spinazzola, & van der Kolk, 2012). Interpersonal traumas, such as bullying, erode victims' abilities to form social and emotional attachments to others such as an inability to successfully attach to a peer group or to school (Popp & Peguero, 2012; Smokowski & Kopasz, 2005); further, bullying threatens the physical well-being of victims, who often report feeling afraid and helpless.

Bullying victimization is a form of humiliation and interpersonal trauma that makes forming and sustaining relationships difficult for the victim. The negative relationship effects of bullying are not isolated to victims. Bullying episodes and the humiliation engendered disrupt social cohesion in the school and classroom. Although the majority of youth are not directly involved in the bullying dynamic, witnessing the ongoing humiliation of a classmate erodes bystanders' feelings of safety and security and leaves them constantly wondering 'Will I be next?' The fear of becoming the next victim and suffering the same type of humiliation they have witnessed makes it unlikely that bystanders will intervene to help victims. Instead, youth often passively watch the bullying or support the bully. The desire to maintain power encourages bullies to continue bullying and the fear of being humiliated sustains bystanders' complicit silence.

Indeed, the fear of humiliation "… appears to be one of the most powerful motivators of individual and collective human behavior" (Klein, 1991, p. 96). The fear of becoming a victim creates an atmosphere of trepidation and mistrust that further erodes relationships and disrupts social cohesion.

Highly emotional and personally significant events, such as being bullied, tend to be remembered in great detail (van der Kolk, 1997). Traumatic events are often stored at a somatosensory level, that is, highly emotional, personal events are stored as visual images or sensations related to the trauma and those visual images persist over time (van der Kolk, 1994). Indeed, "… recurrent observations about the nature of traumatic memories have given rise to the notion that traumatic memories may be encoded differently than memories for ordinary events …" (van der Kolk, 1997, p. 248). Moderate amounts of stress, such as that present in bullying encounters, actually facilitate memory (Siegel, 2012). This assertion has been supported by research suggesting that adults who were bullied during childhood continue to vividly remember the details of their victimization experiences years later (Carlisle & Rofes, 2007; Russell, 2010).

For example, a retrospective study using a sample of 60 adults (mean age 29.7 years) who were bullied as children due to their perceived sexual orientation, asked participants about their bullying victimization (Rivers, 2001). Questions included who bullied them, how they were bullied, where and when the bullying occurred, and who they told about the bullying. Participants also answered questions about the age at which they first knew they were gay, lesbian, or bisexual. Participants were reinterviewed 12–14 months later and were asked the same questions. The majority of the answers about being bullied at Time 1 were highly and significantly correlated with answers at Time 2. Specifically, participants consistently recalled the forms of bullying they endured as well as the specific location where the bullying occurred, indicating the vividness with which these humiliating memories were recalled. However, participants did not exhibit the same level of memory recall for subsequent events, including who the victim told about the bullying and at what age the person developed awareness of his or her sexual orientation. These later events were recalled with less consistency and were not significantly correlated between Time 1 and Time 2 (Rivers, 2001). These findings highlight that events that caused less humiliation were not recalled with as much vividness as the memories of events that caused high levels of humiliation, including being bullied. Further, adults who were victimized as children have an increased risk for depression and anxiety (Gladstone, Parker, & Malhi, 2006; Ttofi, Farrington, Losel, & Loeber, 2011), suggesting that memories of bullying are persistent and negatively influence victims' mental health in adulthood.

In summary, bullying victimization is a form of humiliation and can be considered an interpersonal trauma. Bullying is used to create a hierarchy of social status in which bullies reside on the top and victims are relegated to a lower social position. The presence of bullying in schools erodes social cohesion because bullying fuels a pervasive intimidating fear of becoming the next victim and of being publicly humiliated. Viewing bullying victimization as a form of humiliation highlights why the memories of bullying victimization are persistent and can affect adult outcomes.

2.5 Implications for Practitioners

Practitioners can use the theories and information presented above to gain a more comprehensive understanding of what might be motivating the bully's behavior and how this behavior might impact the victim. Understanding the inherent scramble for social capital, power, and control over social networks is critically important so that practitioners can determine how, when, and where to intervene to have the greatest impact.

Social capital development is about access to information, resources, relationships, and roles. Practitioners can help guide healthy social network formation by understanding sociometric functioning and actively facilitating group formation, especially during early group development (i.e., at the beginning of middle school or first semester of ninth grade). Structured group activities can greatly facilitate positive social network formation, rather than allowing leaderless jockeying of group members for control. Diverse subgroups of students should be brought together to learn about each other and broaden social group development. This is especially helpful for introverted students who tend to withdraw, raising their risk for isolation and victimization. Indeed, practitioners can help these students find valued roles to play in social groups (i.e., the marching band, the school newspaper), encouraging them towards active participation rather than marginalization.

Dominance theory helps frame interactions in terms of power, control, and subjugation. Practitioners are commonly socialized to see power inequities; however, disparities are often seen in terms of race, ethnicity, class, gender, and sexual orientation. While respecting the importance of these categories, practitioners handling bullying situations also must consider differences in power due to physical features, interpersonal skills, social disability, and other characteristics that set one child apart from other children. Children may become targets for victimization due to being too short, too tall, too heavy, too skinny, too smart, not smart enough, and for many other attributes. Practitioners should identify students who are quiet, self-conscious, isolated, and on the margins of social groups. These victims and potential victims should be brought into welcoming social groups, linked to higher functioning children or adult mentors to nurture friendships, and given the opportunity to play some type of role in the school community to develop pride in their social contribution. In short, practitioners should seek out children on the margins of the social ecology and find ways for them to participate.

Bullies often desire power and are willing to use antisocial strategies, such as humiliation, to obtain their goal. Recognizing this underlying need, practitioners can help bullies find less destructive, prosocial ways in which to gain a feeling of power and confidence. Like victims, bullies may feel that they are on the margins of prosocial peer groups; however, they cope by creating antisocial subgroups of their own, generating "antisocial" capital rather than positive social capital. Recognizing this, practitioners can help bullies gain respect and control in positive ways through access to prosocial roles and in cultivating friendships that are not based on power and control. Humiliation experiences should be dealt with quickly and with clear consequences; perpetrators should be disciplined and victims coping with public humiliation should be offered trauma-informed treatment. Given that humiliation experiences have serious and far-reaching impacts on the emotional life of the child, practitioners should help the child express his or her feelings and continue to engage with other students. It is unhealthy for the victim to withdraw from social participation and internalize the humiliation experience.

Youth might not be aware of the mechanisms underlying the bullying dynamic and educating youth about the causes and consequences of bullying might help them understand their experiences with bullying. Helping victims verbalize their feelings of humiliation and supporting them in acquiring self-confidence is clearly a vital element of enabling victims to heal from bullying and might help combat the onset of depression and anxiety. Finally, practitioners must remember that bullying affects the entire school community. While intervening in and attempting to change individual bullying dynamics is important, the whole climate and culture of the school must be altered in order to totally extinguish bullying.

2.6 Conclusions

The bullying dynamic includes several roles: the bully, the victim, the bully-victim (who are both victimized and victimize others), and the bystanders who aligns with the bully (negative bystanders) or stands up to help the victim (prosocial bystanders) or passively witnesses the bullying event. These roles are reinforced by childhood peer relationship hierarchies in which some youth are considered popular for either prosocial or antisocial reasons, others are controversial in being both liked and disliked, others are rejected by peer groups for being aggressive or being withdrawn, and others are neglected or ignored by their peers. Popular-antisocial and rejected-aggressive youth are at highest risk for becoming bullies. They often seek dominance and status in peer groups without showing empathy or cooperation with others. Rejected-withdrawn and neglected children are at risk for becoming victimized, having low status and few resources or friends to defend themselves. Other popular-prosocial, controversial, and average-status children witness bullying as bystanders and have to decide to respond in a negative or positive way, supporting the bully or the victim, or doing nothing. These playground politics are explained by evolutionary psychology, social capital, and dominance theories by a drive within bullies to seek power and dominance at the expense of victims, who concomitantly lose status through the deleterious effects of humiliation and loneliness.

References

Adler, P. A., Kless, S. J., & Adler, P. (1992). Socialization to gender roles: Popularity among elementary school boys and girls. *Sociology of Education, 65*, 169–187.

Anderson, K. B., & Graham, L. M. (2007). Hostile attribution bias. In R. F. Baumesiter & K. D. Vohs (Eds.), *Encyclopedia of social psychology* (pp. 445–446). Thousand Oaks, CA: Sage Publications.

Asendorpf, J. (1990). Beyond social withdrawal: Shyness, unsociability, and peer avoidance. *Human Development, 33*, 250–259.

Asher, S., & Coie, J. (1990). *Peer rejection in childhood.* New York, NY: Cambridge University Press.

Asher, S., & Parker, J. (1989). Significance of peer relationship problems in childhood. In B. H. Schneider, G. Attili, J. Nadel, & R. P. Weissberg (Eds.), *Social competence in developmental perspective (5-23). NATO Advanced Science Institute series. Series D: Behavioral and social sciences* (Vol. 51). Dordrecht: Kluwer Academic.

Asher, S. R., & Paquette, J. (2003). Loneliness and peer relations in childhood. *Current Directions in Psychological Science, 12*, 75–78.

Atlas, R. S., & Pepler, D. J. (1998). Observations of bullying in the classroom. *Journal of Educational Research, 92*(2), 86–99.

Bacallao, M., & Smokowski, P. R. (2010). Sociometric Status and bullying in school: Peer relationships, power, and victimization. In N. A. Ramsay & C. Morrison (Eds.), *Youth violence and juvenile justice: Causes, intervention and treatment programs.* Hauppauge, NY: Nova Science Inc.

Bagwell, C. L., & Schmidt, M. E. (2011). *Friendships in childhood and adolescence.* New York, NY: Guilford Press.

Bell-Dolan, D., Foster, S., & Sikora, D. (1989). Effects of sociometric testing on children's behavior and loneliness in school. *Developmental Psychology, 25*, 306–311.

Bergin, G. (1986). Sociometric status and social interaction: Are the neglected children socially less active? *Perceptual and Motor Skills, 63*, 823–830.

Beugelsdijk, S., & Smulders, S. (2003). *Bridging and bonding social capital: Which type is good for economic growth?* Paper submitted to European Regional Science Association. Retrieved from http://www-sre.wuwien.ac.at/ersa/ersaconfs/ersa03/cdrom/papers/517.pdf

Bierman, K., Smoot, D., & Aumiller, K. (1993). Characteristics of aggressive-rejected, aggressive-nonrejected, and rejected-nonaggressive boys. *Child Development, 64*, 139–151.

Bronfenbrenner, U. (1943). A constant frame of reference for sociometric research. *Sociometry, 6*, 363–397.

Cadwallader, T. (2000/2001). Sociometry reconsidered: The social context of peer rejection in childhood. *International Journal of Action Methods, 53*(3/4), 99–118.

Cairns, R., Cairns, B., Neckerman, H., Gest, S., & Gariepy, J.-L. (1988). Social networks and aggressive behavior: Peer support or peer rejection. *Developmental Psychology, 24*, 815–823.

Cairns, R. B., & Cairns, B. D. (1994). *Lifelines and risks: Pathways of youth in our time.* New York, NY: Cambridge University Press.

Cairns, R. B., Leung, M., Buchanan, L., & Cairns, B. D. (1995). Friendships and social networks in childhood and adolescence: Fluidity, reliability, and interrelations. *Child Devlopment, 66*(5), 1330–1345.

Camodeca, M., & Goossens, F. A. (2005). Aggression, social cognitions, anger, and sadness in bullies and victims. *Journal of Child Psychology and Psychiatry, 46*(2), 186–197.

Camodeca, M., Goossens, F. A., Terwogt, M. M., & Schuengel, C. (2002). Bullying and victimization among school-age children: Stability and links to proactive and reactive aggression. *Social Development, 11*, 332–345.

Carlisle, N., & Rofes, E. (2007). School bullying: Do adults survivors perceive long-term effects? *Traumatology, 13*(1), 16–26.

Cillessen, A., van IJzendoorn, H., van Lieshout, C., & Hartup, W. (1992). Heterogeneity among peer-rejected boys: Subtypes and stabilities. *Child Development, 63*, 893–905.
Cillessen, A. H. N., & Mayeux, L. (2004). From censure to reinforcement: Developmental changes in the association between aggression and social status. *Child Development, 75*(1), 147–163.
Cillessen, A. H. N., & Rose, A. (2006). Understanding popularity in the peer system. *Current Directions in Psychological Science, 14*(2), 102–105.
Coie, J., Dodge, K., & Coppotelli, H. (1982). Dimensions and types of social status: A cross-age perspective. *Developmental Psychology, 18*, 557–570.
Coie, J., Dodge, K., & Kupersmidt, J. (1990). Peer group behavior and social status. In S. R. Asher & J. D. Coie (Eds.), *Peer rejection in childhood* (pp. 17–59). Cambridge: Cambridge University Press.
Coie, J., & Kupersmidt, J. (1983). A behavioral analysis of emerging social status in boys' groups. *Child Development, 54*, 1400–1416.
Coie, J. D., Lochman, J. E., Terry, R., & Hyman, C. (1992). Predicting early adolescent disorder from childhood aggression and peer rejection. *Journal of Consulting and Clinical Psychology, 60*, 783–792.
Coleman, J. S. (1988). Social capital in the creation of human capital. *American Journal of Sociology, 94*, S95–S120.
Copeland, W. E., Wolke, D., Angold, A., & Costello, E. J. (2013). Adult psychiatric outcomes of bullying and being bullied by peers in childhood and adolescence. *JAMA Psychiatry, 70*, 419–426.
Copeland, W. E., Wolke, D., Lereya, S. T., Shanahan, L., Worthman, C., & Costello, E. J. (2014). Childhood bullying involvement predicts low-trade system inflammation into adulthood. *Proceedings of the National Academy of Sciences of the United States of America, 111*(21), 7570–7575.
Crick, N. R., & Grotpeter, J. K. (1995). Relational aggression, gender, and social-psychological adjustment. *Child Development, 66*(3), 710–722.
Czeschlik, T., & Rost, D. (1995). Sociometric types and children's intelligence. *British Journal of Developmental Psychology, 13*, 177–189.
D'Andrea, W., Ford, J., Stolbach, B., Spinazzola, J., & van der Kolk, B. A. (2012). Understanding interpersonal trauma in children: Why we need a developmental appropriate trauma diagnosis. *American Journal of Orthopsychiatry, 82*, 187–200.
de Bruyn, E. H., Cillessen, A. H. N., & Wissink, I. B. (2010). Associations of peer acceptance and perceived popularity with bullying and victimization in early adolescence. *The Journal of Early Adolescence, 3D*, 543–566.
Dubin, R. (1978). *Theory building*. Jor Bagh: Social Sciences Press.
Dunn, J. C., Dunn, J. G. H., & Bayduza, A. (2007). Perceived athletic competence, sociometric status, and loneliness in elementary school children. *Journal of Sport Behavior, 30*(3), 249–269.
Ellis, B. J., Bianchi, J. M., Griskevicius, V., & Frankenhuis, W. E. (2017). Beyond risk and protective factors: An adaptation-based approach to resilience. *Perspectives on Psychological Science, XX*, 1–27.
Ellis, B. J., Volk, A. A., Gonzalez, J. M., & Embry, D. D. (2016). The meaningful roles intervention: An evolutionary approach to reducing bullying and increasing prosocial behavior. *Journal of Research on Adolescence, 26*, 622–637.
Evans, C. B. R., & Smokowski, P. R. (2015). Prosocial bystander behavior in bullying dynamics: Assessing the impact of social capital. *Journal of Youth and Adolescence, 44*(12), 289–307.
Evans, C. B. R., Smokowski, P. R., Rose, R., Mercado, M. C., & Marshall, K. (2018). Cumulative bullying experiences, adolescent behavioral and mental health, and academic achievement: An integrative model of perpetration, victimization, and bystander behavior. *Journal of Child & Family Studies., 27*, 1–14.
Feldman, E., & Dodge, K. (1987). Social information processing and sociometric status: Sex, age, and situational effects. *Journal of Abnormal Child Psychology, 15*, 211–217.

Fergusson, D. M., Swain-Campbell, N. R., & Horwood, L. J. (2002). Deviant peer affiliations, crime and substance use: A fixed effects regression analysis. *Journal of Abnormal Child Psychology, 30*, 419–430.
Fersch, E. F. (Ed.). (2006). *Thinking about psychopaths and psychopathy: Answers to frequently asked questions with case examples*. Lincoln, NE: iUniverse.
Fine, G. A. (1987). *With the boys: Little league baseball and preadolescent culture*. Chicago, IL: University of Chicago Press.
Fitness, J. (2001). Betrayal, rejection, revenge, and forgiveness: An interpersonal script approach. In M. Leary (Ed.), *Interpersonal rejection* (pp. 73–103). New York, NY: Oxford University Press.
Fitness, J., & Fletcher, G. J. O. (1993). Love, hate, anger, and jealousy in close relationships: A prototype and cognitive appraisal analysis. *Journal of Personality and Social Psychology, 65*(5), 942–958.
Franz, D., & Gross, A. (2001). Child sociometric status and parent behaviors: An observational study. *Behavior Modification, 25*, 3–20.
Fraser, M. W., Kirby, L. D., & Smokowski, P. R. (2004). Risk and resilience in childhood. In M. W. Fraser (Ed.), *Risk and resilience in childhood: An ecological perspective* (2nd ed., pp. 13–66). Washington DC: NASW Press.
French, D. (1990). Heterogeneity among peer-rejected girls. *Child Development, 61*, 2028–2031.
French, D., & Waas, G. (1985). Behavior problems of peer-neglected and peer-rejected elementary age children: Parent and teacher perspectives. *Child Development, 56*, 246–252.
Frey, N., & Fisher, D. (2008). The under-appreciated role of humiliation in the middle school. *Middle School Journal, 39*, 4–12.
Gladden, R. M., Vivolo-Kantor, A. M., Hamburger, M. E., & Lumpkin, C. D. (2014). *Bullying surveillance among youths: Uniform definitions for public health and recommended data elements, Version 1.0.* Atlanta, GA: National Center for Injury Prevention and Control, Centers for Disease Control and Prevention and U.S. Department of Education.
Gladstone, G. L., Parker, G. B., & Malhi, G. S. (2006). Do bullied children become anxious and depressed adults? A cross-sectional investigation of the correlates of bullying and anxious depression. *The Journal of Nervous and Mental Disease, 194*(3), 201–208.
Guerin, S., & Hennessy, E. (2002). Pupils' definitions of bullying. *European Journal of Psychology and Education, 17*(3), 249–261.
Hanish, L. D., & Guerra, N. G. (2002). A longitudinal analysis of patterns of adjustment following peer victimization. *Development and Psychopathology, 14*, 69–89.
Harrist, A., Zaia, A., Bates, J., Dodge, K., & Petit, G. (1997). Subtypes of social withdrawal in early childhood: Sociometric status and social-cognitive differences across four years. *Child Development, 68*, 278–294.
Hartling, L. M., & Luchetta, T. (1999). Humiliation: Assessing the impact of derision, degradation, and debasement. *Journal of Primary Prevention, 19*(4), 259–278.
Hawkins, D. L., Pepler, D. J., & Craig, W. M. (2001). Naturalistic observations of peer interventions in bullying. *Social Development, 10*(4), 512–527.
Hawkins, J. D., & Weis, J. G. (1985). The social development model: An integrated approach to delinquency prevention. *Journal of Primary Prevention, 6*(2), 73–97.
Hawley, P. H. (2003). Prosocial and coercive configurations of resource control in early adolescence: A case for the well-adapted Machiavellian. *Merrill-Palmer Quarterly, 49*(3), 279–309.
Howard, A. M., Landau, S., & Pryor, J. B. (2013). Peer bystanders to bullying: Who wants to play with the victim? *Journal of Abnormal Child Psychology, 42*, 265–276.
Jackson, M. A. (1999). *Distinguishing shame and humiliation* (Doctoral Dissertation). Retrieved from ProQuest Dissertation and Thesis Database. (UMI Number 9968089).
Juffer, F., Stams, G. J. M., & van IJzendoorn, M. H. (2004). Adopted children's problem behavior is significantly related to their ego resiliency, ego control, and sociometric status. *Journal of Child Psychology and Psychiatry, 45*, 697–706.
Juvonen, J., Graham, S., & Schuster, M. A. (2003). Bullying among young adolescents: The strong, the weak, and the troubled. *Pediatrics, 112*, 1231–1237.

Kaplow, J. B., Curran, P. J., Dodge, K. A., & The Conduct Problems Prevention Research Group. (2002). Child, parent, and peer predictors of early-onset substance use: A multisite longitudinal study. *Journal of Abnormal Child Psychology, 30*, 199–216.

Klein, D. C. (1991). The humiliation dynamic: An overview. *The Journal of Primary Prevention, 12*(2), 93–121.

Kosciw, J. G., Greytak, E. A., Palmer, N. A., & Boesen, M. J. (2014). *The 2013 national school climate survey: The experiences of lesbian, gay, bisexual and transgender youth in our nation's schools*. New York, NY: GLSEN.

Krappmann, L. (1996). Amicitia, drujba, shin-yu, philia, freundschaft, friendship: On the cultural diversity of a human relationship. In W. M. Bukowski, A. F. Newcomb, & W. W. Hartup (Eds.), *The company they keep: Friendship in childhood and adolescence* (pp. 19–40). New York, NY: Cambridge University Press.

Kupersmidt, J., Coie, J., & Dodge, K. (1990). The role of poor peer relationships in the development of disorder. In S. R. Asher & J. D. Coie (Eds.), *Peer rejection in childhood*. Cambridge: Cambridge University Press.

Kupersmidt, J. B., & Coie, J. D. (1990). Preadolescent peer status, aggression, and school adjustment as predictors of externalizing problems in adolescence. *Child Development, 61*, 1350–1362.

LaFontana, K. M., & Cillessen, A. H. N. (2002). Children's perceptions of popular and unpopular peers: A multimethod assessment. *Developmental Psychology, 38*, 635–647.

Langman, P. (2009a). Rampage school shooters: A typology. *Aggression and Violent Behavior, 14*, 79–86.

Langman, P. (2009b). Columbine, bullying, and the mind of Eric Harris. *Psychology Today*. Retrieved from https://www.psychologytoday.com/blog/keeping-kids-safe/200905/columbine-bullying-and-the-mind-eric-harris

Lin, N. (2001). *Social capital: A theory of social structure and action*. New York, NY: Cambridge University Press.

Lin, N., Cook, K., & Burt, R. S. (2001). *Social capital: Theory and research*. New Brunswick, NJ: Transaction Publishers.

Lindner, E. G. (2001a). *Towards a theory of humiliation: Somalia, Rwanda/Burundi, and Hitler's Germany* (Doctoral Dissertation). University of Regensburg, Germany. Retrieved from http://www.humiliationstudies.org/documents/evelin/HumiliationBook2.pdf

Lindner, E. G. (2001b). Humiliation and the human condition: Mapping a minefield. *Human Rights Review, 2*(2), 46–63. https://doi.org/10.1007/s12142-001-1023-5

Lindner, E. G. (2003). *The theory of humiliation: A summary. Human dignity and humiliation studies*, 1–56. Unpublished manuscript. Retrieved from http://www.humiliationstudies.org/documents/evelin/HumiliationTheorySummary.pdf

Lindner, E. G. (2006). *Making enemies: Humiliation and international conflict*. Westport, CT: Praeger Security International.

Lindner, E. G. (2007). In times of globalization and human rights: Does humiliation become the most disruptive force? *Journal of Human Dignity and Humiliation Studies, 1*(1), 1–30. Retrieved from http://www.humilliationstudies.upeace.org/

Lonczak, H. S., Huang, B., Catalano, R. F., Hawkins, J. D., Hill, K. G., Abbott, R. D., & Kosterman, R. (2001). The social predictors of adolescent alcohol misuse: A test of the social development model. *Journal of Studies on Alcohol, 62*, 179–189.

Long, J. D., & Pellegrini, A. D. (2003). Studying change in dominance and bullying with linear mixed models. *School Psychology Review, 32*(3), 401–417.

Meltzer, H., Vostanis, P., Ford, T., Bebbington, P., & Dennis, M. S. (2011). Victims of bullying in childhood and suicide in adulthood. *European Psychiatry, 26*, 498–503.

Menesini, E., Modena, M., & Tani, F. (2009). Bullying and victimization in adolescence: Concurrent and stable roles and psycholgical health symptoms. *Journal of Genetic Psychology, 170*(2), 115–134.

Miller-Johnson, S., Coie, J. D., Maurmary-Gremaud, A., Lochman, J., & Terry, R. (1999). Relationship between childhood peer rejection and aggression and adolescent delinquency severity and type amont African American youth. *Journal of Emotional and Behavioral Disorders, 7*, 137–146.

Miller-Johnson, S., Coie, J. D., Maumary-Gremaud, A., Bierman, K., & The Conduct Problems Prevention Research Group. (2002). Peer rejection and aggression and early starter models of conduct disorder. *Journal of Abnormal Child Psychology, 30*, 217–230.

Mishna, F. (2012). *Bullying: A guide to research, intervention, and prevention*. New York, NY: Oxford University Press.

National Center for Education Statistics. (2015). *School crime supplement to the national crime victimization survey 2015 Questionaire*. Washington, DC: U.S. Department of Commerce Economics and Statistics Administration. Retrieved from https://nces.ed.gov/programs/crime/student_questionnaires.aspcrime/pdf/student/SCS2015.pdf

National Center for Educational Statistics. (2011). *Student reports of bullying and cyber-bullying: Results from the 2009 school crime supplement to the National Crime Victimization Survey*. Washington, DC: Author. Retrieved from http://nces.Ed.gov/pubs2011/2011336.pdf

Nelson, S. E., & Dishion, T. J. (2004). From boys to men: Predicting adult adaptation from middle childhood sociometric status. *Development and Psychopathology, 16*(2), 441–459.

Newcomb, A. F., & Bukowski, W. M. (1983). Social impact and social preference as determinants of children's peer group status. *Developmental Psychology, 19*(6), 856–867.

Newcomb, A., Bukowski, W., & Pattee, L. (1993). Children's peer relations: A meta-analytic review of popular, rejected, neglected, controversial, and average sociometric status. *Psychological Bulletin, 113*, 99–128.

Parker, J. G., & Asher, S. R. (1993). Friendship and friendship quality in middle childhood: Links with peer group acceptance and feelings of loneliness and social dissatisfaction. *Developmental Psychology, 29*, 611–621.

Parker, J. G., Rubin, K. H., Erath, S. A., Wojslawwowicz, J. C., & Buskirk, A. R. (2006). Peer relationships, child development, and adjustment: A developmental psychopathology perspective. In D. Cicchetti & D. J. Cohen (Eds.), *Developmental psychopathology* (2nd ed., pp. 419–493). Hoboken, NJ: John Wiley & Sons.

Parkhurst, J., & Asher, S. (1992). Peer rejection in middle school: Subgroups differences in behavior, loneliness, and interpersonal concerns. *Developmental Psychology, 28*, 231–241.

Parkhurst, J., & Hopmeyer, A. (1998). Sociometric popularity and peer-perceived popularity: Two distinct dimensions of peer status. *Journal of Early Adolescence, 18*, 125–144.

Pellegrini, A. D. (2002). Bullying, victimization, and sexual harassment during the transitions to middle school. *Educational Psychologist, 37*, 151–163.

Pellegrini, A. D., & Bartini, M. (2001). Dominance in early adolescent boys: Affiliative and aggressive dimensions and possible functions. *Merrill-Palmer Quarterly, 47*(1), 142–163.

Pellegrini, A. D., Bartini, M., & Brooks, F. (1999). School bullies, victims, and aggressive victims: Factors relating to group affiliation and victimization in early adolescence. *Journal of Educational Psychology, 91*, 216–224.

Peskin, M. F., Tortolero, S. R., & Markham, C. M. (2006). Bullying and victimization among Black and Hispanic adolescents. *Adolescents, 41*(163), 467–484.

Popp, A. M., & Peguero, A. A. (2012). Social bonds and the role of school-based victimization. *Journal of Interpersonal Violence, 27*(17), 3366–3388.

Poulin, F., & Dishion, T. J. (2008). Methodological issues in the use of peer sociometric nominations with middle school youth. *Social Development, 17*, 908–921.

Prinstein, M. J., & Cillessen, A. H. N. (2003). Forms and functions of adolescent peer aggression associated with high levels of peer status. *Merrill-Palmer Quarterly, 49*(3), 310–342.

Puhl, R. M., Luedicke, J., & Heuer, C. (2011). Weight-based victimization toward overweight adolescents: Observations and reactions of peers. *Journal of School Health, 81*(11), 696–703.

Putallaz, M. (1983). Predicting children's sociometric status from their behavior. *Child Development, 54*, 1417–1426.

Putallaz, M., & Wasserman, A. (1990). Children's entry behaviors. In S. R. Asher & J. D. Coie (Eds.), *Peer rejection in childhood*. New York, NY: Cambridge University Press.
Putnam, R. (1995). Bowling alone: America's decline in social capital. *Journal of Democracy, 6*, 65–78.
Putnam, R. D. (2000). *Bowling alone: The collapse and revival of American community*. New York, NY: Simon & Schuster.
Reijntjes, A., Vermande, M., Olthof, T., Goossens, F. A., van de Schoot, R., Aleva, L., & van der Meulen, M. (2013). Costs and benefits of bullying in the context of the peer group: A three wave longitudinal analysis. *Journal of Abnormal Child Psychology, 41*, 1217–1229.
Rieffe, C., Villanueva, L., & Meerum Terwogt, M. (2005). Use of trait information in the attribution of intentions by popular, average, and rejected children. *Infant and Child Development, 14*, 1–10.
Rivers, I. (2001). Retrospective reports of school bullying: Stability of recall and its implications for research. *British Journal of Developmental Psychology, 19*, 129–142.
Rodkin, P. C., & Berger, C. (2008). Who bullies whom? Social status asymmetries by victim gender. *International Journal of Behavioral Development, 32*, 473–486.
Rodkin, P. C., Farmer, T. W., Pearl, R., & Van Acker, R. (2000). Heterogeneity of popular boys: Antisocial and prosocial configurations. *Developmental Psychology, 36*, 14–24.
Rose, A. J. (2002). Co-rumination in the friendships of girls and boys. *Child Development, 73*, 1830–1843.
Rose, A. J., Swenson, L. P., & Waller, E. M. (2004). Overt and relational aggression and perceived popularity: Developmental differences in concurrent and prospective relations. *Developmental Psychology, 40*, 378–387.
Rubin, K. H. (2002). *The Friendship Factor: Helping our children navigate their social world—And why it matters for their success and happiness*. New York, NY: Viking Penguin.
Rubin, K. H., Chen, X., Coplan, R., & Buskirk, A. A. (2005). Peer relationships in childhood. In M. Bornstein & M. Lamb (Eds.), *Developmental science: An advanced textbook* (5th ed., pp. 469–512). New York, NY: Psychology Press.
Russell, J. (November 28, 2010). *World of misery left by bullying*. Boston, MA: The Boston Globe. Retrieved from http://www.boston.com/news/local/massachusetts/articles/2010/11/28/a_world_of_misery_left_by_bullying/
Ryalls, B. O., Gull, R. E., & Ryalls, K. R. (2000). Infant imitation of peer and adult models: Evidence for a peer model advantage. *Merrill-Palmer-Quarterly, 46*, 188–202.
Salmivalli, C. (2010). Bullying and the peer group: A review. *Aggression and Violent Behavior, 15*, 112–120.
Salmivalli, C., Lappalainen, M., & Lagerspetz, K. M. J. (1998). Stability of change behavior in connection to bullying in schools: A two-year follow-up. *Aggressive Behavior, 24*, 205–218.
Scholte, R. H. J., Overbeek, G., ten Brink, G., Rommes, E., de Kemp, R. A. T., Goossens, L., & Engles, R. C. M. E. (2008). The significance of reciprocal and unilateral friendships for peer victimization in adolescence. *Journal of Youth and Adolescence, 89*, 89–100.
Sidanius, J., & Pratto, F. (1999). *Social dominance: An intergroup theory of social hierarchy and oppression*. New York, NY: Cambridge University Press.
Siegel, D. J. (2012). *The developing mind*. New York, NY: Guilford Press.
Simmons, R. (2002). *Odd girl out*. New York, NY: Houghton Mifflin Harcourt Publishing.
Smith, D. (2001). Organizations and humiliation: Looking beyond Elias. *Organization, 8*(3), 537–560.
Smokowski, P. R., & Bacallao, M. (2010). *Becoming bicultural: Risk and resilience in Latino youth*. New York, NY: New York University Press.
Smokowski, P. R., & Kopasz, K. H. (2005). Bullying in school: An overview of types, effects, family characteristics, and intervention strategies. *Children and Schools, 37*(2), 101–110.
Thornberg, R., Tenenbaum, L., Varjas, K., Meyers, J., Jungert, T., & Vanegas, G. (2012). Bystander motivation in bullying incidents: To intervene or not to intervene? *The Western Journal of Emergency Medicine, 13*(3), 247–252.

Ttofi, M. M., Farrington, D. P., Losel, F., & Loeber, R. (2011). Do victims of school bullies tend to become depressed later in life? A systematic review and meta-analysis of longitudinal studies. *Journal of Aggression, Conflict, and Peace Research, 3*(11), 63–73.

U.S. Department of Education. (2016). *Student reports of bullying: Results from the 2015 School Crime Supplement to the National Crime Victimization Survey*. Washington, DC: National Center for Education Statistics. Retrieved from https://nces.ed.gov/pubs2017/2017015.pdf

Vaillancourt, T., Hymel, S., & McDougall, P. (2003). Bullying is power: Implications for school-based intervention strategies. *Journal of Applied School Psychology, 19*(2), 157–176.

van der Kolk, B. A. (1994). The body keeps the score: Memory and the evolving psychobiology of postraumtic stress. *Harvard Review Psychiatry, 1*(5), 253–265.

van der Kolk, B. A. (1997). Traumatic memories. In P. S. Apelbaum, L. A. Uyehara, & M. R. Elin (Eds.), *Trauma and memory: Clinical and legal controversies* (pp. 243–260). New York, NY: Oxford University Press.

Véronneau, M.-H., & Vitaro, F. (2007). Social experience with peers and high school graduation: A review of theoretical and empirical research. *Educational Psychology, 27*, 419–445.

Volk, A., Camilleri, J., Dane, A., & Marini, Z. (2012a). If, when, and why bullying is adaptive. In T. Shackelford & V. Shackelford (Eds.), *Oxford handbook of evolutionary perspectives on violence, homicide, and war* (pp. 270–290). New York, NY: Oxford University Press.

Volk, A., Camilleri, J., Dane, A., & Marini, Z. (2012b). Is adolescent bullying an evolutionary adaptation? *Aggressive Behavior, 38*, 222–238.

Volk, A. A., Dane, A. V., & Marini, Z. A. (2014). What is bullying? A theoretical redefinition. *Developmental Review, 34*, 327–343.

Williams, B., & Gilmour, J. (1994). Sociometry and peer relationships. *Journal of Child Psychology and Psychiatry and Allied Disciplines, 35*, 997–1013.

Chapter 3
Consequences of Bullying in Childhood, Adolescence, and Adulthood: An Ecological Perspective

3.1 Introduction

The news is replete with stories of youth bullied to death: children and adolescents who endured physical and verbal harassment day in and day out who eventually could not take it anymore and chose death over continuing to suffer at the hands of their peer group. Bullied youth of all ages have resorted to suicide: A 7-year-old boy in Detroit hung himself on his bunk bed due to constant bullying at school; 11-year-old Ty Smalley shot himself with a 0.22 caliber pistol after repeatedly being shoved into lockers and tormented from name calling; 13-year-old Ryan Halligan hung himself after enduring years of bullying; 15-year-old Amanda Cummings threw herself in front of a bus following ongoing bullying and cyberbullying; and 17-year-old Tyler Long hung himself in his bedroom closet after his classmates repeatedly spit in his food, called him "faggot," and stole his possessions. No matter the age, victims of bullying are at risk for serious negative consequences.

The Process–Person–Context–Time model, the third phase of Bronfenbrenner's (1979) ecological systems theory (Rosa & Tudge, 2013), helps organize and make sense of the negative outcomes associated with bullying involvement. Bullying is an intensely negative social interaction between peers; the social *Process* of bullying can prevent victims from engaging in positive social relationships and results in overall negative peer relationships. Other negative outcomes of bullying victimization occur at the individual *Person* level including poor mental health and disrupted neurobiological processes. Further, because bullying usually occurs in the school *Context*, victims often have negative perceptions of school. Finally, bullying that happens over *Time* is most detrimental, thus considering how the duration of bullying impacts victim outcomes in the short- and long-term is important.

According to ecological systems theory (Bronfenbrenner, 1979), human development is impacted by multiple environments (e.g., home, school/work, community) and the social interactions (i.e., proximal processes) that occur within and between these environments (Bronfenbrenner, 1994). Ecological systems theory

© Springer Nature Switzerland AG 2019

P. R. Smokowski, C. B. R. Evans, *Bullying and Victimization Across the Lifespan*, https://doi.org/10.1007/978-3-030-20293-4_3

was revised throughout the course of Bronfenbrenner's career and the third and final version, the Process–Person–Context–Time (P-P-C-T) model, is also referred to as bioecological theory and the bioecological model of human development. This model provides a framework for understanding human development over time by highlighting the interactions between the developing individual and his/her context (Bronfenbrenner, 2005; Rosa & Tudge, 2013). The P-P-C-T model differs from the previous iterations of ecological systems theory primarily in its focus on proximal processes (i.e., social interactions or processes) as opposed to the environment (Bronfenbrenner & Morris, 2006). *Process* refers to interactions between the individual and his/her environment including social interactions with family and peers referred to as proximal processes; these processes are the main catalyst of development but vary depending upon characteristics of the individual person. Thus, *Person* refers to individual attributes (e.g., mental health, neurobiology) that impact development; *Context* includes the surrounding environment such as family, school, or work; and *Time* refers to age, events, or historical factors that impact developmental outcomes (Bronfenbrenner & Morris, 2006; Rosa & Tudge, 2013). Although Bronfenbrenner delineated the process–person–context–time organization of the model to emphasize the paramount importance of Process interactions, we modify the presentation to discuss person–process–context–time in that order because this follows an ecological path from individual attributes to interpersonal relationships embedded within context and developing over time (i.e., working from what is most proximal to the child through increasingly distal environmental layers; see Fig. 3.1).

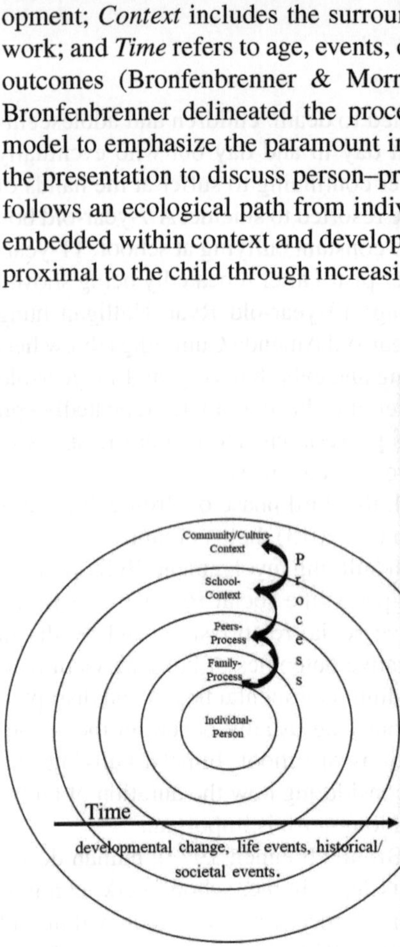

	Victims	Bullies
PERSON	Sex: females (relational, cyber); males (physical) Race/Ethnicity Appearance Disability Status Anxiety Depression Low Self Esteem Introversion Learned helplessness	Sex: females (relational, cyber); males (physical) Anxiety Depression ADHD Self Esteem (sometimes high) Suicidality? Hostile attribution bias
PROCESS	Low social skills Few friendships Sociometric rejection and neglect by peers	Seek power and control in relationships Exposure to domestic and community violence Seen as popular but not liked, antisocial behavior
CONTEXT	Varies by country, state in US, school settings, families	Varies by country, state in US, school settings, families
TIME	Age, grade (highest in middle school), cumulative victimization	Age, grade, developmental stage guides targets (peers, dating partners, spouses)

Fig. 3.1 Person–process–context–time model for bullying victimization and perpetration—bio-ecological model

Using this model, it is possible to map out some of the most salient negative outcomes associated with bullying at each ecological level. Figure 3.1 illustrates the model and summarizes victim and perpetrator risk factors at each level.

3.2 Person: Individual Attributes

The *Person* level of the P-P-C-T model refers to individual characteristics and we begin our discussion with individual attributes that might impact the bullying dynamic. The discussion of the prevalence of bullying in Chap. 1 showed that the bullying dynamic varies for females versus males. Victims are also targeted due to personal attributes, such as appearance, weight, height, religious background, socio-economic status, race/ethnicity including immigrant status, and presence of a disability, among other traits. Any personal characteristic that singles a child out from the normative peer group can be used by a strategic bully; the bully's power lies in identifying the victim's vulnerability and magnifying it to cause social damage that separates that child from the normative peer group. For example, a sixth grade boy who has not experienced puberty may be sensitive that he is shorter than his peers. The strategic bully who is taller and heavier may use the power differential to physically beat the smaller child but also may psychologically torture his victim by labeling him "wittle Willie Wilcox," a nickname the victim has to bear through high school and still irritates him 20 years later as an adult with below average height. Conversely, if William Wilcox was not sensitive about his small stature, the bully's power is reduced and the resulting damage may be minimal. A Puerto Rican female fifth grader described how her bully magnified personal attributes in this way.

> Some people pick on me because I'm big, 'cause I'm Puerto [Rican], I'm Hispanic, from where I come from, when you're young you have a lot of hair on your arms, so she picks on me 'cause of [my arm hair] and my weight and I'm working on it. She picks on me because of my arm hair and the way I dress. I sometimes dress like, um, a boy, 'cause when I dress like a tomboy she doesn't recognize who I am. She doesn't recognize and mess with me. I don't tell my mom things because she has mental problems, she has strokes. I don't want to stress her out, so I don't tell her, but the girl bullying me keeps on and on and on.

All human beings have personal attributes that may cause them to be vulnerable. The constellation of personal characteristics makes each of us unique but also provides fodder for perpetrators who want to point out that someone does not fit into the dominant group. Victims are usually sensitive about some type of personal attribute; manipulation and social humiliation around the area of vulnerability often precipitates an extreme emotional reaction and long-term memories. For example, nearly 30 years ago, Graydon Carter, an editor of Vanity Fair magazine, described Donald Trump in Spy magazine as a "short-fingered vulgarian" (Shapiro, 2016). President Trump, arguably one of the most powerful people in current society, has a particular sensitivity related to the size of his hands. Since 1988, Mr. Trump has sent pictures of himself back to Mr. Carter with his hands circled in gold sharpie to show they are a normal size. This issue continued to irritate Trump on the 2016 presidential campaign trail in derisive exchanges with "Little Marco Rubio." This is an example of how immature playground politics are easily manifested in national politics but also illustrates how magnification of a personal vulnerability damages self-esteem even in the context of massive resources and strength in other areas. Social humiliation around personal attributes is particularly powerful in combination with other mental health factors, such as anxiety and depression, that we will discuss below.

3.3 Person: Mental Health and Neurobiological Impacts of Bullying

In addition to the physical individual attributes discussed above, personality attributes also impact bullying. In general, individual characteristics impact development; although development is impacted by outside forces, the relationship is bidirectional. More specifically, individual characteristics of youth elicit differing responses during social interactions, which then shapes their development. For example, a depressed child may present with a flat affect, speak in a quiet, monotone voice, and be withdrawn; such a child would not likely easily engage others in conversation and might therefore sit alone at lunch and have few friends. In contrast, an outgoing and energetic child might be inclined to smile and make eye contact, initiate conversation, and seek out social companions; this child might have many friends and be constantly engaged in positive social interactions. These children would have very different developmental trajectories in part due to their individual presentations and personalities and how the outside world responds to them. The individual characteristics of mental health and neurobiology will be discussed as related to bullying involvement.

If the medical community could invent a vaccine to prevent kids from becoming enmeshed in the bullying dynamic as a perpetrator, victim, or both, children and adolescents would be happier and healthier. Indeed, such a vaccine would protect youth from the devastating mental health consequences associated with involvement in bullying. Across the board, youth who avoid involvement in the bullying dynamic consistently report better mental health outcomes compared to victims, perpetrators, or youth who fill both roles (e.g., Lester, Cross, & Shaw, 2012; Menesini, Modena, & Tani, 2009; Pollastri, Cardemil, & O'Donnell, 2009). Although any sort of involvement in the bullying dynamic, even witnessing bullying, is harmful, victims and bully-victims appear to suffer the most.

3.3.1 Person: Mental Health Impact of Bullying on Victims and Bully-Victims

Imagine for a moment that you are a seventh-grade girl and you desperately want to be popular, but for some reason the queen bee, who was your best friend last year, does not want you in her group anymore. At lunch, you can hear your name being whispered followed by quiet snickers. In the hallway, the queen bee and her followers ignore you and refuse to even acknowledge your existence. You find a list of superlatives lying on the classroom floor and you were voted "Most Likely to Never Have a Boyfriend." Rumors that you still sleep with your childhood teddy bear start circulating and now everyone seems to avoid you like the plague. On the weekend, photos are posted on Facebook of a sleepover you were not invited to. At age 13, how do you cope with this?

Imagine now that you are a tenth-grade boy and when you walk down the hallway, an upper classman shoves you as he walks by and hisses, "faggot" under his breath. Some days only one person does this, but other days it seems like every 3 ft someone is calling you a "fag" or a "fairy." At lunch, no one will sit with you. And in the locker room after gym class, people steal your clothes and hide them so you are forced to wear your gym shorts for the rest of the day. At age 16, how do you handle this day in and day out? The quote below describes the experience of an 11-year-old Caucasian sixth grade boy who had been bullied for three months. He tells of his process of becoming a bully-victim.

> This boy named [Eddie], he's always tryin' to push me and trip me with my necklace. He tried to grab my necklace around my neck and pulled to trip me. Every time I tell him to leave somebody else alone, he calls me bunny rabbit cause the top of my teeth are like pushed out, pushed out further. Umm, feels bad. I tell the teacher, but she doesn't really do anything. So that's when I take things into my own hands. I end up fightin'. At the beginning of this year, he kept on talkin' about my mom and then I started, tellin' him about his, I went to the teacher and told her, then he was still talking about me, and then I started talkin' about his daddy and then he pushed me and that's when I got mad and I started swingin' at him. I hit him like a bunch of times. We both went to in-school suspension. Sometimes I actually fake like I'm sick to stay out of school. Like, at least once or twice every week … I talk to my Mom. She tells me to stand up for myself and if they, like hit me first, go tell the teacher, if they still do it, and they hit me again, just hit 'em back … If you're bullied, it can lead to you being the bully. 'Cause, you get so tired of it and then you try to be like the other bullies so they'll stop. I was getting' picked on so much that I started picking on my friends.

Thinking about what victims of bullying experience, it is no wonder that in general, victims are insecure and anxious, have low self-esteem, a negative self-image, and high rates of depression (Aluede, Adeleke, Omoike, & Afen-Akpaida, 2008; Nazir & Piskin, 2015; Turner, Exum, Brame, & Holt, 2013). It follows that victims and bully-victims reported higher rates of depression, anxiety, and withdrawal compared to bullies and noninvolved youth. For example, one study of 1874 middle- and high-school youth found that compared to non-victimized youth, victimized youth were significantly more likely to report depression and suicidal ideation (Turner et al., 2013). Another study assessed anxious/depressed symptoms among 1278 youth ages 13–20 and found substantial/significant differences in the mean scores across groups. Specifically, researchers found that victims had a mean score of 9.35 for anxious/depressed symptoms and bully-victims had a mean score of 8.08, whereas perpetrators had a mean score of 5.49 and noninvolved youth had a mean score of 6.41 (Menesini et al., 2009). Similarly, in a sample of 1985 sixth grade students from 11 public middle schools in Los Angeles, victims had the highest levels of depression, social anxiety, and loneliness, followed by bully-victims; noninvolved youth and perpetrators had the lowest levels (Juvonen, Graham, & Schuster, 2003). Notably, other researchers have found the worst mental health outcomes are among bully-victims, followed by victims, and then bullies. In a sample of 16,410 Finish adolescents ages 14–16 years, depression was most common among adolescents who were bully-victims (i.e., odds ratio [OR] = 6.3), followed by victims (OR = 4.2), and then bullies (OR = 2.8; Kaltiala-Heino, Rimpela, Marttunen, Rimplea, & Rantanen, 1999). In other words, bullies were nearly three times more likely to report depression compared to non-involved youth; victims were more than four times more likely; and bully-victims were more than six times more likely to report depression than non-involved youth.

Anxiety and depression are understandable responses to bullying victimization, especially in the context of social humiliation experiences that magnify personal vulnerabilities. Victims face verbal and physical harassment day after day and often do not know when the next attack will come, leaving them on high alert, constantly waiting for the next slap or mean comment. This state of high alertness often follows an experience of trauma and is called hypervigilance and is commonly a sign of post-traumatic stress disorder (American Psychiatric Association, 2013; National Institute of Mental Health, n.d.). When an adverse event like bullying happens on an intermittent schedule, meaning that it is unpredictable and can occur at any time, the child's stress response system remains activated in anticipation of the next event. This constant state of high alert leaves victims feeling anxious and on edge, with racing adrenaline, attention scanning the environment, and thoughts preoccupied with bullying scenarios. Not knowing when the next attack will occur creates an ongoing state of vulnerability and stress. An 11-year-old Latina fifth grader was bullied over the course of three years. This is how she described her experience:

> I'm missin' a lot of work just because one person is bullying me. And I'm missin' my education just because one person is bullying me. I don't feel good. I just pretend to be sick just to go home so I don't have to deal with it no more. Cause it comes the next day and it just starts all over again. I just stay away from her as far as I can, but everywhere I go, she's right there … And it makes me feel like I shouldn't be in school, I should be in some … in jail, locked up, just cause somebody's makin me feel like that. And I'm thinkin it's not right that I have to put up with all of this and my mom said that my self-esteem has gone down. I'm usually excited to go places. But one girl just keeps messin with me and it's like [my excitement's all gone], I'm not gonna actually have fun because I have all of this to worry about. When we go back to school she's gonna go all over again … In class when I start to write, my hand starts to shake that somebody's gonna come behind me and just hit me in the head. And when she gets near me, that's how I feel, I start to shake, and I can't control when I start shakin my hands. When she gets near me, I start shakin my hands and when she goes away, they stop. It's like when she comes near me, I start getting tense.

This constant state of stress is akin to what scientists refer to as chronic stress and it has serious negative physical and emotional consequences such as "learned helplessness" (Peterson, Maier, & Seligman, 1995). Chronic stress causes the muscles in the body to remain tense, which can result in tension headaches or migraines (American Psychological Association, 2017). Normally the body's stress response system turns off once the stressor is removed. However, with chronic stress, such as bullying, the stressor is constant and thus the stress response system stays turned on, overexposing the body to cortisol and other stress hormones and thus increasing the risk for many negative outcomes including anxiety, depression, digestive problems, headaches, sleep problems, and impaired concentration and memory (Mayo Clinic, 2016). It follows that compared to bullies and noninvolved youth, victims and bully-victims reported a higher likelihood of sleep problems, tension, fatigue, and dizziness (Gini, 2008). These symptoms are in part likely a result of the chronic stress caused by victimization. In addition, constantly being verbally and/or physically attacked (especially around one's personal vulnerabilities) damages youths' self-esteem, and causes them to feel sad, down, and lonely. It is no wonder that victimized youth feel depressed. Bullying can become such an all-encompassing experience and the ensuing depression can become so severe that youth choose death over dealing with the pain of ostracism and social rejection. Figure 3.2 elegantly illustrates this point with a simple drawing by a sixth grader. The black eye in the drawing certainly hurts, but there is clearly a sense from the red halo of shame and humiliation around his head that the psychological consequences are even more damaging.

To understand even more fully why being bullied is painful and results in such profound depression and anxiety, we must consider the social exclusion that is at the core of bullying. Human beings are biologically programmed to be social beings; belonging to a social group provides us with protection, support, and nurturance. This is the evolutionary perspective discussed in Chap. 2. Bullying excludes the victim from social networks, which is incredibly painful given our innate, human desire to belong and have social connections. Social belonging and connection is

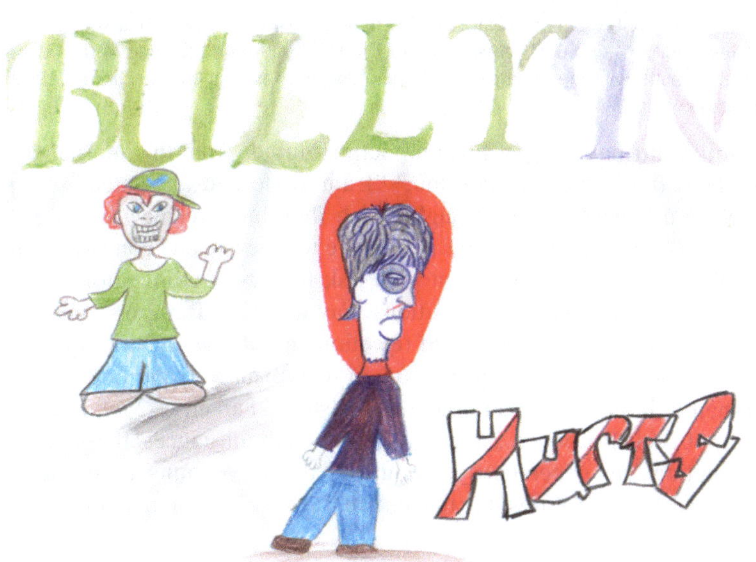

Fig. 3.2 "Bullying hurts" drawing by sixth grade male

particularly important for adolescents as this vulnerable age group is in the processes of forming their identity and gaining independence from parents and caregivers. Further, bullying is often done in a very public venue so that victims are humiliated in front of their peers. Indeed, bullying is considered a form of humiliation (Meltzer, Vostanis, Ford, Bebbington, & Dennis, 2011; Simmons, 2002). The humiliation that results from being bullied violates the fundamental human need for respect, recognition, and social connection and can often cause intense anger (Evans & Smokowski, 2016). If this anger is internalized, depression can result. However, this anger can also be externalized in the form of retaliation, which explains how youth become bully-victims (Evans & Smokowski, 2016). In light of the intense humiliation engendered by bullying victimization, it is understandable why victimized youth have low self-esteem; social ostracism leaves youth feeling worthless and alone. Indeed, given that the bullying dynamic functions to form a social hierarchy with empowered bullies and powerless victims, the major risk for victims is internalizing bullying messages that they are unwanted, unneeded, unacceptable, unloved, flawed beyond repair in some way, and rejected by others. The pain of this social rejection is registered in the brain by the same receptors that signal physical pain (See Eisenberger, 2012 for a review; See Tchalova & Eisenberger, 2017 for a review). Below, one victim discusses how the bullying impacted her stress, self-esteem, sleep, and eating habits:

> Like, during 3rd period or wherever she [the bully] sees me. "Oh look at her, she's so big. Oh look at this, she's so ugly." And when I come home it's like I've been at a job all day. Sometimes I don't even do my homework. I just fall right to sleep. And I wake up in the middle of the night and can't go back to sleep 'cause I feel like the next day I won't be able to go back to school. My mom thinks that when I'm stressed out, I eat a lot, yes that's true. That is true and she tries to control it, but I can't even control myself. And when I get real mad, only my brothers can calm me down, or my mom … I feel like a volcano exploding, I just want to…explode [whispers]. So, I'm just waitin until the end of the year when she does something, I'm gonna just blow me up, soon as we get out of school … Probably a hurricane of me.

The cognitive attributions that form in victims' minds from the internalized bullying messages (e.g., "People hate me," "I am alone and unwanted," "Why even try?") create a negative lens through which they interpret new experiences and interactions. Consequently, victims may move to a new social context by changing schools, for example, but remain at high risk for new victimization experiences. The power of these negative attributions may cause a disempowered worldview wherein victims anticipate continued rejection and ultimately stop trying to forge positive relationships. This helps to explain why damage from the childhood bullying dynamic lasts far into adulthood (Gladstone, Parker, & Malhi, 2006; Ttofi, Farrington, Losel, & Loeber, 2011a). In extreme circumstances, these intense negative attributions can generate psychological pain that prompts victims to consider suicide or make plans for revenge that end in tragedy, as seen in incidents of school shootings.

3.3.2 Person: Mental Health Impact of Bullying on Perpetrators

It is easy to vilify youth who bully others. Perpetrators choose to be cruel to their peers so they are at fault, right? On the one hand the answer is yes, because youth need to take responsibility for their behavior, however, there are often underlying social and emotional problems that are at the root of bullying behavior. While adults might be inclined to malign bullying perpetrators, it is important to try and figure out what is motivating their behavior. Although one large-scale study mentioned above (Kaltiala-Heino et al., 1999) found that victims and bully-victims had the highest rates of depression, bullies showed the highest risk of suicidal ideation (OR = 4.0), followed by bully-victims (OR = 2.5), and then victims (OR = 2.1), indicating that bullies are at a higher risk for suicidal ideation than previously thought.

This suggests that youth who bully might suffer from poor mental health, but rather then become victims, these youth channel their poor mental health into harming others. Indeed, a large scale study of parent report data from 63,997 youth ages 6–17 who participated in the 2007 National Survey of Children's Health study, found that youth diagnosed with a mental health disorder were significantly more likely to bully others compared to youth without a mental health diagnosis. Specifically, 13% of youth with no mental health issues were identified as bullies compared to 30% of youth with a mental health diagnosis. Youth diagnosed with depression, anxiety, and Attention Deficit Hyperactivity Disorder (ADHD) had almost three times the odds of being identified as a bully compared to those without these diagnosis (Benedict, Vivier, & Gjelsvik, 2015). These findings highlight the fact that although it is easy to vilify youth who perniciously bully their peers, they might actually be suffering themselves and are in need of support. This is not meant to excuse their egregious behavior, but simply meant to highlight the fact that adults should delve into the reasons why youth are bullying others.

Youth who bully others might also be victims or witnesses of domestic and community violence. These youths might bully others because they are reenacting the violence they have experienced and/or witnessed at home or in the community. Indeed, youth exposed to domestic violence have increased rates of internalizing and externalizing behavior (e.g., anxiety, depression, conduct problems, aggression; Bauer et al., 2006) that can translate into bullying others. For example, in one study of 700 fifth grade students, 61% of bullies and 59% of bully-victims witnessed domestic violence and violent community attacks; higher percentages than victims and non-involved youth (Holt, Finkelhor, & Kaufman Kantor, 2007). Another study of 1059 Italian elementary- and middle-school students found that witnessing domestic violence was significantly associated with bullying behavior (Baldry, 2003). Therefore, it is possible that youth who engage in bullying others, are actually victims in their homes and/or communities. Perhaps bullying is a way for them to regain a feeling of power after being abused by a parent or caregiver.

It is also possible that self-esteem and confidence plays a role in bullying perpetration. Research is inconsistent on how bullying others relates to self-esteem, but self-esteem might impact youths' proclivity to bully others. One thought is that perpetrators have healthy self-esteem levels on par with youth not involved in the bullying dynamic (Pollastri et al., 2009). If this is the case, perhaps robust self-esteem gives perpetrators the confidence to dominate their weaker classmates as a way of gaining additional power and prestige and maintaining their self-esteem. The profile of perpetrators with high self-esteem might include popular youth who bully others as a means of securing their social power and gaining respect from their peers. Other researchers have found that perpetrators had higher levels of peer self-esteem (e.g., self-esteem regarding popularity with peers) compared to the youth they victimize and non-involved youth, but lower general self-esteem compared to non-involved youth (Karatzias, Power, & Swanson, 2002). If this is the case, perhaps youth who bully feel threatened by those non-involved youth who appear confident and self-assured and bully to gain more social power than these non-involved youth. It is also possible that some perpetrators feel insecure and have low self-esteem; bullying then becomes an avenue for them to subjugate their less powerful peers and perhaps gain a feeling of confidence. Relegating someone else to a lower social position in the social hierarchy could give these insecure perpetrators a feeling of power. Given the elevated rates of exposure to domestic and community violence bullies experience, bullying others may also be an attempt to have victims feel pain and suffer like the bullies have. This is speculative because few childhood bullies articulate psychologically sophisticated reasoning for their bullying.

We can extend the discussion of cognitive attributions given above for victims to bullying perpetrators. Given that bullies are often exposed to domestic or community violence, they may have formed a social cognitive lens for seeing the world filled with hostility and interpersonal conflict. This "hostile attribution bias" is common in children and adolescents with conduct problems (See Crick & Dodge, 1994 for a review), leaving them interpreting new experiences and social stimuli with a framework that sees the world as a violent and unforgiving place. Based on their past experiences, fighting for power and control in the social hierarchy through coercion rather than collaboration is a foregone conclusion, the result of learning from past adversities. Similar to the victimization template that victims may use in moving from context to context, the hostility and power template that bullies may form also guides their new experiences and social choices, raising the risk of long-term behavior problems with lasting consequences.

To summarize, bullying involvement negatively impacts all participants, however, victims and bully-victims are the most negatively affected as evidenced by their high rates of anxiety and depression. Bully perpetrators also often suffer from poor mental health especially increased rates of depression, anxiety, and ADHD, which could explain their high rates of suicidal ideation. Further, experiences of domestic and/or community violence might fuel bullying behavior highlighting the fact that although it is easy to vilify perpetrators, they are often victims in other contexts and might be in need of support. It is possible that bullying victimization impacts mental health because the experience of victimization might actually impact brain structure and function.

3.3.3 *Person: Neuroscience-How Trauma and Stress Impact the Brain and Neurobiology*

Bullying victimization has recently been studied as a form of interpersonal trauma (D'Andrea, Ford, Stolbach, Spinazzola, & van der Kolk, 2012). Indeed, the ongoing humiliation engendered by bullying, and the intense emotional response victims have, highlight the importance of labeling bullying as a trauma. Bullying is not a rite of passage that kids must endure. It is not a normal part of growing up. It does not toughen kids up. It is not a box that needs to be checked off on the way to adulthood. Bullying is traumatic. In light of the devastating consequences of bullying discussed above, and the fact that other traumatic experiences such as childhood maltreatment impact brain structure and function, it follows that being bullied might also have an impact on the brain. The brain is an organ with plasticity, meaning that it is malleable and constantly impacted by experiences, especially trauma. Although research on how bullying victimization specifically impacts the brain is nascent, research on other traumatic events in general suggests that bullying might also alter certain structures of the brain.

Given recent advances in neuroimaging, it has become possible to use functional magnetic resonance imaging (fMRI) to study brain structure and function. This technology has recently been used to compare the brain structure and function in individuals who have experienced adverse childhood experiences (e.g., child abuse and neglect, trauma, poverty) with the brains of those who have not experienced adverse childhood experiences. While the majority of this research has examined adverse childhood experiences other than bullying, this research suggests that traumatic interpersonal experiences such as bullying might lead to structural and functional changes in the brain.

In general, researchers have focused on investigating if and how adverse childhood experiences impact the hippocampus, amygdala, and prefrontal cortex. The hippocampus and amygdala are part of the limbic system, a set of structures responsible for memory, emotion, and motivation. Specifically, the hippocampus is vital in the process of converting short-term memories into long-term memories and the amygdala is the center for emotions, emotional behavior, and motivation. The prefrontal cortex is involved in forming plans and strategies as well as personality development (Carlson, 2002). One meta-analysis of 15 studies found that individuals who had experienced childhood adversity (i.e., any difficult or unpleasant experience in childhood including trauma, abuse, neglect, poverty, or more general measures of adversity and early life stress) had decreased hippocampal volume compared to those without childhood adversity; there were no differences in terms of the amygdala (Calem, Bromis, McGuire, Morgan, & Kempton, 2017). However, the difference in hippocampal size diminished when gender was controlled for and the association differed depending upon whether participants with psychopathology were included (Calem et al., 2017). A comprehensive review article found 37 studies reporting on hippocampal size in adults with histories of childhood maltreatment, and 30 of the studies found one or more significant differences between maltreated and non-maltreated groups, or an inverse correlation between severity of maltreatment and hippocampal volume. The authors also found 27 studies examining the amygdala in subjects with and without maltreatment histories; eight studies reported a significant reduction in the size of the amygdala, 13 studies reported no significant size difference, and four reported a significant increase (Teicher & Samson, 2016). Another study found that children who experienced early life stress had smaller left amygdalae and those who were specifically physically abused or from a low socioeconomic status had smaller hippocampi relative to comparison children (Hanson et al., 2015). Another study of maltreated and non-maltreated adults found that childhood maltreatment was associated with smaller left and right hippocampal volumes (Chaney et al., 2014) and a study of college age students found that self-reported childhood maltreatment was associated with decreased gray matter volumes within the medial prefrontal cortex and the left hippocampus (Gorka, Hanson, Radtke, & Hariri, 2014). Although the findings are mixed, in general, childhood trauma in the form of abuse, maltreatment, or poverty seems to diminish the size of the hippocampus, amygdala, and prefrontal cortex. Researchers have also begun to examine how bullying experiences might impact the brain. Figure 3.3 summarizes the effects of social defeat as a form of PTSD on neurobiological processes.

In an attempt to specifically understand how social rejection (a form of relational bullying that adolescents often experience) impacts brain functioning, one group of

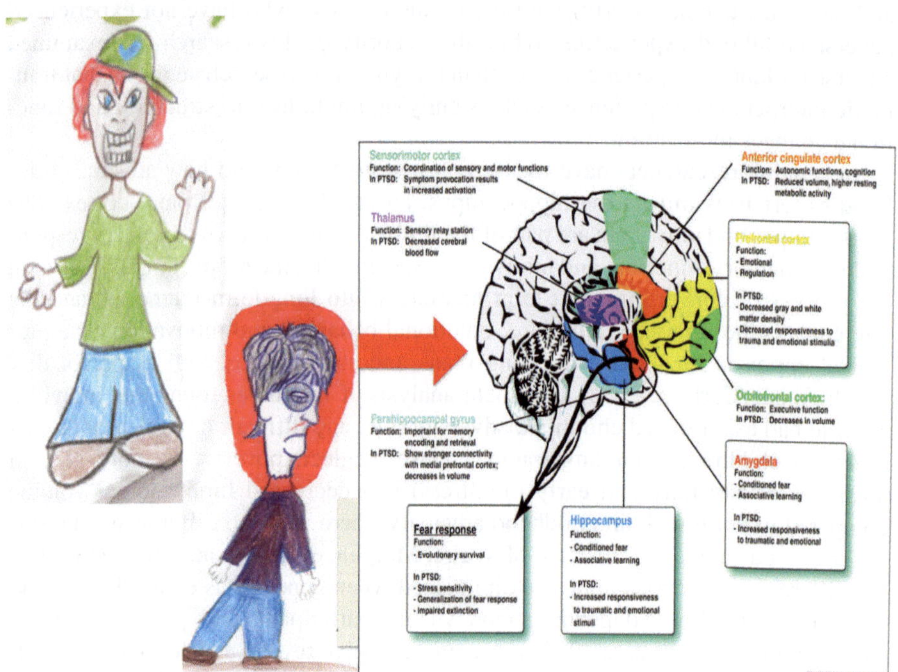

Fig. 3.3 Neurobiological response to bullying—social defeat and PTSD

researchers (Sebastian et al., 2011) compared fMRIs from 19 female adolescents ages 14–16 to the fMRIs of 16 female adults. Participants engaged in the Cyberball social paradigm; a virtual game of catch where participants are excluded from the game at certain points. Findings indicated that across all participants, social exclusion (as compared to social inclusion) triggered responses in regions of the brain associated with social evaluation, processing of negative affect, and affect regulation (i.e., the bilateral medial prefrontal cortex [mPFC], ventral and subgenual anterior cingulate cortex, medial orbitofrontal cortex, and left ventrolateral PFC [vlPFC]). Notably, regulation of rejection-related distress has been associated with activity in the right vlPFC in previous studies; however, in the Sebastian et al., 2011 study, the activity in the right vlPFC was much weaker in adolescents compared to adults. This finding indicated that the adolescent brain is not as adept at handling social rejection as the adult brain, which highlights why relational bullying can be particularly devastating to teenagers.

Other studies of the brain highlight the fact that bullying and physical pain might be processed in the same areas in the brain. Bullying is a form of social pain; social pain refers to actual or potentially damaged social connections via rejection or exclusion (Eisenberger, 2012). Neurobiological research suggests that experiences of social pain include some of the same neurobiological substrates connected to physical pain (see Eisenberger, 2012 for a review). This means that certain regions of the brain related to physical pain are also activated when we experience social rejection, which partially explains why social rejection is such a physically uncomfortable and distressing experience. Ongoing research is needed to more fully establish if and how bullying involvement impacts the brain, but preliminary research suggests that this form of social exclusion has the power to impact brain structure and function.

In addition to alterations in brain structure and function, the trauma of bullying also disrupts the body's neurobiological response to stress. The hypothalamic-pituitary-adrenal (HPA) axis is one of the central neuroendocrine systems that respond to stress in humans and animals. The HPA axis is activated in response to perceived physical or psychological threat, triggering the release of multiple hormones. First, the hypothalamus releases corticotropin releasing factor (CRF), which elicits the pituitary to release adrenocorticotropic hormone (ACTH) into the bloodstream, and finally ACTH triggers the adrenal cortex to release glucocorticoids (GCs) such as cortisol (Lupien et al., 2005). In the absence of stress, cortisol patterns usually show a circadian rhythm, with levels highest in the morning and then decreasing throughout the day (Kirschbaum & Hellhammer, 1989). The term Cortisol Awakening Response (CAR) refers to the increase in cortisol about 20–30 min after waking, which is the peak in the diurnal patterns and then cortisol levels gradually decrease throughout the day (Knack, Jensen-Campbell, & Baum, 2011). However, the secretion of cortisol can be disrupted by stress and the form of disruption depends upon the nature of the stress. A meta-analysis of 107 independent studies of 8521 individuals who experienced chronic stress (e.g., war, abuse, assault, natural disasters) found that overall, chronic stress was associated with significantly lower concentrations of morning cortisol ($d = -0.08$), higher concentrations of afternoon/evening cortisol

($d = 0.18$), a flatter diurnal rhythm ($d = 0.39$), and a higher daily volume of cortisol output ($d = 0.31$). Stress in the form of physical threat had a similar pattern with lower morning cortisol ($d = -0.16$), higher afternoon/evening cortisol ($d = 0.22$), and higher daily output ($d = 0.46$). However, stress in the form of social threat resulted in a slightly different pattern where morning cortisol levels were higher ($d = 0.27$), afternoon/evening levels were higher ($d = 0.26$), and the volume of daily output was lower ($d = 0.04$; Miller, Chen, & Zhou, 2007). Both increased and decreased levels of cortisol are damaging (Miller et al., 2007), indicating that cortisol disruptions caused by chronic stress in general and specific forms of stress such as physical or social threats, are problematic. Given that bullying is a form of chronic stress and often involves both physical and social threats, it follows that bullying could disrupt the body's stress response.

Indeed, researchers have begun examining how the stress of bullying impacts cortisol levels. A cross sectional study of a 154 12-year-old youth found that occasional and frequent verbal peer victimization was associated with lower secretion of cortisol. However, sex moderated the relationship between occasional verbal victimization and cortisol such that for girls, occasional exposure was associated with lower cortisol while for boys it was associated with higher cortisol (Vaillancourt et al., 2008). This same group of researchers then followed 168 12-year-old youth over 2 years and collected data at four time points. Results indicated that peer victimization at Time 1 predicted elevated symptoms of depression at Time 2, which predicted lower morning and evening cortisol levels at Time 3 and resulted in decreased memory at Time 4 (Vaillancourt et al., 2011). Another study of 12-year-old youth found that, compared to non-maltreated or non-bullied youth, those who had been maltreated and/or bullied showed a lower HPA axis reactivity to stress in the form of lower cortisol excretion following a stress test; non-maltreated or non-bullied children showed an expected increase in cortisol after a stress test while the maltreated or bullied youth did not. This lower cortisol response was also associated with more social and behavioral issues among the maltreated or bullied group (Ouellet-Morin, Odgers, et al., 2011). This finding was replicated in 35 monozygotic twin pairs discordant for bullying victimization. Bullied twins displayed the blunted cortisol response following a stress test compared to their non-bullied twin who showed the expected increase in cortisol (Ouellet-Morin, Danese, et al., 2011). The finding was also replicated in a sample of 107 12-year-old youth; peer victimization predicted a flattened CAR, which was in turn linked to health problems. Specifically, non-victimized youth showed a peak in cortisol level about 30 min after waking with a subsequent decrease throughout the day while victimized youth had lower levels of cortisol 30 min after waking and 20 min before bed (Knack et al., 2011). Taken together, findings indicate that bullying results in blunted cortisol response in victims. This decrease in cortisol might play a role in the behavioral and social difficulties displayed by victims (Ouellet-Morin, Odgers, et al., 2011).

To summarize, Person attributes are critically important to the bullying dynamic because they serve as risk factors that heighten the victim's chances of being selected for abuse and increase vulnerability if an area of personal sensitivity is magnified during social humiliation. Mental health issues, such as anxiety, depression, and chronic stress reactivity, can also play a major role in making the bullying dynamic deleterious for both victims and bullies.

3.4 Process: Peer Relationships

Process refers to the social interactions that occur across the ecological levels of adolescent development. These social interactions include interactions with parents, siblings, friends, peers, teachers, neighbors, and other community members and play a central role in child and adolescent development by impacting development across the lifespan. Although all social interactions are important, social interactions with peers are vital to the bullying dynamic and will therefore be the focus of this section. The act of bullying is an intensely negative social interaction that occurs between peers. Given that social interactions (i.e., proximal processes) are viewed as a central catalyst of development (Bronfenbrenner & Morris, 2006), it follows that a negative social interaction like bullying would have severe negative consequences on development, including damaged peer relationships.

3.4.1 Process: Victims' Peer Relationships

Victims of bullying often have problematic peer relationships due in part to their decreased levels of social competence. Social competence refers to a child's capacity to form and maintain positive peer relationships through his or her mastery of social skills (e.g., emotion regulation, cooperation) and by responding appropriately to constantly changing social stimuli (Bierman, 2004). In one study, low social competence significantly predicted victimization, whereas higher social competence significantly predicted bullying (Nation, Vieno, Perkins, & Santinello, 2008). Decreased social competence leads to difficulties navigating peer relationships (e.g., negotiating conflicts, making friends), which in turn, leads to victims having few friends (Bagwell & Schmidt, 2011; Scholte et al., 2008), feeling lonely and excluded (Kvarme, Helseth, Saeteren, & Natvig, 2010), and perceiving low levels of peer support (Demaray & Malecki, 2003; Furlong, Chung, Bates, & Morrison, 1995; Holt & Espelage, 2007). A negative feedback loop ensues whereby low social competence makes youth prime targets for bullying, and then ongoing bullying further damages youths' confidence in their social competence and prevents them from increasing their social competence through positive social interactions. Once bullying begins, it can be difficult for victims to escape because they lack the social skills to navigate this complex social dynamic and garner little support from friendly peers. Further, victims might become classroom pariahs of sorts and classmates could be reticent to interact with them for fear of also becoming victimized or being viewed as "uncool" for hanging out with them. In this regard, bullying becomes an impediment to increasing social competence and forming positive social connections. One way social competence increases is through practice with ongoing positive social interactions; being bullied not only constantly exposes youth to negative and dysfunctional peer interactions but also prevents victims from engaging in positive social interactions because prosocial classmates might shun their victimized peers. Thus, victimized youth do not often have the opportunity to engage in and practice prosocial interactions.

However, this is not to imply that all victims are totally without friends. Indeed, some victims have friends, although fewer friends than youth not involved in bullying (Scholte et al., 2008) and when victims' friends are not involved in the bullying dynamic, such friendships serve as a protective factor that inhibits victimization. However, when victims are friends with other victims, friendship does not serve as a buffer against bullying (Pellegrini, Bartini, & Brooks, 1999). Victims' friends are often less well-adjusted compared with the friends of bully-victims and noninvolved youth. Moreover, friends of victims often report feelings of loneliness and rejection (Scholte et al., 2008), which might indicate they are also victims and therefore unable to provide themselves or their friends with protection from bullies. Victims are consistently engaged in dysfunctional social processes either with the youth who bully them, or with their few friends, who may also have poor social skills and low social competence. Given this constant exposure to stressful social interactions, it follows that in addition to having poor peer relationships, victims often also have poor mental health outcomes as a result of being bullied. The social humiliation that often comes with the bullying dynamic has profound impacts on a victim's self-esteem and individual psychology.

Outside of peer relations, victims often close themselves off from supportive relationships out of self-consciousness, shame, and embarrassment. Parents and teachers are not told about the bullying because victims might think adult involvement will only make it worse or they are too embarrassed to ask for help. Some youth find adult involvement ineffective. One victim described her attempts at soliciting teacher support as follows:

> When I go tell the teacher sometimes, all they do is tell her to stop and that's it. They don't do nothin' else about it. And then, when I go tell again, they just act like they forgot. But one of my teachers, her name is Ms. Horvath, when I tell her, she handles it. She steps them out into the hallway, she tells 'em, "if you mess with one more person you are getting written up for bullying." So, she stops for a little while, but then she start back up bullying me and she keeps sayin' that she's going to get her cousins to jump me. Then I get scared to go to school. So I tell my mom. Sometimes I pretend to be sick just to stay home. And I can't hit her 'cause I know that I'm gonna get in trouble, so I don't hit her or touch her in any kind of way. I just kinda have to take it.

Even though social support can buffer the negative impact of the victimization, many victims cope by withdrawing from social interactions and focusing inward, a choice that keeps them isolated, stressed, lonely, and preoccupied with the negative events.

3.4.2 *Process: Bullies' Peer Relationships*

As noted in Chap. 2, youth who bully others also have complex peer relationships and are often disliked by their classmates but are viewed as popular (Cillessen & Mayeux, 2004; Prinstein & Cillessen, 2003). This seemingly contradictory finding actually makes sense because there is a difference between being liked and being viewed as popular. Being liked by classmates indicates that they enjoy your company, want to spend time with you, and generally like your personality. Popularity on the other hand, centers on power and social status. Thus, a child can be viewed as powerful with a high social status (i.e., popular) but disliked by classmates. Research suggests that youth who engage in relational aggression and bullying (e.g., rumor spreading) are viewed as popular but are disliked (Cillessen & Mayeux, 2004). Classmates likely fear these bullies and view them as powerful which equates with popularity but simultaneously dislike their mean behavior.

Social status and popularity allow perpetrators to accrue social capital, which refers to the benefits gained from social relationships (Putnam, 2000). Although they might be disliked by classmates, the popularity that bullying behavior garners allows perpetrators access to what social capital theorists argue are four beneficial resources (Lin, 2001; Lin, Cook, & Burt, 2001): (1) *Information*—being popular puts youth in contact with popular peers who can provide information about opportunities, such as after school social engagements, that provide the opportunity to further strengthen bonds with the popular crowd; (2) *Influence*—being popular and connected to the popular crowd might allow bullies to influence other people in power and get a cadre of bullies together who "rule the school"; (3) *Social Credentials*—being socially connected to certain individuals provides access to social resources (e.g., by bullying and gaining social status, perpetrators then gain access to the social resource of popularity and the connection to other popular classmates who can help maintain their status); (4) *Identity Reinforcement*—social relationships reinforce an individual's identity and sense of self-worth; bullying others and gaining social status could provide bullies with a sense of power and belonging. In summary, the social status and popularity that often comes with bullying provides youth with social capital and the four aforementioned benefits that serve to fuel and encourage ongoing bullying behavior.

Finally, the friendships of aggressive youth who might be prone to bullying are qualitatively different than friendships between non-aggressive youth. In fact, the friendships between aggressive youth were rated as having more intense negative affect during conflict and were perceived as engaging in more frequent rule breaking than nonaggressive friend dyads (Bagwell & Coie, 2004). This finding suggests that when bullies are friends they might feed off of each other, creating an antisocial dynamic. Indeed, the friendships of aggressive youth generally seem to lack the positive interactions and mutuality of nonaggressive friendships (Bagwell & Schmidt, 2011).

3.5 Context: School Experiences

In the P-P-C-T model, *Context* refers to the environments that impact development, sometimes referred to as macrosystems. While there are multiple environments across the lifespan that impact development such as home, school, work, and neighborhood, the school context is most central to the child and adolescent bullying dynamic. Indeed, given that bullying victimization commonly occurs in the school setting, it follows that victims often report negative school experiences and dislike the school context.

3.5.1 Context: Negative Impact of Bullying Victimization on Victims' School Experiences

For victims, school is viewed as a dangerous and unsafe place. As compared with non-victimized youth, victims reported lower school connectedness (You et al., 2008) and higher levels of school dissatisfaction (Dulmus, Sowers, & Theriot, 2006). These findings appear to hold worldwide; a study of more than 200,000 youth 11–15 years old from 40 countries showed negative school perceptions were significantly related to victimization (Harel-Fisch et al., 2011). Specifically, victims of bullying perceived school as unsafe and viewed their peers as unsupportive and unaccepting. One reason victims have negative perceptions of school stems from their perceptions of teachers as unable to protect them from bullying (Cunningham, 2007). Further, although peer bystanders are present for almost 90% of bullying episodes (Atlas & Pepler, 1998; Hawkins, Pepler, & Craig, 2001), peers rarely intervene to support victims. A 2-year longitudinal study of 189 adolescents found that when participants were in sixth grade, only 17% of bystanders intervened to defend the victim. By eighth grade, this rate had increased slightly, but only 20% of eighth-grade bystanders intervened to support the victim (Salmivalli, Lappalainen, & Lagerspetz, 1998). This lack of support leads victims to think of school as an unsupportive and hostile environment, resulting in social disengagement that might explain, at least in part, victims' and bully-victims' lower achievement scores and their reports of decreased feelings of school belonging (Glew, Fan, Katon, Rivara, & Kernic, 2005).

3.5.2 Context: Negative Impact of Bullying on Bullies' School Experiences

Youth who bully others also suffer from negative school experiences. Along with victims, bully-victims and bullies also reported lower levels of school bonding, less perceived monitoring by adults, and higher perceived rates of school aggressiveness compared to the perceptions of youth not involved in the bullying dynamic (Totura et al., 2009). These negative perceptions of school adversely impact perpetrators' academic performance and compared with victims and noninvolved youth, bullies have poorer academic outcomes (Totura et al., 2009). It follows that youth who bully others are at an increased risk of dropping out of school (Vanderbilt & Augustyn, 2010). While temporal order is unclear (i.e., does the bullying behavior cause youth to become disengaged from school and have poor academic outcomes and low school bonding? Or do poor academic outcomes and low school bonding promote bullying behavior?), this body of research indicates that bullies are in need of support to ensure that they stay engaged in school. Improving bullies school experiences could be one avenue to help them become connected to academics and the school community and stop their bullying behavior.

3.5.3 *Context Outside of School*

Along with schools, there are other important contexts that influence on the bullying dynamic. As shown in Chap. 1, bullying is a universal problem; however, some countries (i.e., contexts) foster more of this behavior than other countries. The larger macrosystem includes culture, norms, values, politics, policies, rules, and all types of messages that can exacerbate or limit the bullying dynamic. Some societies and cultural institutions (e.g., churches, organizations, schools) are more inclusive than others, allowing the proliferation of bullying against minority groups that are not valued. Discrimination against racial minorities, homosexuals, Jewish people, immigrants, Christians, individuals with a disability, women, and many other disempowered groups is common in certain contexts that are guided by exclusionary messages, hierarchical conflicts, and norms that emphasize power and control. We will discuss how social contexts enable or discourage the bullying dynamic in Chap. 11.

3.6 Time: Cumulative Bullying Victimization

Time is the final element of the P-P-C-T model. As related to bullying, time should be considered in terms of when bullying happens and how long bullying continues. Cumulative bullying victimization, victimization that occurs year after year, is particularly damaging and can have a long-term negative impact on victims that can endure throughout adolescence and into adulthood. Victimization can be cumulative in two ways. First, experiences of victimization can accumulate over time, meaning that youth are bullied year after year. While it is possible that a victim could be bullied repeatedly over one specific year of school and then the next year the bullying could stop, other youth could be victimized repeatedly year after year; this is cumulative victimization. Second, victimization can be cumulative in terms of types of victimization; youth can suffer from multiple forms of bullying. Some youth might simply be the victim of relational bullying and have rumors spread about them. However, like Ty Smalley mentioned in the introduction who was stuffed into lockers (physical bullying) and called mean names (verbal bullying), youth are often bullied in multiple ways. Cumulative victimization is particularly pernicious as the victimization experiences cumulate over the years resulting in negative consequences that are more severe than when the bullying is experienced over a shorter time period. Or, in the case of youth who experience cumulative bullying through multiple types of bullying, the various forms of bullying experienced serve to traumatize and emotionally harm the victims. The concept of a "dose–response" relationship helps explain why cumulative victimization is so harmful.

The term "dose–response" indicates that different degrees of exposure (i.e., dose) to a stimulus will result in varying outcomes (i.e., responses; Waddell, 2010). Although this term is most commonly used in scientific research (Waddell, 2010), it has more recently been used in social sciences research on interpersonal trauma (e.g., Freer, Whitt-Woosley, & Sprang, 2010; Kelleher et al., 2013). Cumulative exposure to stress and/or trauma results in increased psychological impairment: "Sequential stressors can have a cumulative effect … Chronic and unpredictable stress may be more likely to … disrupt an individual's basic sense of trust in relationships and confidence in the future" (McFarlane & de Girolamo, 1996, pp. 132, 138). In other words, the higher the dose of victimization (e.g., the more victimization is experienced either in duration or type), the worse the developmental outcomes. Indeed, bullying researchers have confirmed a dose response relationship between bullying victimization and negative outcomes such that increased bullying over time or experiencing more types of bullying are related to worse developmental outcomes.

For example, a cross sectional study of 856 Norwegian youth ages 13–15 found that those who reported more frequent bullying victimization also reported increased physical (i.e., headache, stomach, backache, dizziness) and psychological (i.e., feeling low, irritable, nervous) symptoms compared to their counterparts who were not victimized or were victimized less frequently (Natvig, Albreksten, & Qvarnstrom, 2001). A longitudinal study using a nationally representative sample of 1112 youth ages 13–16 years found that the more types of bullying victimization an adolescent endorsed (e.g., relational, verbal, having things stolen) at baseline, the higher the odds of psychotic symptoms at 3- and 12-month follow-ups. Specifically, adolescents who endorsed three or more types of victimization on the six-item scale had an odds ratio (OR) of 7.94 for psychotic experiences at the 12-month follow-up compared to those who endorsed two items (OR = 4.14) or those who endorsed one item (OR = 3.80; Kelleher et al., 2013). Another longitudinal study of 2426 adolescents in middle and high school confirmed a dose–response relationship in terms of both duration and type of bullying. Youth who were both traditionally and electronically bullied every year over the 3-year study window had the worst outcomes including increased depression, anxiety, aggression, and school hassles and decreased self-esteem, future optimism, school satisfaction, and perceived discrimination. Outcomes gradually improved as the duration of the bullying decreased and for youth who only experienced one form of bullying (traditional or electronic; Evans, Smokwoski, & Cotter, 2014).

Figure 3.4 illustrates the dose–response relationship between years of victimization and developmental problems. In a 6-year panel study of more than 10,000 ethnically diverse adolescents living in rural areas and attending 38 middle and high schools in North Carolina, 41% of participants reported never being victimized, 29% reported 1 year of victimization, 17% reported 2 years, 8% 2 years, 4% 4 years, and 1% were victimized every year for 5 years. It is shocking that both 59% of adolescents were victimized at some point in time, and 13% were bullied for at least 3 years. In other words, more than one in every ten youth in this study was abused by their peers for at least half of their adolescent developmental stage from middle school through high school (Evans et al., 2014).

In the same study, 31.4% of youth reported bullying others; 22% for 1 year, 7% for 2 years, 2% for 3 years, and 0.4% for 4 years. These perpetrators often have multiple victims. In addition, 42% of adolescents in this longitudinal study reported negative bystander behavior (i.e., cheering the bully on, helping with the victimization) for 1 or 2 years while, on an optimistic note, 81% reported helping victims at some point. Figure 3.5 depicts a longitudinal model using the cumulative exposure to roles in the bullying dynamic to predict behavioral, mental health, and academic outcomes at the end of the 5-year panel study (Evans, Smokowski, Rose, Mercado, & Marshall, 2018). Cumulative bullying victimization was significantly associated with increased levels of aggression and internalizing symptoms and decreased levels of self-esteem and future optimism. Cumulative bullying perpetration was significantly associated with increased levels of aggression and decreased levels of future optimism. Cumulative negative bystander behavior was significantly associated with increased aggression and internalizing symptoms and decreased academic achievement and future optimism. Cumulative prosocial bystander behavior was significantly associated with increased levels of internalizing symptoms, academic achievement, self-esteem, and future optimism.

These findings make sense. The longer youth endure bullying, the greater the negative impact bullying has on their mental health and developmental outcomes. Although enduring bullying for 1 year of school is devastating, if the bullying stops,

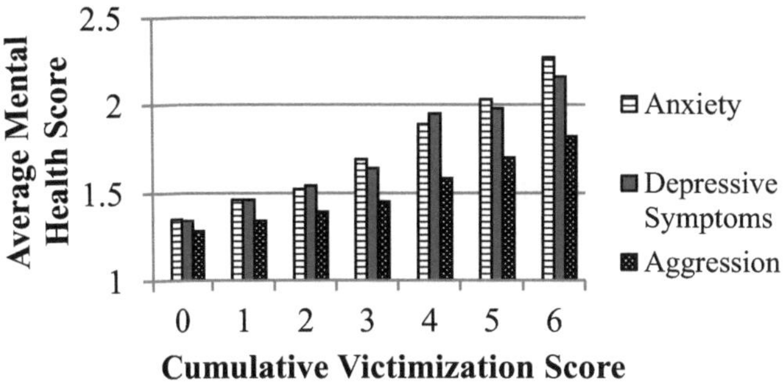

Fig. 3.4 Cumulative victimization and mental health outcomes

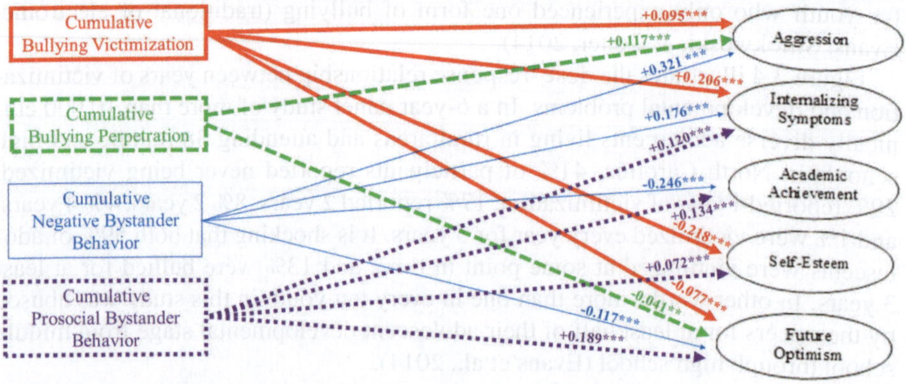

Fig. 3.5 Longitudinal model of cumulative effects of bullying dynamics. Note: $*p < 0.05$; $**p < 0.01$; $***p < 0.001$. CFI = 0.995, TLI = 0.994, RMSEA = 0.033

victims have time to heal, recover, and make positive social connections that might help resolve some of the negative feelings lingering in the aftermath of the bullying. Once the bullying stops, victims have the opportunity to regain self-confidence and to form positive social bonds. However, if the bullying continues over time, year after year, youth have no respite and no time to increase their self-esteem or feel a part of the social fabric of the classroom and school. Youth who endure multiple forms of bullying also receive no break from the bullying as they might face physical and verbal bullying at school and then be hit with electronic bullying via nasty text messages and Facebook posts when they go home. Overall, the longitudinal consequences of cumulative exposure to bullying are quite negative. As Fig. 3.5 shows, victims become more aggressive, depressed, and anxious, with decreased self-esteem and future optimism. Bullies become more aggressive and report lower future optimism. Negative bystanders who help bullies, reported more aggression, depression, and anxiety as well as lower academic achievement and future optimism. The heroic actions of prosocial bystanders who help victims are the only positive effects; these adolescents reported higher academic achievement, self-esteem, and future optimism. Yet they also report increased anxiety (Evans et al., 2018). These results underscore the importance of preventing cumulative exposure to bullying and training adolescents to be prosocial bystanders.

3.7 Time: The Longitudinal Impact of Bullying

3.7.1 Victimization

Time should also be considered in terms of the duration of the negative impact of bullying. Although school based bullying occurs in childhood and adolescence, the negative impact of bullying can endure long after the bullying has ended. A meta-analysis of 29 studies found that bullying victimization in childhood resulted in increased rates of depression that endured for up to 36 years post-victimization, with an average of 6.9 years post-victimization (Ttofi et al., 2011a). Adult victims of childhood bullying are also at an increased risk for other internalizing disorders such as anxiety (Gladstone et al., 2006). Another meta-analysis of 51 reports of 28 longitudinal studies found that childhood victimization was associated with aggressive (e.g., fighting) and violent behavior (e.g., assault, robbery, rape) an average of 6 years following victimization (Ttofi, Farrington, & Losel, 2012). This finding suggests that victimization often results in subsequent violent behavior years later, heightening the risk for engagement with the juvenile justice system, criminality, and in some instances school shootings planned as revenge. The risk for all of these antisocial outcomes could be decreased with a strong societal emphasis on prevention of initial victimization. A retrospective study of 72 adults found that those who recalled being victimized in childhood had poorer psychosocial outcomes as adults as evidenced by significantly higher anxiety and fear of negative evaluation and significantly lower self-esteem and life satisfaction compared to adults who were bullies, bully-victims, bystanders, or uninvolved in bullying as children (Blood & Blood, 2016). Using data from the National Child Development Study, researchers analyzed bullying and mental health service utilization data from 9242 participants. Findings indicated that compared to those who were not bullied in childhood, participants who endure frequent bullying were significantly more likely to use mental health services in childhood and adolescence (Odds ratio [OR] = 2.53, CI 1.88–3.40) and in midlife (i.e., age 50; OR = 1.3, CI 1.10–1.55; Evans-Lacko et al., 2017). These findings highlight that bullying causes emotional distress at the time it occurs, but this distress lingers long into adulthood, causing victims to seek mental health support. Taken together, research on the longitudinal impact of bullying highlights the fact that even once childhood bullying stops, the scars endure for decades.

3.7.2 *Bullying*

Youth engaged in bullying perpetration also have negative long-term outcomes. For example, a meta-analysis of 28 studies that compared childhood bullies with non-bullies found that bullies displayed increased levels of criminal offending up to 11 years post-bullying (Ttofi, Farrington, Losel, & Loeber, 2011b). This finding suggests that the aggressive and antisocial behavior in which bullies engage, can become a somewhat permanent part of their behavior that endures years after school ends. Further, the behavior escalates from harassing peers to actual criminal offending. Overall, these longitudinal findings indicate that both victimization and bullying are associated with a host of long-term negative consequences (e.g., depression, anxiety, aggression, violence), highlighting the necessity of putting a stop to this harmful behavior.

3.8 Conclusions

The person–process–context–time model provides a convenient framework for examining the negative bioecological impact of the bullying dynamic. Bullying itself is a negative social process that leads to disrupted peer relationships. At the person level, victims commonly suffer from a variety of negative mental health outcomes, which could cause changes in brain structure and function and/or disruptions in the body's stress response. Because bullying commonly takes place in the context of school, victims have negative views of school and low levels of school connectedness. Finally, considering time, cumulative bullying is particularly harmful and the effects of bullying endure long after the dynamic ends.

References

Aluede, O., Adeleke, F., Omoike, D., & Afen-Akpaida, J. (2008). A review of the extent, nature, characteristics, and effects of bullying behaviour in schools. *Journal of Instructional Psychology, 35*, 151–158.

American Psychiatric Association. (2013). *Diagnostic and statistical manual of mental disorders* (5th ed.). Arlington, VA: American Psychiatric Publishing.

American Psychological Association. (2017). *Stress effects on the body*. Washington, DC: Author. Retrieved from http://www.apa.org/helpcenter/stress-body.aspx

Atlas, R. S., & Pepler, D. J. (1998). Observations of bullying in the classroom. *Journal of Educational Research, 92*(2), 86–99.

Bagwell, C. L., & Coie, J. D. (2004). The best friendships of aggressive boys: Relationship quality, conflict management, and rule-breaking behavior. *Journal of Experimental Child Psychology, 88*, 5–24.

Bagwell, C. L., & Schmidt, M. E. (2011). *Friendships in childhood and adolescence*. New York, NY: Guilford Press.

Baldry, A. C. (2003). Bullying in schools and exposure to domestic violence. *Child Abuse & Neglect, 27*, 713–732.

Bauer, N. S., Herrenkohl, T. I., Lozano, P., Rivara, F. P., Hill, K. G., & Hawkins, D. (2006). Childhood bullying involvement and exposure to intimate partner violence. *Pediatrics, 118*(2), e235–e242.

Benedict, F. T., Vivier, P. M., & Gjelsvik, A. (2015). Mental health and bullying in the United States among children aged 6 to 17 years. *Journal of Interpersonal Violence, 30*(5), 782–795.

Bierman, K. L. (2004). *Peer rejection: Developmental processes and intervention strategies*. New York, NY: Guilford.

Blood, G. W., & Blood, I. M. (2016). Long-term consequences of childhood bullying in adults who stutter: Social anxiety, fear of negative evaluation, self-esteem, and satisfaction with life. *Journal of Fluency Disorders, 50*, 72–84.

Bronfenbrenner, U. (1979). *The ecology of human development: Experiments by nature and design*. Cambridge, MA: Harvard University Press.

Bronfenbrenner, U. (1994). Ecological models of human development. In *International encyclopedia of education* (Vol. 3, 2nd ed.). Oxford: Elsevier. Reprinted in M. Guavain, & M. Cole (Eds.), Readings on the development of children (2nd edn.; pp. 37–43). New York, NY: Freeman.

Bronfenbrenner, U. (2005). *Making human beings human*. Thousand Oaks, CA: Sage.

Bronfenbrenner, U., & Morris, P. A. (2006). The bioecological model of human development. In W. Damon (Series Ed.) & R. M. Lerner (Vol. Ed.), *Handbook of child psychology: Theoretical models of human development* (pp. 793–828). New York, NY: Wiley.

Calem, M., Bromis, K., McGuire, P., Morgan, C., & Kempton, M. J. (2017). Meta-analysis of associations between childhood adversity and hippocampus and amygdala volumes in non-clinical and general population samples. *Neuroimage: Clinical, 14*, 471–479.

Carlson, N. R. (2002). *Foundations of physiological psychology* (5th ed.). Boston, MA: Allyn and Bacon.

Chaney, A., Carballedo, A., Amico, F., Fagan, A., Skokauskas, N., Meaney, J., & Frodl, T. (2014). Effect of childhood maltreatment on brain structure in adult patients with major depressive disorder and healthy participants. *Journal of Psychiatry and Neuroscience, 39*(1), 50–59.

Cillessen, A. H. N., & Mayeux, L. (2004). From censure to reinforcement: Developmental changes in the association between aggression and social status. *Child Development, 75*(1), 147–163.

Crick, N. R., & Dodge, K. A. (1994). A review of reformulation of social information-processing mechanisms in children's social adjustment. *Psychological Bulletin, 115*(1), 74–101.

Cunningham, N. J. (2007). Level of bonding to school and perception of the school environment by bullies, victims, and bully victims. *The Journal of Early Adolescence, 27*, 457–478.

D'Andrea, W., Ford, J., Stolbach, B., Spinazzola, J., & van der Kolk, B. A. (2012). Understanding interpersonal trauma in children: Why we need a developmental appropriate trauma diagnosis. *American Journal of Orthopsychiatry, 82*, 187–200.

Demaray, M. K., & Malecki, C. K. (2003). Perceptions of the frequency and importance of social support by students classified as victims, bullies, and bully/victims in an urban middle school. *School Psychology Review, 32*(3), 471–489.

Dulmus, C. N., Sowers, K. M., & Theriot, M. T. (2006). Prevalence and bullying experiences of victims and victims who become bullies (bully-victims) at rural schools. *Victims and Offenders, 1*(15), 15–31.

Eisenberger, N. I. (2012). The pain of social disconnection: Examining the shared neural underpinnings of physical and social pain. *Nature Reviews Neuroscience, 13*, 421–434.

Evans, C. B. R., & Smokowski, P. R. (2016). Theoretical explanations for bullying in school: How ecological processes propagate perpetration and victimization. *Child and Adolescent Social Work Journal, 33*(4), 365–375.

Evans, C. B. R., Smokowski, P. R., Rose, R., Mercado, M. C., & Marshall, K. (2018). Cumulative bullying experiences, adolescent behavioral and mental health, and academic achievement: An integrative model of perpetration, victimization, and bystander behavior. *Journal of Child and Family Studies., 27*, 1–14.

Evans, C. B. R., Smokwoski, P. R., & Cotter, K. L. (2014). Cumulative bullying victimization: An investigation of the dose-response relationship between victimization and the associated mental health outcomes, social supports, and school experiences of rural adolescents. *Children and Youth Services Review, 44*, 256–264.

Evans-Lacko, S., Takizawa, R., Brimblecombe, N., King, D., Knapp, M., Maughan, B., & Arsenault, L. (2017). Childhood bullying victimization is associated with use of mental health services over five decades: A longitudinal nationally representative cohort study. *Psychological Medicine, 47*, 127–135.

Freer, B. D., Whitt-Woosley, A., & Sprang, G. (2010). Narrative coherence and the trauma experience: An exploratory mixed-methods analysis. *Violence and Victims, 25*(6), 742–754.

Furlong, M. J., Chung, L. A., Bates, M., & Morrison, R. L. (1995). Who are the victims of school violence? A comparison of student non-victims and multi-victims. *Education & Treatment of Children, 18*(3), 282–298.

Gini, G. (2008). Associations between bullying behavior, psychosomatic complaints, emotional and behavioral problems. *Journal of Pediatrics and Child Health, 44*, 492–497.

Gladstone, G. L., Parker, G. B., & Malhi, G. S. (2006). Do bullied children become anxious and depressed adults? A cross-sectional investigation of the correlates of bullying and anxious depression. *The Journal of Nervous and Mental Disease, 194*(3), 201–208.

Glew, G., Fan, M., Katon, W., Rivara, F. P., & Kernic, M. A. (2005). Bullying, psychosocial adjustment, and academic performance in elementary school. *Archives of Pediatric Adolescence, 159*, 1026–1031.

Gorka, A. X., Hanson, J. L., Radtke, S. R., & Hariri, A. R. (2014). Reduced hippocampal and medial prefrontal gray matter mediate the association between reported childhood maltreatment and trait anxiety in adulthood and predict sensitivity to future life stress. *Biology of Mood Anxiety Disorders, 4*, 1–10.

Hanson, J. L., Nacewicz, B. M., Sutterer, M. J., Cayo, A. A., Schaefer, S. M., Rudolph, K. D., … Davidson, R. J. (2015). Behavioral problems after early life stress: Contributions of the hippocampus and amygdala. *Biological Psychiatry, 77*, 314–323.

Harel-Fisch, Y., Walsh, S. D., Fogel-Grinvald, H., Amitai, G., Picket, W., Molcho, M., … Members of the HBSC Violence and Injury Prevention Focus Group. (2011). Negative school perceptions and involvement in school bullying: A universal relationship across 40 countries. *Journal of Adolescence, 34*, 639–652.

Hawkins, D. L., Pepler, D. J., & Craig, W. M. (2001). Naturalistic observations of peer interventions in bullying. *Social Development, 10*(4), 512–527.

Holt, M., Finkelhor, D., & Kaufman Kantor, K. (2007). Hidden victimization in bullying assessment. *School Psychology Review, 36*, 345–360.

Holt, M. K., & Espelage, D. L. (2007). Perceived social support among bullies, victims, and bully-victims. *Journal of Youth and Adolescence, 36*, 984–994.

Juvonen, J., Graham, S., & Schuster, M. A. (2003). Bullying among young adolescents: The strong, the weak, and the troubled. *Pediatrics, 112*, 1231–1237.

Kaltiala-Heino, R., Rimpela, M., Marttunen, M., Rimplea, A., & Rantanen, P. (1999). Bullying, depression, and suicidal ideation in Finnish adolescents: School survey. *British Journal of Medicine, 319*, 348–351.

Karatzias, A., Power, K. G., & Swanson, V. (2002). Bullying and victimization in Scottish secondary schools: Same or separate entities? *Aggressive Behavior, 28*, 45–61.

Kelleher, I., Keeley, H., Corcoran, P., Ramsay, H., Wasserman, C., Carli, V., … Cannon, M. (2013). Childhood trauma and psychosis in a prospective cohort study: Cause, effect, and directionality. *The American Journal of Psychiatry, 170*(7), 734–741.

Kirschbaum, C., & Hellhammer, D. H. (1989). Salivary cortisol in psychobiological research: An overview. *Neuropsychobiology, 22*, 150–169.

Knack, J. M., Jensen-Campbell, L. A., & Baum, A. (2011). Worse than sticks and stones? Bullying is associated with altered HPA axis functioning and poorer health. *Brain and Cognition, 77*(2), 183–190.

Kvarme, L. G., Helseth, S., Saeteren, B., & Natvig, G. K. (2010). School children's experience of being bullied-and how they envisage their dream day. *Scandinavian Journal of Caring Sciences, 24*, 791–798.

Lester, L., Cross, D., & Shaw, T. (2012). Problem behaviors, traditional bullying and cyberbullying among adolescents: Longitudinal analysis. *Emotional and Behavioral Difficulties, 17*(3-4), 435–447.

Lin, N. (2001). *Social capital: A Theory of social structure and action*. New York, NY: Cambridge University Press.

Lin, N., Cook, K., & Burt, R. S. (2001). *Social capital: Theory and research*. New Brunswick, NJ: Transaction Publishers.

Lupien, S. J., Fiocco, A., Wan, N., Maheu, F., Lord, C., Schramek, T., & Tu, M. T. (2005). Stress hormones and human memory function across the lifespan. *Psychoneuroendocrinology, 30*, 225–242.

Mayo Clinic. (2016). *Stress management: Chronic stress pubs your health at risk*. Rochester, MN: Author. Retrieved from http://www.mayoclinic.org/healthy-lifestyle/stress-management/in-depth/stress/art-20046037

McFarlane, A. C., & de Girolamo, G. (1996). The nature of traumatic stressors and the epidemiology of posttraumatic reactions. In B. A. van der Kolk, A. C. McFarlane, & L. Weisaeth (Eds.), *Traumatic stress: The effects of overwhelming experience on mind, body, and society* (pp. 129–154). New York, NY: Guilford Press.

Meltzer, H., Vostanis, P., Ford, T., Bebbington, P., & Dennis, M. S. (2011). Victims of bullying in childhood and suicide in adulthood. *European Psychiatry, 26*, 498–503.

Menesini, E., Modena, M., & Tani, F. (2009). Bullying and victimization in adolescence: Concurrent and stable roles and psychological health symptoms. *Journal of Genetic Psychology, 170*(2), 115–133.

Miller, G. E., Chen, E., & Zhou, E. S. (2007). If it goes up, must it come down? Chronic stress and the hypothalamic-pituitary-adrenocortical axis in humans. *Psychological Bulletin, 133*, 25–45.

Nation, M., Vieno, A., Perkins, D. D., & Santinello, M. (2008). Bullying in school and adolescent sense of empowerment: An analysis of relationships with parents, friends, and teachers. *Journal of Community & Applied Social Psychology, 18*(3), 211–232.

National Institute of Mental Health. (n.d.). *Post-traumatic stress disorder (PTSD)*. Bethesda, MD: Author. Retrieved from https://www.nimh.nih.gov/health/publications/post-traumatic-stress-disorder-ptsd/ptsd-508-05172017_38054.pdf

Natvig, G. K., Albreksten, G., & Qvarnstrom, U. (2001). Psychosomatic symptoms among victims of school bullying. *Journal of Health Psychology, 6*, 365–377.

Nazir, T., & Piskin, M. (2015). School bullying: Effecting child's mental health. *The International Journal of Indian Psychology, 2*(4), 130–135.

Ouellet-Morin, I., Danese, A., Bowes, L., Shakoor, S., Ambler, A., Pariante, C. M., … Arseneault, L. (2011). A discordant monozygotic twin design shows blunted cortisol reactivity among bullied children. *Journal of the American Academy of Child and Adolescent Psychiatry, 50*(6), 574–582.

Ouellet-Morin, I., Odgers, C. L., Danese, A., Bowes, L., Shakoor, S., Papadopoulos, A. S., … Arseneault, L. (2011). Blunted cortisol responses to stress signal social and behavioral problems among maltreated/bullied 12-year-old children. *Biological Psychiatry, 70*, 1016–1023.

Pellegrini, A. D., Bartini, M., & Brooks, F. (1999). School bullies, victims, and aggressive victims: Factors relating to group affiliation and victimization in early adolescence. *Journal of Educational Psychology, 91*(2), 216–224.

Peterson, C., Maier, S. F., & Seligman, M. (1995). *Learned helpless: A Theory for the age of personal control*. New York, NY: Oxford University Press.

Pollastri, A. R., Cardemil, E. V., & O'Donnell, E. H. (2009). Self-esteem in pure bullies and bully/victims: A longitudinal analysis. *Journal of Interpersonal Violence, 25*, 1489–1502.

Prinstein, M. J., & Cillessen, A. H. N. (2003). Forms and functions of adolescent peer aggression associated with high levels of peer status. *Merrill-Palmer Quarterly, 49*(3), 310–342.

Putnam, R. D. (2000). *Bowling alone: The collapse and revival of American community*. New York, NY: Simon & Schuster.

Rosa, E. M., & Tudge, J. (2013). Urie Bronfenbrenners's theory of human development: Its evolution from ecology to bioecology. *Journal of Family Theory & Review, 5*(4), 243–258.

Salmivalli, C., Lappalainen, M., & Lagerspetz, K. M. J. (1998). Stability of change behavior in connection to bullying in schools: A two-year follow-up. *Aggressive Behavior, 24*, 205–218.

Scholte, R. H. J., Overbeek, G., ten Brink, G., Rommes, E., de Kemp, R. A. T., Goossens, L., & Engles, R. C. M. E. (2008). The significance of reciprocal and unilateral friendships for peer victimization in adolescence. *Journal of Youth and Adolescence, 89*, 89–100.

Sebastian, C. L., Tan, G. C. Y., Roiser, J. P., Viding, E., Dumontheil, I., & Blakemore, S. (2011). Developmental influences on the neural bases of responses to social rejection: Implications of social neuroscience for education. *Neuroimage, 51*(3), 686–694.

Shapiro, E. (March 4 2016). The history behind the Donald Trump 'Small Hands' insult. ABC News Retrived from https://abcnews.go.com/Politics/history-donald-trump-small-hands-insult/story?id=37395515

Simmons, R. (2002). *Odd girl out*. New York, NY: Houghton Mifflin Harcourt Publishing.

Tchalova, K., & Eisenberger, N. I. (2017). The shared neural substrates of physical and social pain. In K. D. Williams (Ed.), *Ostracism, exclusion, and rejection* (pp. 61–80). New York, NY: Taylor & Francis.

Teicher, M. H., & Samson, J. A. (2016). Annual research review: Enduring neurobiological effects of childhood abuse and neglect. *Journal of Child Psychology and Psychiatry, 57*(3), 241–266.

Totura, C. M. W., Mackinnon-Lewis, C., Gesten, E. L., Gadd, R., Divine, K. P., Dunham, S., & Kamboukos, D. (2009). Bullying and victimization among boys and girls in middle school: The influence of perceived family and school contexts. *Journal of Early Adolescence, 29*, 571–609.

Ttofi, M., Farrington, D. P., & Losel, F. (2012). School bullying as predictor of violence later in life: A systematic review and meta-analysis of prospective longitudinal studies. *Aggression and Violent Behavior, 17*, 405–418.

Ttofi, M. M., Farrington, D. P., Losel, F., & Loeber, R. (2011a). Do victims of school bullies tend to become depressed later in life? A systematic review and meta-analysis of longitudinal studies. *Journal of Aggression, Conflict, and Peace Research, 3*(11), 63–73.

Ttofi, M. M., Farrington, D. P., Losel, F., & Loeber, R. (2011b). The predictive efficiency of school bullying versus later offending: A systematic/meta-analytic review of longitudinal studies. *Criminal Behavior and Mental Health, 21*, 80–89.

Turner, M. B., Exum, M. L., Brame, R., & Holt, T. J. (2013). Bullying victimization and adolescent mental health: General and typological effects across sex. *Journal of Criminal Justice, 41*(1), 53–59.

Vaillancourt, T., Duku, E., Becker, S., Schmidt, L., Nicol, J., Muir, C., & MacMillan, H. (2011). Peer victimization, depressive symptoms, and high salivary cortisol predict poor memory in children. *Brain and Cognition, 77*, 191–199.

Vaillancourt, T., Duku, E., deCatanzaro, D., MacMillan, H., Muir, C., & Schmidt, L. A. (2008). Variation in hypothalamic-pituitary-adrenal axis activity among bullied and non-bullied children. *Aggressive Behavior., 34*, 294–305.

Vanderbilt, D., & Augustyn, M. (2010). The effects of bullying. *Pediatrics and Child Health, 20*(7), 315–320.

Waddell, W. J. (2010). History of dose–response. *The Journal of Toxicological Sciences, 35*(1), 1–8.

You, S., Furlong, M. J., Felix, E., Sharkey, J. D., Tanigawa, D., & Green, J. G. (2008). Relations among school connectedness, hope, life satisfaction, and bully victimization. *Psychology in the Schools, 45*(5), 446–460.

Chapter 4
To Intervene or Not Intervene? That Is the Question: Bystanders in the Bullying Dynamic

The world is dangerous not because of those who do harm, but because of those who look at it without doing anything. Nothing that I can do will change the structure of the universe. But maybe by raising my voice I can help the greatest of all causes—goodwill among men and peace on earth.
—Albert Einstein

4.1 Introduction

Imagine for a moment that you are walking down a crowded high school hallway in between classes. Everyone is rushing to their next class, greeting friends, laughing, and talking. Out of the corner of your eye you see a boy from your biology class get pushed into a locker by two upper classmen who laugh and then walk away. It takes only a few seconds and the older boys move on, but the boy from your biology class looks stunned. You think this must be a one-time event, so you keep walking. But the next day, and the day after that, and the day after that you see something similar. What do you do? Now think about being in middle school gym class. There is a girl who is overweight and every day the popular girls in your class whisper and snicker whenever she runs. Sometimes they try and trip her or whisper "fatty," when she walks by. How do you respond? Next, you are a junior in high school. Your neighborhood is changing and a family from Pakistan moved in down the block. You've heard kids snicker about the long black dresses and scarves the new girl wears. A popular girl you grew up with says she will look the new girl up on Facebook and tell her to go back to her own country. Her friends add that they are probably terrorists. Once again, what do you do?

Bystanders have to weigh multiple factors when deciding how to respond and your response to these situations would result from a split-second appraisal of many elements. For example, are you friends with the perpetrators? If so, perhaps that gives you the courage to stand up to them knowing they are your friends and will respect your decision to protect the victim. But conversely, you might be worried that standing up to them could make them angry and could damage your friendship. If you are not friends with the perpetrators maybe that increases the likelihood that

© Springer Nature Switzerland AG 2019

P. R. Smokowski, C. B. R. Evans, *Bullying and Victimization Across the Lifespan*, https://doi.org/10.1007/978-3-030-20293-4_4

they would turn on you and you would become the next victim. Have you been victimized by these perpetrators or other perpetrators in the past? If you have, you might be hesitant about putting yourself out there to protect another victim for fear of being victimized yourself. The bad memories of your own victimization come into your mind as you weigh whether or not to help someone else. How popular and well liked are you at school? If you have many friends and are popular, the fear of being victimized is likely diminished because you know your friends will support you if the perpetrators turn on you. Conversely, if you are unpopular, that might decrease your courage to stand up to the perpetrators. Are other bystanders present? How are they behaving? What are classroom, school, and teacher expectations about bystander behavior? Are you an empathetic person? If so, you might readily feel the pain the victim is feeling and be inclined to help, if not, you could be totally unaffected by witnessing someone else's plight. How severe is the bullying? Do you think your intervention could help? All of these questions run through your mind and you have a split second to act. What do you do?

In the above examples, you are the bystander. You are not directly involved in the bullying as the bully or victim, but you are part of the dynamic simply by witnessing the bullying. There are three basic options as a bystander: (1) Act as a negative bystander and support the actions of the person bullying by verbally encouraging him/her or by directly joining in the taunting or physical harassment; (2) Act as a passive bystander and take no action or wait until the bullying ends and then possibly comfort the victim; or (3) Act as a prosocial bystander and directly confront the bully, intervene to support the victim, or get a teacher. Researchers have coined slightly different terms to discuss bystander behavior. Negative bystanders are referred to as reinforcers (e.g., those who encourage the bully) or assistants (e.g., those who assist the bully by holding the victim); passive bystanders are called outsiders (e.g., they refrain from taking any action, simply serving as witnesses); and prosocial bystanders are referred to as defenders (e.g., trying to stop the bullying and protect the victim; Salmivalli, Lagerspetz, Bjorkqvist, Osterman, & Kaukiainen, 1996). For the purposes of this chapter, the terms negative, passive, and prosocial bystander will be used.

Recently, the word "upstander" has been used to describe the actions of a prosocial bystander. The term upstander was coined by US Ambassador to the United Nations Samantha Power in 2002 when she was discussing her Pulitzer Prize-winning book *A Problem from Hell: America and the Age of Genocide*. Powers used the word "upstander" to describe people who spoke up against atrocities and injustices such as genocide (Facing History and Ourselves, 2017). In 2013, two seniors at Watchung Hills Regional High School in New Jersey, Monica Mahal and Sarah Decker, were writing an anti-bullying speech and noticed that spell-check did not recognize the word "upstander." Mahal and Decker decided to rectify this problem and created a petition at change.org to add upstander to the dictionary (Zimmer, 2016). This term is gradually becoming common nomenclature in bullying research.

An upstander is someone who chooses to make a difference in the world by standing up to injustice and creating positive change (Facing History and Ourselves, 2017); acting as a Prosocial bystander is synonymous with being an upstander.

Bystanders have tremendous power in the bullying dynamic and their behavior often dictates if the bullying continues or stops. Thus, increasing upstander behavior is one key mechanism to decreasing rates of school bullying. Understanding what motivates bystanders to behave in certain ways when witnessing bullying situations is vital to increasing upstander behavior. Figure 4.1 captures the strength of upstander behavior in a drawing made by an eighth grader. In this drawing, a concerned bystander finds a teacher by the lockers to help a classmate who is being bullied inside a classroom. This chapter will provide an overview of bystander research with a discussion of motivating factors in bystander behavior and a focus on how to increase prosocial bystander behavior as well as a discussion of how bystanders are impacted by witnessing bullying behavior.

4.2 Prevalence of Bystanders and Their Behavior in Bullying Dynamics

School bullying commonly takes place in public spaces such as the classroom, hallway, bus, gym locker room, lunch room, or library. This means that bystanders are ubiquitous during episodes of school-based bullying. It is partially the presence of these bystanders that makes bullying so painful for the victim: public humiliation. However, bystanders are not always present and research varies in regards to what percentage of the time bystanders are actually present. Small scale observational research studies in elementary and middle school indicate that bystanders are present for 85–88% of bullying episodes (Atlas & Pepler, 1998; Hawkins, Pepler, & Craig, 2001). A more recent nationally representative sample of 791 victimized

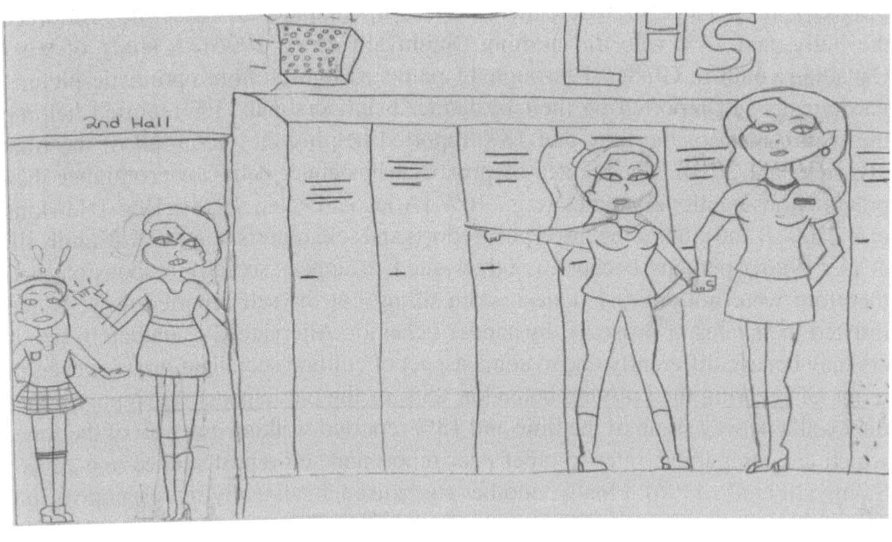

Fig. 4.1 Illustration of bystander behavior

youth ages 10–20 found that these victims reported that bystanders were present for 80% of bullying incidents (Jones, Mitchell, & Turner, 2015). A larger scale study of 9397 youth in Grade 4–11 found that 68% of youth self-reported being a bystander (Trach, Hymel, Waterhouse, & Neale, 2010). Another study of 2002 middle and high school-aged youth found that 30% reported being bystanders only, 15% reported being bystanders and victims, 7% bystanders and perpetrators, and 11% bystanders, victims, and perpetrators; that means in this study 63% of youth reported being bystanders at some point in time (Rivers & Noret, 2010). Furthermore, in this study, 34% of youth reported playing multiple roles in the bullying dynamic (i.e., bystander, perpetrator, victim at different times). This highlights the churning whirlpool of peer relations. While research differs slightly on the exact proportion of bullying episodes witnessed by bystanders, it appears that bystanders are present between 80% and 88% of bullying episodes and between 63% and 68% of youth report having been a bystander. Given the public nature of many bullying episodes, it follows that the majority of incidents are witnessed by bystanders. The behavior of these bystanders is vital in terms of determining whether or not the bullying behavior continues; however, the majority of youth refrain from supporting the victim and do not engage in upstander behavior.

For example, in one study of 60 videotaped bullying episodes of first through sixth graders, researchers coded bystanders as intervening to help the victim only 10% of the time (Atlas & Pepler, 1998). In a similar study, 306 videotaped bullying episodes were coded and bystanders assisted the victim 19% of the time (Hawkins et al., 2001). A third observational study of youth ages 5–12 examined 360 h of video tapes over a 3-year period. Findings indicated that 54% of the time bystanders were passive, 21% of the time they supported the bully, and 25% of the time the supported the victim (O'Connell, Pepler, & Craig, 1999). Studies using self- and peer-report surveys of bystander behavior mirror these results. In a sample of 573 Finnish sixth graders, 17% defended the victim, compared to 20% who reinforced the bully, and 24% who did nothing (Salmivalli et al., 1996). A study of 9397 Canadian youth in Grades 4 through 11 paints a slightly more optimistic picture. Participants self-reported on their bystander behaviors and 31% reported helping the victim most of the time and 18% reported helping the victim all of the time (Trach et al., 2010). These rates of prosocial bystander behavior are higher than previous observational studies (e.g., 10% [Atlas & Pepler, 1998]; 19% [Hawkins et al., 2001]) and studies that used peer reports and self-reports (e.g., 17% [Salmivalli et al., 1996]) perhaps because youth wanted to appear socially responsible and therefore were not entirely honest when filling out the self-reported surveys and inflated their rates of prosocial bystander behavior. Alternately, Canadian bystanders may behave differently due to some aspect of cultural socialization. However, in terms of ignoring the bullying behavior, 28% of the participants self-reported that they walked away some of the time and 13% reported walking away all of the time, which are comparable rates to other peer-report and self-report studies (e.g., 24%; Salmivalli et al., 1996). Finally, another study used a nationally representative survey of 791 victims ages 10–20 from the Technology Harassment and Victimization Survey, who reported on their victimization experiences by discussing how bystanders behaved when they were being bullied. Victims indicated that in 70% of bullying incidents a bystander tried to make the victim feel better or went and got a teacher; over half of the time a bystander said they were sorry the bullying happened (55%) or told the perpetrator to stop (53%). However, bystanders also commonly avoided the perpetrator (58%), came closer to see the bullying happen (51%), or left (43%). In about one quarter of the bullying incidents (24%), bystanders joined in the harassment or laughed at the victim (Jones et al., 2015). These findings suggest that bystanders might intervene more frequently to support the victim than past research has suggested, but the majority of the time victims are left to fend for themselves.

Overall, the prevalence rates of prosocial bystander behavior are fairly low and ranged from 10% to 31% but could rise as high as 70% according to one study. Given that Prosocial Bystander behavior decreases the frequency of bullying, this overall low rate is problematic because it indicates that the vast majority of bystanders do nothing to assist the victim, allowing the bullying behavior to continue. When bystanders defended the victim, the bullying stopped 57% of the time (Hawkins et al., 2001). In another study of 6762 Finnish children ages 9–11, prosocial bystander behavior in the form of defending the victim was significantly associated with decreased levels of classroom bullying ($b = -0.35$, $p < 0.05$) while negative bystander behavior in the form of reinforcing the bullying was significantly associated with increased bullying in the classroom ($b = 2.05$, $p < 0.001$; Salmivalli, Voeten, & Poskiparta, 2011). Further, victim outcomes were worse in classrooms where bystanders supported the bully; for example, in a study of 6980 youth in Grades 3–5, rejected and anxious students had an increased risk for victimization in classrooms where bystanders often supported the perpetrators; however, the risk for victimization decreased when bystanders commonly defended victims (Karna, Voeten, Poskiparta, & Salmivalli, 2010). This finding highlights the moderating impact of bystander behavior such that rejected and anxious children at risk of being bullied are more at risk when there are higher rates of negative bystander behavior (Karna et al., 2010). Taken together, this research highlights the influence that bystander behavior has on rates of classroom bullying behavior; the more bystanders intervene to support and defend the victim, the less bullying there is. Conversely, increased bystander support of the bully increases rates of classroom bullying. The bottom line is that bystanders have the power to shape the culture and climate of the classroom and school.

Bystanders who join in the bullying add fuel to the bullying fire, allowing a conflagration to ensue. Although standing by silently is preferable to supporting the bully, taking no action sends the message that the bullying behavior is acceptable and this inaction allows the bullying to continue. It is critical for bystanders to understand that passively watching is not a neutral message, especially from the victim's perspective. The victim sees passive bystanders as giving silent sanction to the bullying behavior. In contrast, protecting the victim, either by directly confronting the bully or getting a teacher, sends the message that bullying is not acceptable. Comforting the victim after the bullying has ended does little to alter bullying behavior on the classroom or schoolwide scale but can have a tremendously positive impact on the victim. However, increasing upstander behavior in the form of prosocial bystander behavior is vital to decreasing rates of bullying. It follows that decreasing rates of bullying will not only protect children from the negative outcomes associated with direct bullying involvement (i.e., being a bully, a victim, or a bully-victim) but could also protect bystanders from the negative impact of witnessing bullying.

4.3 The Impact of Witnessing Bullying on Bystanders

Figure 4.2 depicts a bullying incident with multiple bystanders. What is the impact of witnessing this event on these bystanders? Is there a difference between the impact on the girl in the green shirt, who appears to be ambivalent—covering her mouth while also confronting the bully, and the girl in the red shirt who appears to be smiling with her arms folded? The negative consequences of bullying involvement for bullies, victims, and bully-victims are well documented (e.g., Aluede, Adeleke, Omoike, & Afen-Akpaida, 2008; Gini, 2008; Kaltiala-Heino, Rimpela, Marttunen, Rimplea, & Rantanen, 1999; Nansel et al., 2001). Less research has examined how bystanders are affected by witnessing bullying; however, the existing research suggests that witnessing bullying as a bystander can have damaging effects. In a qualitative study of eight bystanders ages 12 and 13, some participants reported

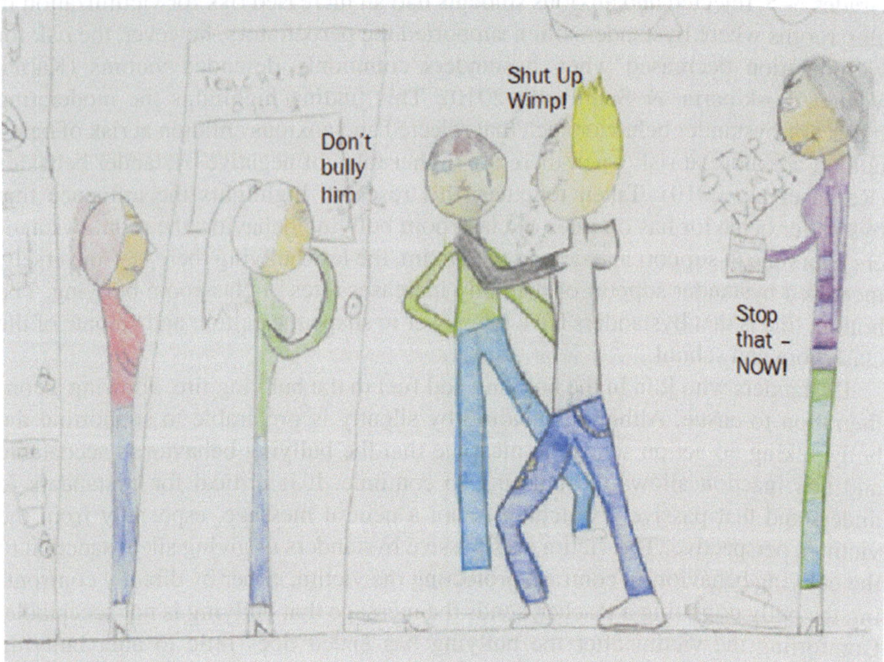

Fig. 4.2 Bystander behavior during physical bullying drawn by a 6th grade male

feeling guilty for failing to defend their victimized classmates, but the fear of becoming the next victim kept them silent (Hutchinson, 2012); other researchers confirm that bystanders indeed experience guilt (Obermann, 2011). Many of the interviewed children reported feeling upset and angry when witnessing the bullying, a few had empathetic responses (i.e., "… imagine that it was me …"; Hutchinson, 2012, p. 433), and many reported feeling very alone while watching the situation. Indeed, bystanders may be traumatized by witnessing bullying.

One group of researchers (Janson & Hazler, 2004) randomly assigned 79 college students (mean age of 21) to discuss a memory of being victimized or a memory being a bystander while measuring heart rate (HR) and skin conductance (SC). Participants also filled out the Impact of Event Scale—Revised (IES-R), a scale that assesses the physiological and psychological impacts of a traumatic event (Weiss, 2004). Although not all of the memories discussed involved bullying victimization or witnessing bullying, memories of direct bullying victimization and witnessed bullying victimization were common. When asked how they felt at the time of the event, victims reported higher levels of distress as compared to bystanders (as indicated by elevated IES-R scores); however, both groups did not differ significantly on present levels of distress. In fact, both groups reported current IES-R scores that fell into the elevated clinical range, indicating levels of distress experienced by emergency service workers and individuals suffering from psychotic breaks. Further, bystanders and victims did not differ significantly in regards to HR or SC when they recounted memories of the experienced or witnessed victimization, indicating that discussing and reliving a memory of being a bystander was just as traumatizing as discussing one's own victimization (Janson & Hazler, 2004). These findings highlight the traumatic nature of being a bystander.

The trauma associated with being a bystander to bullying may erode mental health functioning. For example, bystanders are at a slightly elevated risk of experiencing suicidal ideation compared to youth not involved in the bullying dynamic (i.e., youth who did not witness bullying). Further, females who had the dual role of victim and bystander, were at a particularly high risk for endorsing life ending thoughts as compared to pure bystanders and uninvolved youth (Rivers & Noret, 2010). Even when controlling for having been a victim or perpetrator, being a bystander was associated with poor mental health outcomes including elevated levels of anxiety, paranoid ideations, and depression (Rivers, Poteat, Noret, & Ashurst, 2009). Future bystander research should focus on whether the amount of bullying witnessed by bystanders impacts their mental health outcomes. In line with a dose–response relationship discussed in Chap. 3 (i.e., increased exposure to a stimulus results in varying outcomes; Waddell, 2010), it seems plausible that more exposure to bullying as a bystander would result in worse outcomes; however, this has not been tested.

Witnessing bullying is traumatic for a few reasons. First, witnessing someone else be traumatized can itself be a traumatizing experience. The criteria for Post Traumatic Stress Disorder (PTSD) note that witnessing a trauma (e.g., seeing someone else exposed to actual or threatened serious injury) can result in symptoms of PTSD (American Psychiatric Association, 2013). Bystanders directly witness victims being exposed to actual physical and emotional injury, which could be traumatizing for the bystander especially if he/she has high levels of empathy. If bystanders are empathetic, they might be more able to internalize the experiences of the victim and, in a sense, feel what the victim is going through, which would increase their own distress. In cognitive neuroscience, there is the emerging concept of "mirror neurons" which fire in the brain both when an action is taken and when the animal observes the same action performed by another (Arbib, 2006; Keysers & Gazzola, 2006; Molenberghs, Cunnington, & Mattingley, 2009). Proponents of this concept suggest that mirror neurons may help us understand the actions of other people, learn new skills by imitation, and feel emotions such as empathy. Although most of this research has been done with primates and remains controversial, it is intriguing to consider neural brain mechanisms that would help to explain bystander behavior, or lack thereof, and consequences of witnessing traumatizing events.

Second, bystanders might worry that they could become the next victim, resulting in increased anxiety and hyperarousal. Witnessing bullying reminds bystanders that at any time the perpetrator could turn on them and they could experience the pain of social humiliation. This worry might put bystanders on high alert as they constantly scan their environment for potential threats. As discussed in Chap. 3, humans are innately social beings who will do almost anything to avoid social isolation. If bystanders appraise a bullying situation and deem that protecting the victim might put their own social connections in harm's way, they could opt to avoid social humiliation rather than stand up for the victim. Third, bystanders might feel guilty that they are not taking any action to help the victim, which could contribute to feelings of depression, despair, inadequacy, or helplessness. In summary, although direct involvement in the bullying dynamic is most harmful, bystanders suffer from immediate and long-lasting feelings of guilt and psychological discomfort such as depression and anxiety. In extreme cases, bystanders could also be traumatized from witnessing bullying. Perhaps if bystanders were able to take action to end the bullying this could minimize the negative impact of witnessing bullying; it is thus important to consider what factors impact bystanders' decisions to behave as an upstander or to engage in negative or passive bystander behavior.

4.4 To Defend or Not Defend?: Factors Influencing Bystander Behavior

Given that prosocial bystanders who support the victim may interrupt the bullying dynamic, it is vital for researchers to gain insight into what influences children and adolescents to defend their victimized peers. There are a variety of factors that impact bystander responses such as emotional and physiological responsiveness to witnessing bullying, classroom sociometric status/perceived popularity, and situational factors such as what type of bullying is witnessed. Understanding the personal characteristics of prosocial bystanders is important in order to create interventions to increase bystander defending behavior.

4.4.1 *Emotional and Physiological Responsiveness*

Researchers have begun to investigate why certain children support the victim and other children do not (e.g., Barhight, Hubbard, & Hyde, 2013). In one study, 845 fourth and fifth grade students filled out surveys assessing victimization experiences, self-efficacy in confronting peers (e.g., "Stand up for yourself when you feel you are being treated unfairly"), empathy (e.g., "My friend's unhappiness does not make me feel anything"), emotional expressiveness (e.g., "I am emotional and show my feelings") and bystander behavior (i.e., students nominated peers who try and stop bullying). A random sample of 79 children were also selected to view six short videotaped bullying vignettes while their heart rate was monitored. Following the videos, participants rated how sad, mad, and scared they felt when watching the bullying episodes. Using Latent Profile Analysis (LPA), two groups of students emerged: the Emotional Group (i.e., 43% of the sample who reported high levels of negative emotions and displayed increased heart rate while watching the bullying vignettes) and the Unemotional Group (i.e., 57% of the sample who reported low levels of negative emotions and a decelerating heart rate). The Emotional Group reported significantly higher rates of victimization (Cohen's $d = 0.46$; which indicates a moderate-sized relationship) and emotional expressiveness (Cohen's $d = 0.47$) compared to the Unemotional Group. Further, a marginally significant trend indicated that peers were more likely to nominate participants from the Emotional Group as bystanders who intervened to help victims compared to participants from the Unemotional Group (Cohen's $d = 0.34$, $p = 0.14$). Group membership (i.e., Emotional versus Unemotional) significantly predicted bystander behavior and the Emotional group was more likely to protect victims when witnessing bullying (Barhight et al., 2013).

These results suggest that children may not intervene in the bullying dynamic because they are not emotionally and physiologically affected by witnessing a bullying event. Some youth have a low capacity to feel empathy and thus see no need to help the victim. The Unemotional Group was less likely to intervene perhaps because they were not bothered by the bullying behavior and did not realize how upset the victim might be. The fact that over half of the sample was labeled as Unemotional indicates that this is a common trait rather than indicative of pathological cruelty or insensitivity (Barhight et al., 2013). Given the high rates of bullying in US schools (Nansel et al., 2001; Wang, Iannotti, & Nansel, 2009) and general violence in the media, this lack of arousal may indicate habituation. Many children may not be emotionally upset by bullying because they witness it so frequently. Perhaps bullying has become the norm and does not evoke a strong emotional response; the decelerating heart rate displayed by the Unemotional Group is indicative of habituation. If children are not emotionally or physiologically upset by witnessing bullying, they will not be motivated to intervene. Conversely, the Emotional Group was more likely to intervene to help victims, possibly motivated by the emotional and physiological upset they experienced upon witnessing bullying. This emotional upset was demonstrated by increasing heart rate and higher levels of self-reported feelings of being mad, sad, and scared after watching a bullying vignette. The Emotional Group likely felt empathy for the victims, which could motivate them to engage in prosocial bystander behavior. Clearly, bullying interventions in schools should focus on teaching children about the severity of bullying in an attempt to increase emotional and physiological responses to this social dynamic, which could increase supportive bystander interventions. Increasing youth's empathy is a key to increasing prosocial bystander behavior.

Indeed, another study confirmed that empathy plays a critical role in impacting prosocial bystander behavior but perhaps only for boys. In a sample of 318 Italian middle school-aged children, empathetic responsiveness was significantly and positively associated with actively assisting victimized classmates and significantly and negatively associated with pro-bullying behavior. However, this relationship was not present for girls (Gini, Albiero, Benelli, & Altoe, 2007). In summary, personal characteristics, such as empathy, dictate if and how bystanders are impacted by witnessing bullying and these characteristics will either increase or decrease the likelihood that they support the victim.

4.4.2 Sociometric and Perceived Popularity

Social standing in the classroom has a profound effect on whether youth engage in prosocial bystander behavior. If youth feel adequately supported by a cadre of friends or feel that they are popular and have social power in the classroom, they might be more willing to stand up to the perpetrator and actively support the victim. Youth with social support know that even if the bully turns on them, their friends will have their back. Conversely, youth who have few or no friends or are unpopular, might be more reticent to protect the victim and thus put themselves in the potential position to become victimized.

As discussed in Chap. 2, sociometric popularity, also referred to as acceptance, is the extent to which an individual is liked or disliked by his or her peer group (Asher, Parker, & Walker, 1996). One method of assessing sociometric popularity uses peer rating scales that ask youth to nominate or choose the peers they like most and like least (e.g., Bell-Dolan, Foster, & Sikora, 1989; Fontaine et al., 1999). Other researchers have used Likert scales, ranging from 3-point to 7-point scales, that ask participants to rate how much they like each of their classmates (e.g., Parker & Asher, 1993). Perceived popularity differs from sociometric popularity in that perceived popularity is a measure of who students think their classmates perceive as popular, while sociometric popularity is measured with like-most/like-least nominations (Parkhurst & Hopmeyer, 1998). Sociometric and perceived popularity do not necessarily align. For example, it is possible for youth to have low sociometric popularity (i.e., they are disliked by classmates) but have high perceived popularity (i.e., they are viewed as popular). Conversely, youth could be liked by their classmates (i.e., high sociometric popularity) but be viewed as only mildly popular or even unpopular (i.e., low perceived popularity).

Popular-prosocial youth are well-liked (i.e., high sociometric and perceived popularity), tend to accurately read social situations, and behave according to perceived social norms (Dodge, Pettit, McClaskey, & Brown, 1986). This illustrates the "social savvy" (Bierman, 2004, p. 19) that well-liked children possess and suggests that they may have an advanced theory of mind, which means they are able to take the perspective of another more easily than other children (Bagwell & Schmidt, 2011). This ability to take the perspective of another, may result in increased feelings of empathy when witnessing bullying victimization, which may spur children to intervene on behalf of the victim. This is one possible explanation for why popular and well-liked children are more likely to display positive bystander behavior and support the victim. Another reason, cited above, is that popular and well-liked youth might feel protected by their friends and secure in the fact that they will not become the next victim. Popular-prosocial children are often seen as leaders in the class and are commonly aligned with teachers and other authority figures. Revisiting the drawing in Fig. 4.1, the prosocial bystander pointing to the bullying is very close in appearance and stature to the teacher next to her. Intervening in bullying by alerting teachers may enhance her popular-prosocial status and deepen her relationships with authority figures.

Indeed, research supports this assertion and sociometrically popular children are more likely to defend victims compared to sociometrcially unpopular children. In a sample of 573 Finnish sixth graders, both males and females who defended the victim were categorized as sociometrically popular-prosocial (i.e., they received many like-most nominations and few like-least nominations). These positive bystanders were highly accepted in the classroom and had low levels of rejection. Females who engaged in negative bystander behavior (e.g., reinforced the bully by laughing, shouting encouragements, gathering others to come see the bullying, holding the victim or directly joining in on the bullying; see Fig. 3.1 for a depiction of many negative bystanders) scored low on social acceptance (i.e., few like-most nominations) and high on social rejection (i.e., many like-least nominations), indicating that they were socially rejected children and had low sociometric popularity. However, males who supported the bully showed the opposite trend and scored high on acceptance (i.e., many like-most nominations) and low on rejection (i.e., few like-least nominations) indicating that they were categorized as sociometrically popular-antisocial. Males who assisted the bully were sociometrically average; they scored close to average on both acceptance and rejection (i.e., received equal numbers of like-most and like-least nominations). Male and female passive bystanders scored low on both like-most and like-least nominations (Salmivalli et al., 1996), placing them in the sociometrically neglected category. To summarize, popular-prosocial youth tended to defend the victim while popular-antisocial boys supported the bully. Socially rejected girls and sociometrically average boys were negative bystanders. Sociometrically neglected girls and boys tended to be passive bystanders who witnessed and did nothing. See Table 2.2 for definitions of sociometric categories.

The gender differences in these findings are interesting: female bystanders who supported the bully by reinforcing or assisting had low sociometric popularity, but the male reinforces had high sociometric popularity. The social expectations of females and males are different and it is generally more socially acceptable for males to behave aggressively. Perhaps males who supported the bully were accepted due to classroom norms of male aggression, while aggressive females were rejected because it is not socially acceptable for females to behave aggressively and there were classroom norms of non-aggressive female behavior.

The fact that prosocial bystanders were well-liked may indicate that sociometric popularity provides children with the confidence to defend victims (i.e., the popular-prosocial subgroup). However, this was a cross sectional study and causation cannot be established, thus it is also possible that children who defend victims gain sociometric popularity and acceptance due to their altruistic behavior. However, researchers have posited that popularity and social acceptance provide children with a secure social position, reducing the possibility of victimization and enabling socially successful children to stand up for victimized classmates (Salmivalli, Karna, & Poskiparta, 2011). Therefore, sociometric popularity (i.e., being liked by your classmates) likely precedes prosocial bystander behavior, but further longitudinal research is needed to confirm this relationship.

Perceived popularity also plays a role in bystander behavior and the relationship between sociometric popularity, perceived popularity, and bystander behavior may be influenced by age. Specifically, perceived popularity (i.e., student nominations of the most popular children in the class—popular-prosocial children) was positively associated with defending behavior in a group of 266 Italian elementary school children (i.e., ages 8 through 10), but this association was not present in a group of 195 Italian middle school children (i.e., ages 11–14). However, sociometric popularity (i.e., like-most and like-least nominations) was positively associated with defender behavior across both age groups (Caravita, Di Blasio, & Salmivalli, 2009). The sociometric popularity of prosocial bystanders appears to be stable across age groups, while the perceived popularity of prosocial bystanders is high in elementary school and then decreases in middle school, suggesting that in later grades being liked impacts bystander behavior more than being viewed as popular.

The body of literature discussing the connections between sociometric popularity, perceived popularity, and bystander behavior points to the importance of encouraging and empowering students with high social status to intervene on the victim's behalf. This is particularly important given the findings that prosocial bystanders often effectively stop bullying (Hawkins et al., 2001; Salmivalli, Voeten, & Poskiparta, 2011). These findings highlight the necessity of establishing bullying interventions to teach and reinforce prosocial bystander behavior, especially to students with high social status.

4.4.3 Situational Factors

Research suggests that bystander behavior is impacted by situational factors including the form and severity of the bullying, victim reaction, the presences of other bystanders, and bystanders' history of past bullying or victimization. Bystander behavior appears to be impacted by the form of bullying that is witnessed. For example, when bystanders witnessed direct relational aggression they supported the perpetrator 30% of the time; when indirect verbal or indirect relational aggression were witnessed youth supported the aggressor 39% and 38% of the time respectively. However, when direct physical or direct verbal aggression was witnessed, support of the perpetrator dropped to 17% and 12% respectively (Tapper & Boulton, 2005). Perhaps direct physical and verbal aggression is so forceful, bystanders do not feel the need to join in as additional aggression seems unnecessary. However, with more indirect forms of aggression bystanders supported the perpetrator a higher percentage of the time, perhaps because they felt additional aggression was warranted. Alternately, relational aggression by gossiping or excluding may happen in a small group of one's friends where it is harder not to join in. Relational aggression may also be considered less harmful because there is no physical damage, making it more fun and less daunting to join in the negative group dynamic.

In another study, 298 college students were asked to recall a time when they had witnessed bullying and to provide various details about the event. Findings indicated that when bystanders recalled witnessing multiple types of bullying (e.g., physical, verbal, social) they were less likely to support the victim than when only physical bullying was present. The presence of multiple forms of bullying could seem more threatening to bystanders, thereby decreasing their defense of the victim (Oh & Hazler, 2009). In a qualitative study of 24 bystanders from Taiwan, participants indicated that they were willing to intervene in a serious bullying incident but were likely to refrain if it was not serious (Chen, Chang, & Cheng, 2016). This finding suggests that when bystanders perceive victims to be in serious danger they are more likely to intervene than when the bullying is milder and does not seem very harmful. This is a dangerous finding because the extent of damage from bullying can only be fully assessed by the victim; bystanders cannot accurately assess the extent of the victim's suffering because much of the damage is psychological rather than physical. While bloody noses or bruises may be obvious, bystanders cannot tell how a victim of relational aggression is fully impacted by the event, especially when victims work very hard to hide their emotional reactions.

Other important situational factors include the response of the victim. Victims who got angry elicited negative bystander reactions while sad victims increased bystanders desire to intervene. Victims who responded with confidence caused bystanders to view the bullying as less severe (Sokol, Bussey, & Rapee, 2015). Further, bystanders reported wanting to help victims who appeared to have done nothing to elicit the bullying, as opposed to victims who had somehow annoyed the perpetrator and "made a mistake" which resulted in their being bullied (Chen et al., 2016). These findings highlight bystanders' inclination to blame the victim when victims respond aggressively or seem to have caused their own bullying; blaming the victim would decrease bystanders' desire to help the victim.

Further, the presence of other bystanders and past experiences with bullying impacts bystander behavior. For example, when other bystanders were present, past engagement in bullying others decreased the probability that a bystander would defend the victim (Song & Oh, 2017). Perhaps youth who have bullied in the past wanted to be viewed as tough and strong by their classmates and therefore refrained from helping victims when others were present. However, when no other bystanders were present, past victimization was associated with an increased probability of defending the victim. These past victims had high levels of empathy towards the current victim and therefore intervened to help, but only when no other bystanders were present. However, the power of social conformity usurped their empathy and these bystanders did not support the victim when their classmates were present (Song & Oh, 2017). The relationship between the bystander and the victim and perpetrator is also important to consider. The closer the bystander was with the victim and the more distant he/she was with the perpetrator and the higher the bystander's popularity, the greater the probability that the bystander would defend the victim (Song & Oh, 2017). Taken together, research suggests that there are multiple situational factors that bystanders take into consideration as they contemplate what action to take.

4.5 Ways to Improve Prosocial Bystander Behavior

One method for increasing upstander behavior among youth who witness bullying is to implement school-based curricula focused on increasing prosocial bystander behavior. A meta-analysis of 12 school-based programs involving 12,874 students found that overall programs were successful at improving bystander behavior with modest (but important) effectiveness (Polanin, Espelage, & Pigott, 2012). However, interestingly, the interventions did not have a significant impact on bystander empathy (i.e., bystanders intervened more but did not feel more empathic towards the victims). There were larger effects for high school youth compared to elementary and middle school youth (Polanin et al., 2012). Two programs from the meta-analysis are reviewed below as well as an online campaign used to increase upstander behavior.

4.5.1 Steps to Respect

Steps to Respect is an anti-bullying intervention for grades three through six that targets behaviors such as joining groups, social-emotional skill building to foster positive peer relationships, being a responsible bystander, and differentiating reporting from tattling (Frey et al., 2005). The program emphasizes avoiding destructive bystander responses to bullying by promoting socially responsible behavior through perspective taking, help seeking, and assertive reporting (Frey, Hirshstein, Edstrom, & Snell, 2009). Steps to Respect includes 11 50-min lessons comprised of group discussions, games, and skills practice. Although this program targets bystander behavior, results are mixed in terms of changes in bystander defending behavior at post-test.

In one study of Steps to Respect, six schools were randomly assigned to an intervention or control group ($N = 1023$) and a random sample of 544 children were observed on the playground. Students filled out self-report surveys assessing their participation as a bully, victim, or bystander and teachers also filled out surveys assessing student involvement in the bullying dynamic. Results of the playground observations revealed a near-significant decrease in bystander encouragement of bullying in the intervention group and no significant group differences in terms of rates of victimization. However, there was a significant decrease in observed playground bullying behavior between the control and intervention group between pre-test and post-test, suggesting a decrease in victimization in the intervention group relative to the control group. However, this observed decrease in bullying behavior was not reflected in the self-report measures of bullying behavior (Frey et al., 2005); researchers observed decreased bullying, but students did not report that they were bullying less. Although this intervention targets bystander behavior, there were no noted significant increases in defending behavior yet researchers observed that bullying decreased. These findings suggest that impacting bystander behavior is complex and that, in this study, some other mechanism was responsible for the decrease in bullying behavior other than a change in bystander behavior. Perhaps 11 lessons are not intensive enough to change bystanders' behavior and a longer classroom curriculum is needed.

4.5.2 *KiVa*

While bystander behavior is one component of Steps to respect, KiVa is an anti-bullying intervention focused primarily on bystander behavior. The 20 h of classroom lessons focus on increasing the empathy, self-efficacy, and anti-bullying attitudes of bystanders using discussion, group work, role plays, short films, and an anti-bullying computer game. There is also a focus on teaching bystanders steps for supporting and defending the victim (Karna et al., 2011a).

In one controlled trial study of Kiva involving three waves of data, at Wave 2 (about 7 months into the intervention), bystanders in intervention schools reported significantly higher rates of defending behavior compared to bystanders in control schools, but these effects were nonsignificant by Wave 3. However, at Wave 3, bystanders in intervention schools reported significantly lower levels of assisting and reinforcing the bully compared to bystanders at control schools, which means that 9 months after the KiVa intervention, bystanders in intervention schools reinforced and assisted the bully less than bystanders at control schools. Further, intervention schools had significant decreases in self-reported bullying and victimization and peer-reported victimization compared to control schools (Karna et al., 2011b). Decreased support of the bully may partially explain the decrease in bullying behavior.

Although KiVa successfully increased bystander defending behavior after 7 months of the program, this improvement did not hold over time. The subsequent decrease of defending behavior indicates the need for ongoing reinforcement of positive bystander behavior. It is encouraging that the decreased assisting and reinforcing behavior remained over time; however, if defending behavior had also increased, bullying behavior would have decreased even more in the intervention schools. Given that high sociometric status is associated with defending behavior, perhaps a component should be added to the KiVa intervention that targets popular-prosocial youth in an effort to foster their positive leadership positions in the classroom. This is not to say that students with low social status would be excluded from the intervention, but perhaps additional bystander training for popular/well-liked youth would be beneficial as popular youth often have positions of power in the classroom and could serve as leaders for other students in terms of defending behavior.

There have been numerous controlled trial studies of KiVa conducted in Finland and this intervention is consistently associated with decreased rates of bullying and victimization (Karna et al., 2013; Sainio, Veenstra, Huitsing, & Salmivalli, 2012; Salmivalli, Karna, & Poskiparta, 2011; Williford et al., 2012). The consistent effectiveness of the KiVa intervention in decreasing bullying suggests that a clear focus on increasing bystanders' empathy, self-efficacy, and anti-bullying attitudes through multiple means is an effective way to decrease rates of bullying and victimization. However, the trials of KiVa have been conducted in Finland, which has a much more homogeneous population compared to the USA. Therefore, KiVa might need to be modified for use with US school children.

More information on both the Steps to Respect and KiVa programs is available on the Blueprints for Healthy Youth Development website (blueprintsprograms.com/programs), which considers both programs promising. Despite the promising status, effects for both programs have been modest and KiVa has been implemented and tested in Europe, leaving little information on North American application. The KiVa classroom curricula is more than twice as long as the Steps to Respect curriculum (i.e., 20 h versus 9 h) indicating that changing bullying behavior is a gradual process that requires more intensive participation in anti-bullying curricula. However, researchers need to further examine how to maintain increases in defending behavior over time. Although these programs provide a good start, more options for addressing the bullying dynamic are clearly needed.

4.5.3 Bystander Revolution: Take the Power Out of Bullying

Bystander Revolution is a website dedicated to decreasing bullying behavior by increasing upstander behavior (Bystander Revolution, 2016; http://www.bystanderrevolution.org). The website was launched in 2014 by author and parent MacKenzie Bezos to create a venue to share practical ways to defuse bullying. A number of bullying and violence researchers serve as advisors to the website including Dr. Dorothy Espelage, a renowned bullying researcher; Dr. Philip Zimbardo, psychology professor at Stanford University who studies social influence and conformity; and Gavin de Becker, the world's leading expert on violence prediction and management.

Bystander Revolution currently has 300 videos about personal experiences with being bullied, bullying others, and being a bystander to bullying. The videos are organized by problems (e.g., being a bullying, being the new kid, adults not helping) and by solutions (e.g., don't pass on rumors, interrupt bullying, offer sympathy) as well as a section with videos offering advice for bystanders, people being bullied, and people bullying. A number of celebrities such as Michael J. Fox, Salma Hayek, Demi Lovato, Kevin Spacey, Jason Mraz, and Jared Leto share their experiences and insights in these videos. In addition, teenagers who currently or in the past have had involvement in the bullying dynamic also share their insights. The website also has a section of Solutions, where over 100 contributors have posted advice on how to solve the problem of bullying and be a prosocial bystander. Examples include apologizing, approaching the victim later, sitting with someone new. There is also a section where discussion questions for certain videos have been posted so that youth, teachers, parents, or researchers can begin dialogues about bullying.

Finally, the Weekly Stand provides 52 simple actions that youth can take every week to put an end to bullying. In essence, the Weekly Stand provides concrete steps for youth to take to become upstanders and to generally improve the culture and climate of their school. For example, Week 2 is called Expand Your Circle, and youth are tasked with the job of reaching out to a classmate they have known but never spent time with and ask them to do something like go out for ice cream or pizza. Week 3 is called Shift the Focus and challenges youth to find an opportunity to speak up and engage in prosocial bystander behavior when someone else is being treated unkindly. Week 13 is called Lunch Buddies and asks that once during the week participants ask someone who is sitting alone to sit with them at lunch. Week 36 is called Question the Rumor and challenges youth to stand up to rumors and ask: "How would you feel if someone said that about you?" This website provides practical, concrete, and useful tools that youth can use to become upstanders in their schools and communities. This website provides a large amount of anti-bullying testimony and suggestions; however, the effectiveness in actually lowering the prevalence of the bullying dynamic remains unknown.

4.6 Conclusions

Bystanders are ubiquitous during bullying situations and their behavior has substantial impact on whether the bullying behavior continues or ends. Negative bystanders support the perpetrator through encouragement or by joining in the bullying; passive bystanders take no action or in some cases might wait until the bullying has ended and then comfort the victim; and prosocial bystanders or upstanders support the victim by confronting the perpetrator, removing the victim from the situation, or getting a teacher. Bystander behavior not only has bearing on individual episodes of bullying but also impacts the entire culture and climate of classrooms and the school. Understanding how individual psychology as well as classroom social standing impact bystander behavior is vital in order to create and implement interventions that increase upstander behavior. School-based bullying interventions such as Steps to Respect or KiVa are potential avenues to decrease bullying and increase prosocial bystander behavior. In addition, encouraging youth to visit websites such as Bystander Revolution increases adolescent knowledge about different methods for supporting victims.

References

Aluede, O., Adeleke, F., Omoike, D., & Afen-Akpaida, J. (2008). A review of the extent, nature, characteristics, and effects of bullying behaviour in schools. *Journal of Instructional Psychology, 35*, 151–158.

American Psychiatric Association. (2013). *Diagnostic and statistical manual of mental disorders* (5th ed.). Washington, DC: Author.

Arbib, M. (2006). The mirror system hypothesis on the linkage of action and languages. In M. Arbib (Ed.), *Action to language via the mirror neuron system* (pp. 3–47). Cambridge: Cambridge University Press.

Asher, S. R., Parker, J. G., & Walker, D. L. (1996). Distinguishing friendship from acceptance: Implications for intervention and assessment. In W. M. Burkowksi, A. F. Newcomb, & W. W. Hartfup (Eds.), *The company they keep: Friendship during childhood and adolescence* (pp. 366–405). New York, NY: Cambridge University Press.

Atlas, R. S., & Pepler, D. J. (1998). Observations of bullying in the classroom. *Journal of Educational Research, 92*(2), 86–99.

Bagwell, C. L., & Schmidt, M. E. (2011). *Friendships in childhood and adolescence*. New York, NY: Guilford.

Barhight, L. R., Hubbard, J. A., & Hyde, C. T. (2013). Children's physiological and emotional reactions to witnessing bullying predict bystander intervention. *Child Development, 84*(1), 375–390.

Bell-Dolan, D. J., Foster, S. L., & Sikora, D. M. (1989). Effects of sociometric testing on children's behavior at school. *Developmental Psychology, 25*, 306–311.

Bierman, K. L. (2004). *Peer rejection: Developmental processes and intervention strategies*. New York, NY: Guilford.

Bystander Revolution. (2016). *Bystander Revolution: Take the power out of bullying*. San Francisco, CA: Author. Retrieved from http://www.bystanderrevolution.org/

Caravita, S. C. S., Di Blasio, P., & Salmivalli, C. (2009). Unique and interactive effects of empathy and social status on involvement in bullying. *Social Development, 18*(1), 140–163.

Chen, L., Chang, Y. C. L., & Cheng, Y. (2016). Choosing to be a defender or an outsider in a school bullying incident: Determining factors and the defending process. *School Psychology International, 37*(3), 289–302.

Dodge, K. A., Pettit, G. S., McClaskey, C. L., & Brown, M. M. (1986). Social competence in children. *Monographs of the Society for Prevention Research in Child Development, 51*(2), 1–85.

Facing History and Ourselves. (2017). *What difference can a word make?: Holocaust and Human Behavior*. Brookline, MA: Author. Retrieved from https://www.facinghistory.org/holocaust-and-human-behavior/chapter-12/what-difference-can-word-make

Fontaine, R. G., Yang, C., Burks, V. S., Dodge, K. A., Price, J. M., Pettit, G. S., & Bates, J. E. (1999). Loneliness as a partial mediator of the relation between low social preference in childhood and anxious/depressed symptoms in adolescence. *Development and Psychopathology, 21*, 479–491.

Frey, K. S., Hirschstein, M. K., Snell, J. L., Edstrom, L. V. S., MacKenzie, E. P., & Broderick, C. J. (2005). Reducing playground bullying and supporting beliefs: An experimental trial of steps to respect program. *Developmental Psychology, 41*(3), 479–491.

Frey, K. S., Hirshstein, M. K., Edstrom, L. V., & Snell, J. L. (2009). Observed reductions in school bullying, nonbullying aggression, and destructive bystander behavior: A Longitudinal evaluation. *Journal of Educational Psychology, 101*(2), 466–481.

Gini, G. (2008). Associations between bullying behavior, psychosomatic complaints, emotional and behavioral problems. *Journal of Pediatrics and Child Health, 44*(9), 492–497.

Gini, G., Albiero, P., Benelli, B., & Altoe, G. (2007). Does empathy predict adolescents' bullying and defending behavior? *Aggressive Behavior, 33*, 467–476.

Hawkins, D. L., Pepler, D. J., & Craig, W. M. (2001). Naturalistic observations of peer interventions in bullying. *Social Development, 10*(4), 512–527.

Hutchinson, M. (2012). Exploring the impact of bullying on young bystanders. *Educational Psychology in Practice: Theory, Research, and Practice in Educational Psychology, 18*(4), 425–442.

Janson, G. R., & Hazler, R. J. (2004). Trauma reactions of bystanders and victims to repetitive abuse experiences. *Violence and Victims, 19*(2), 239–255.

Jones, L. M., Mitchell, K. J., & Turner, H. A. (2015). Victim reports of bystander reactions to in-person and online peer harassment: A national survey of adolescents. *Journal of Youth and Adolescence, 44*, 2308–2320.

Kaltiala-Heino, R., Rimpela, M., Marttunen, M., Rimplea, A., & Rantanen, P. (1999). Bullying, depression, and suicidal ideation in Finnish adolescents: School survey. *British Journal of Medicine, 319*, 348–351.

Karna, A., Voeten, M., Little, T. D., Alanen, E., Poskiparta, E., & Salmivalli, C. (2013). Effectiveness of the KiVa antibullying program: Grades 1-3 and 7-9. *Journal of Educational Psychology, 105*(2), 535–551.

Karna, A., Voeten, M., Little, T. D., Poskiparta, E., Alenan, E., & Salmivalli, C. (2011a). Going to scale: A nonrandomized nationwide trial of KiVa antibullying program for grades 1-9. *Journal of Counseling and Clinical Psychology, 79*(6), 796–805.

Karna, A., Voeten, M., Little, T. D., Poskiparta, E., Kaljonen, A., & Salmivalli, C. (2011b). A large-scale evaluation of the KiVa antibullying program: Grades 4-6. *Child Development, 82*(1), 311–330.

Karna, A., Voeten, M., Poskiparta, E., & Salmivalli, C. (2010). Vulnerable children in varying classroom contexts: Bystanders' behaviors moderate the effects of risk factors on victimization. *Merill-Palmer Quarterly, 56*(3), 261–282.

Keysers, C., & Gazzola, V. (2006). Towards a unifying neural theory of social cognition. *Progress in Brain Research, 156*, 379–401.

Molenberghs, P., Cunnington, R., & Mattingley, J. B. (2009). Is the mirror neuron system involved in imitation? A short review and meta-analysis. *Neuroscience and Biobehavioral Reviews, 33*(7), 975–980.

Nansel, T. R., Overpeck, M., Pilla, R. S., Ruan, W. J., Simons-Morton, B., & Scheidt, P. (2001). Bullying behaviors among US youth: Prevalence and association with psychosocial adjustment. *The Journal of the American Medical Association, 285*(16), 2094–2110.

O'Connell, P., Pepler, D., & Craig, W. (1999). Peer involvement in bullying: Insights and challenges for intervention. *Journal of Adolescence, 22*, 437–452.

Obermann, M. (2011). Moral disengagement among bystanders to school bullying. *Journal of School Violence, 10*, 239–257.

Oh, I., & Hazler, R. J. (2009). Contributions of personal and situational factors to bystanders' reactions to school bullying. *School Psychology International, 30*, 291–310.

Parker, J. G., & Asher, S. R. (1993). Friendship and friendship quality in middle childhood: Links with peer group acceptance and feelings of loneliness and social dissatisfaction. *Developmental Psychology, 29*, 611–621.

Parkhurst, J. T., & Hopmeyer, A. (1998). Sociometric popularity and peer-perceived popularity: Two distinct dimensions of peer status. *Journal of Early Adolescence, 18*, 125–144.

Polanin, J. R., Espelage, D. L., & Pigott, T. D. (2012). A meta-analysis of school-based bullying prevention programs' effects on bystander intervention behavior. *School Psychology Review, 41*(1), 47–65.

Rivers, I., & Noret, N. (2010). Participant roles in bullying behavior and their association with thoughts on ending one's life. *Crisis, 31*, 143–148.

Rivers, I., Poteat, V. P., Noret, N., & Ashurst, N. (2009). Observing bullying at school: The mental health implications of witness status. *School Psychology Quarterly, 24*(4), 211–223.

Sainio, M., Veenstra, R., Huitsing, G., & Salmivalli, C. (2012). Same- and other-sex victimization: Are the risk factors similar? *Aggressive Behavior, 38*, 442–455.

Salmivalli, C., Karna, A., & Poskiparta, E. (2011). Counteracting bullying in Finland: The KiVa program and its effects on different forms of being bullied. *International Journal of Behavioral Development, 35*(5), 405–411.

Salmivalli, C., Lagerspetz, K., Bjorkqvist, K., Osterman, K., & Kaukiainen, A. (1996). Bullying as a group process: Participant roles and their relations to social status within the group. *Aggressive Behavior, 22*, 1–15.

Salmivalli, C., Voeten, M., & Poskiparta, E. (2011). Bystanders matter: Associations between Reinforcing, defending, and the frequency of bullying behavior in classrooms. *Journal of Clinical Child & Adolescent Psychology, 40*(5), 668–676.

Sokol, N., Bussey, K., & Rapee, R. (2015). The effect of victims' responses to overt bullying on same-sex peer bystander reactions. *Journal of School Psychology, 53*, 375–391.

Song, J., & Oh, I. (2017). Investigation of the bystander effect in school bullying: Comparison of experiential, psychological, and situational factors. *School Psychology International, 38*(3), 319–336.

Tapper, K., & Boulton, M. J. (2005). Victim and peer group responses to different forms of aggression among primary school children. *Aggressive Behavior, 31*, 238–253.

Trach, J., Hymel, S., Waterhouse, T., & Neale, K. (2010). Bystander responses to school bullying: A cross-sectional investigation of grade and sex differences. *Canadian Journal of School Psychology, 25*, 114–130.

Waddell, W. J. (2010). History of dose response. *The Journal of Toxicological Sciences, 35*(1), 1–8.

Wang, J., Iannotti, R. J., & Nansel, T. R. (2009). School bullying among adolescents in the United States: Physical, verbal, relational, and cyber. *Journal of Adolescent Health, 45*(4), 368–375.

Weiss, D. S. (2004). The impact of event scale-Revised. In J. P. Wilson & T. M. Keane (Eds.), *Assessing psychological trauma and PTSD* (pp. 168–190). New York, NY: Guilford Press.

Williford, A., Boulton, A., Noland, B., Little, T. D., Karna, A., & Salmivalli, C. (2012). Effects of the KiVa anti-bullying program on adolescents' depression, anxiety, and perception of peers. *Journal of Abnormal Child Psychology, 40*, 289–300.

Zimmer, B. (September 9, 2016). How high-school girls won a campaign for 'Upstander'. *Wall Street Journal*. Retrieved from https://www.wsj.com/articles/how-high-school-girls-won-a-campaign-for-upstander-1473436114

Chapter 5
Cyberbullying: Playground Politics (and Worse) in Cyberspace

5.1 Introduction

In 2006, 3 weeks before her 14th birthday, Megan Meier became the first nationally recognized victim of cyberbullying. Meier ended a long and tumultuous friendship with her neighbor, whose mother, Lori Drew, then created a fake MySpace account belonging to a 16-year-old boy and proceeded to befriend Meier online. In order to get back at Meier on behalf of her daughter, Drew began a fake romantic relationship with Meier and then broke up with her, telling her the world would be better off without her. Devastated by the breakup and ensuing hurtful comments, Meier committed suicide by hanging herself. In 2008, a federal judge issued the country's first cyberbullying verdict (Megan Meier Foundation, n.d.; Steinhauer, 2008). Although Meier did not experience this "breakup" in person and read the hurtful words rather than having someone say them to her face, this online harassment was enough to push a fragile teenage girl to end her life and highlighted the devastation that cyberbullying can cause. This story helped launch cyberbullying into the national spotlight where it became a new focus for parents, policy- and law-makers, education officials, mental health providers, and even the first lady of the USA, Melania Trump.

In 2010, Tyler Clementi was an 18-year-old freshman at Rutgers University. He played the violin at an advanced level, even while riding a unicycle, and was working through the coming out process as a gay man. During one of his first dates at college, Tyler's roommate used the webcam on his laptop to record an intimate part of Tyler's date and casted it on the Internet to other students. Tyler viewed his roommate's Twitter feed and was humiliated. He had widely become a topic of ridicule at the University, and many other students watched without offering any help or alerting administrators. Several days later, Tyler Clementi ended his life by jumping off the George Washington Bridge (https://tylerclementi.org).

"Peachy" Costello hated his nickname, attributing it to his buzz haircut that his mother insisted on. Some of his eighth grade classmates said it was also because he was round. His real name was Arnold, which he did not like either. Arnold's life got much worse after guys in his class took pictures of him in the shower after gym class. They posted them on Instagram and debated if he was "Peachy" all over.

Ali had a hard time adjusting to high school. She was elated one day over winter break when a junior asked her out. She fell in love with his blue eyes and dark hair. It seemed to be the thing couples do when he asked her to start sexting. Two months later, he stopped calling her. She later found out it was an upperclassmen prank and all his friends read her texts. She had to change schools and did not date again until she was in college.

© Springer Nature Switzerland AG 2019

P. R. Smokowski, C. B. R. Evans, *Bullying and Victimization Across the Lifespan*, https://doi.org/10.1007/978-3-030-20293-4_5

In 2015, the first author of this book had just started a new job as the Dean of the School of Social Welfare at the University of Kansas. I was on a conference call with researchers from the US Centers for Disease Control when someone loudly pounded on my office door. I opened the door and found a large group of African American students crowded in the hall holding signs. I politely told the leader of the group that I was on a conference call and would come out in fifteen minutes. Closing the door to finish the conference call was one of the worst decisions of my life. Before I walked out to talk to the students ten minutes later, it was already on Facebook and Instagram that "Dean slams door in Black student's face!" It went viral and I received hate messages, calling me a racist and many other unprintable names, for the next seven months. After death threats to my family, I resigned the Deanship.

Growing up in the 1970s, families had landline telephones, possibly one or two per household with 6 ft cords. It was common to have to wait your turn to use the phone and have to talk with no privacy in the middle of a kitchen. Similarly, in 1976, the Internet was born when two computers on different networks were able to talk with one another. Development of the Web was relatively slow with the first search engine invented in 1990 and the first web browser in 1993, which turned into Netscape. In 1993, the first smartphone was also introduced by IBM with a calendar, address book, clock, calculator, notepad, e-mail, and a touchscreen with a QWERTY keyboard. Due to this digital revolution that happened from the 1970s through the 1990s, adolescent development was dramatically different for teenagers growing up when technology was in widespread use.

Today, it is a common to see a group of teenagers sitting around a table at the mall or sprawled across park benches or sitting at a coffee shop, all of them tapping their smartphones as fast as they can. Although youth use their smartphones to generally surf the Internet, check sports scores, or order items online, a large proportion of smartphone and cellphone activity centers around social communication and interaction: texting; checking e-mail; posting photos on Facebook, Instagram, or Snapchat; posting videos on Vine, Musically, or YouTube; posting Tweets on Twitter; or checking up on what friends and family have posted on these various social media sites. It is therefore no surprise that adolescent access to and use of cellphones and the Internet are staggering.

A 2015 nationally representative poll of adolescents ages 13–17 conducted by the Pew Research Center found that 88% of American teenagers have or have access to a mobile phone: 73% have access to a smartphone, 15% have a basic phone, and

Table 5.1 Percentage of adolescents using social media sites

	Total % adolescents	% Girls	% Boys
Facebook	71%	70%	72%
Instagram	52%	61%	44%
Snapchat	41%	50%	31%
Google+	33%	33%	33%
Twitter	33%	37%	30%
Vine	24%	27%	20%
Tumblr	14%	23%	5%

Lenhart (2015)

only 12% reported they had no cell phone access of any type (Lenhart, 2015). This access to cellphones, and smartphones in particular, helps explain why 92% of this age group reported going online daily, with almost one quarter (24%) reporting "almost constant" online use. This online use centers on social media and 89% of adolescents reported using at least one social media site: 71% of youth used Facebook, 52% used Instagram, and 41% used Snapchat (See Table 5.1; Lenhart, 2015). Teenagers also engage in frequent texting and the average girl ages 13–17 sends 79 texts per day while the average boy sends 56 texts per day. Computers are also ubiquitous for US adolescents and 87% have or have access to a desktop or laptop computer, and 58% have or have access to a tablet computer (Lenhart, 2015). Computers and phones are often used for online video game playing and 84% of boys and 59% of girls reported playing video games online or on their phones (Lenhart, 2015).

The widespread adolescent use of smartphones, cellphones, computers, and tablets gives youth unfettered access to texting, the Internet, and the myriad of social media sites the Internet has to offer. Use of these electronic devices, and the access to social media that they provide, has also given rise to increased cyberbullying. Indeed, cyberbullying, using electronic means (e.g., e-mail, instant messaging, chat rooms, websites, gaming sites, cellular phones) to threaten, humiliate, insult, exclude, or intimidate others (Kowalski, Limber, & Agatston, 2012; Raskaukas & Stoltz, 2007) has become a widespread national and international problem (e.g., Kowalski, Giumetti, Schroeder, & Lattanner, 2014; Spears, Taddeo, Daly, Stretton, & Karklins, 2015). According to the 2015 Youth Risk Behavior Surveillance Survey (YRBSS) which assessed a national sample of 15,465 high school youth, about 16% reported being cyberbullied in the year prior to the survey (Centers for Disease Control and Prevention [CDC], 2016a). For the 11 states that provided middle school data, rates were higher and ranged from 18.2% in Delaware ($n = 3033$) to 29.2% in Maine ($n = 5146$; CDC, 2016b). International rates are similar; for example, in a sample of Serbian middle school youth 20% reported being cyberbullied (Popovic-Citic, Djuric, & Cvetkovic, 2011). Other national and international research suggests that rates of cyberbullying range from 4% to as much as 72% depending upon the time frame being assessed (e.g., lifetime, past 6 months), the definition of cyberbullying used, the age and location of the sample, the heterogeneity of the sample, and the frequency rate used to classify someone as a victim (e.g., at least once verses a few times per week; Aboujaoude, Savage, Starcevic, & Salame, 2015; Kowalski et al., 2014). Clearly, cyberbullying is a pernicious issue that impacts hundreds of thousands of adolescents worldwide, highlighting the need to understand this complex topic. This chapter will discuss cyberbullying dynamics by providing a discussion of the nuances of the definition of cyberbullying, the negative impact of cyberbullying on victims and perpetrators, and the relationship between traditional bullying (i.e., any bullying that takes place without the use of an electronic device) and cyberbullying.

5.2 Cyberbullying: Definitions, Roles, and Behaviors

5.2.1 Definition of Cyberbullying

The starting point for any discussion of cyberbullying is first to figure out what exactly is meant by the term cyberbullying? Like our discussion of the definition of traditional bullying in Chap. 1, the definition of cyberbullying is also fraught with a certain amount of ambiguity due in part to the variety of methods used to engage in cyberbullying (e.g., Internet, websites, texting, social media sites; Kowalski et al., 2012). While researchers and practitioners agree that cyberbullying is the use of electronic means (e.g., e-mail, instant messaging, chat rooms, websites, gaming sites, cellular phones) to threaten, humiliate, insult, exclude, or intimidate others (Kowalski et al., 2012; Raskaukas & Stoltz, 2007), applying this definition and identifying cyberbullying is not always straight forward. It can be difficult to ascertain if certain written communication is cyberbullying or simply a normative adolescent argument that occurs over text as opposed to in person. For example, is a heated argument between two acquaintances that occurs over text message or instant messenger cyberbullying or a disagreement using printed instead of spoken words? It depends; did one party overpower the other, intending to harm with humiliation? Further, vocal intonation, facial expression, and body language play a large role in how spoken words are interpreted, and these nonverbal cues are absent in electronic communication, making it possible to misinterpret written comments. In addition, the relationship between the perpetrator and victim should be considered. For example, a teenage girl posts a picture on Facebook of herself covered in mud after a soccer game and a classmate writes, "OMG! You're disgusting!" This comment could be meant in a friendly teasing way as a harmless joke, and if it had been spoken, it would have been accompanied by a friendly smile and laugh, and playful push on the shoulder indicating the innocent and innocuous nature of the comment. However, without these nonverbal cues this comment could be interpreted as mean and spiteful. Further, if the comment was made by a friend, the girl might take it as friendly teasing, but if it was made by someone more popular than the girl or someone who does not like the girl, she might feel threatened and interpret the comment as cyberbullying.

Aftab (2011) followed by Kowalski et al. (2012) discuss how cyberbullying can be both direct and indirect, also referred to as cyberbullying-by-proxy; however, there is some disagreement as to how indirect cyberbullying is defined. Direct cyberbullying occurs when one youth directly sends a message to another youth, such as sending a text message. Indirect cyberbullying involves "using others to help cyberbully the victim, with or without the accomplices knowledge" (Aftab, 2011; as cited in Kowalski et al., 2012; p. 60). For example, a teenage boy could hack into his friend's e-mail or Facebook account by either stealing or being given the password and proceed to send nasty messages to classmates. The owner of the account would be blamed for these messages and could subsequently lose friends and feel embarrassed or humiliated as a result. In this case, there are multiple victims: the people receiving the mean messages are victims; however, the person whose account was hacked is also a victim because he would undoubtedly suffer negative fallout from his "friend" sending nasty messages using his account. The perpetrator could take this indirect cyberbullying a step further and also reset his friend's password so that his friend could no longer access his account.

Other researchers define indirect cyberbullying similarly to how indirect traditional bullying is defined, which is a more covert form of repeated aggression such as relational aggression (e.g., rumor spreading, excluding; Gladden, Vivolo-Kantor, Hamburger, & Lumpkin, 2014; Sumter, Valkenburg, Baumgartner, Peter, & van der Hof, 2015). Following this definition, indirect cyberbullying is measured with items such as this example: in the past 6 months on the internet another child/young person: "… acted like I did not exist," "… excluded me," "… told my secrets to others." According to this definition, indirect cyberbullying occurs when youth are indirectly bullied through electronic means. It seems that researchers need to refer to the first form of "indirect" cyberbullying as cyberbullying-by-proxy to avoid confusion. It follows that indirect cyberbullying would then describe a phenomenon similar to indirect traditional bullying that takes place through electronic devices (e.g., ignoring someone in a chat room, refusing to respond to text messages).

Given the ambiguity that can arise in identifying cyberbullying, establishing a concrete definition is vital, but difficult. Repetition, power imbalance, and intent to harm (Olweus, 1993) were noted in Chap. 1 as the main defining features of traditional bullying. Similarly, based on interviews with 53 focus groups, cyberbullying researchers have established that youth often define cyberbullying according to these three elements: the perpetrator engages in cyberbullying repeatedly, has more power than the cybervictim, and intends to cause harm (Vandebosch & van Cleemput, 2008). Thus, repetition, power imbalance, and intent to harm are also important defining features of cyberbullying. However, the electronic nature of cyberbullying complicates these constructs, especially due to the permanence and publicity of most cyberbullying acts (Fahy et al., 2016).

Cyberbullying can comprise a single act of posting a hurtful comment or photo on a social media website, yet can have severe and far reaching consequences as the comment or photo can remain in cyberspace indefinitely and hundreds of people can access it repeatedly (Evans & Smokowski, 2016; Langos, 2012). Each time the comment or photo is viewed could be counted as an episode of cyberbullying, indicating the presence of repetition (Slonje & Smith, 2008). So, although the perpetrator only engaged in one, single act of posting the comment or photo, the repeated viewing of the harmful online content and the ongoing harm this viewing causes the victim suggests that the isolated act of posting a harmful comment or photo can and should be considered cyberbullying (Evans & Smokowski, 2016). However, the presence of repetition depends on the method of the cyberbullying. As noted above, a perpetrator could post a mean picture of someone only once (no repetition), but because the picture is accessed by hundreds (thousands) of people over and over again, repetition is present. However, considering personal electronic communication complicates the issue. If a nasty text message is sent once, on the surface it does not seem that this is cyberbullying because it was an isolated event and was sent to only one person. However, a text message can survive indefinitely and can be read and reread. Thus, if the victim does not delete the text message, he/she might be repeatedly traumatized by reading it multiple times. Does this mean repetition is present even though the perpetrator engaged in only one act of aggression through electronic means? The physical evidence of cyberbullying endures in a way that damage from traditional physical bullying does not, making it complicated to determine the true salience of repetition. With traditional bullying, repetition is counted as the number of times the perpetrator bullies others. But with cyberbullying, repetition is impacted by the number of bystanders who view (or forward) a post and by the victim's response (e.g., keeping a mean one time text or e-mail versus deleting it). When it comes to defining cyberbullying, establishing a pattern of repeated behavior seems less salient than with traditional bullying because repetition is almost a given when it comes to cyberbullying. Indeed, posts or tweets or comments in chat rooms can be forwarded exponentially, engaging more and more people. The cyberbullying may not be in the original post, but may occur later in the viral string perpetrated by someone the original people posting do not even know.

Power imbalance also becomes tricky when it comes to cyberbullying. Perpetrators who harass their peers online sometimes do so anonymously so it is impossible to know who the perpetrator is. The anonymity of cyberbullying makes elements of power differentials that are pertinent in instances of traditional bullying noted in Chap. 1 (e.g., physical size, age, or social status) insignificant in cyberbullying dynamics (Huang & Chou, 2010). Although it is likely scary and unnerving to not know who the perpetrator is, this anonymity means that physically weak victims with minimal social status could fight back online if they choose because they are not directly confronted with their perpetrator's physical power (Huang & Chou, 2010). However, if the perpetrator is known, then these dimensions of power would certainly become salient, and like traditional bullying, and as we discussed in Chap. 1, their importance would depend on the victim's perception. (e.g., a physically larger and wealthy female cyberbullying a smaller, low-income but popular male—if money and size are intimidating to the boy he would be more likely to view mean online comments made by the girl as cyberbullying; however, if the boy views his popularity and gender as the most salient dimensions of power, the girl's online taunting might be perceived as meaningless). In the absence of physical cues, some aspects of power imbalance to assess are as follows: Is one person more negative, toxic, prolific in writing, or offensive than the other person? Does one person have a group of followers that will magnify the abuse (i.e., negative bystanders)?

It is also important to understand how the anonymity of cyberbullying can become a source of power (Roberts-Pittman, Slavens, & Balch, 2012). The anonymity of the Internet seems to bolster adolescents' courage and decrease their inhibitions, allowing them to make comments or take actions (e.g., posting a mean picture) that they might not engage in in person; in other words, the anonymity of the Internet empowers cyberbullies. This phenomenon has been labeled the online disinhibition effect, whereby spending time on the Internet where rules are less rigid and users can be anonymous and invisible increases user's disinhibition (Suler, 2004). Given that adolescents have a developing prefrontal cortex and parietal brain region, they often behave impulsively (Romer, 2010), and the lawlessness and anonymity of the Internet might therefore be especially enticing for this vulnerable age group. Furthermore, unlike in face-to-face encounters, cyberbullies may not see the pain that their online behavior causes the victim, leaving them with no sense of remorse or empathy.

Other instances of cyberbullying are far from anonymous. Just like in a face-to-face group, individuals may have higher popularity and visibility in virtual spaces, leading to an accumulation of power in cyberspace. For example, President Donald Trump has 20 million Twitter followers with three million actual identified domestic people and businesses using Twitter (many of the rest are foreign, unidentifiable, and bots; Salkowitz, 2017). The president often activates this pool of followers to pile on negativity when he attacks his enemies. Consider the president's repeated tweets against Senator Rand Paul. "Truly weird Senator Rand Paul of Kentucky reminds me of a spoiled brat without a properly functioning brain. He was terrible at DEBATE!" and "Lightweight Senator @RandPaul should focus on trying to get elected in Kentucky—a great state which is embarrassed by him" (Forbes, 2018). Of course, Senator Paul has 67,000 Twitter followers of his own, and this is election campaign toxicity. Yet it clearly rises to the level of cyberbullying based on repetition, power imbalance, and intent to harm.

We believe that power imbalance is clearly present in cyberbullying because of the power of the crowd. Online messages, photos, texts, and other materials can be passed along online so easily that the victim's humiliation can grow exponentially. Thus, the victim remains relatively powerless to make the online abuse stop. The pain of being rejected online is the same as rejection face-to-face, except there is an additional power for the perpetrator in the victim never being able to get away from the online abuse.

Finally, intent to harm can be difficult to establish in cyberbullying. In order to avoid getting into trouble, youth could claim that online comments or text messages were meant as a joke, when in reality they were intended to harm the victim. Without the presence of intonation, body language, and facial expressions, establishing the tone and true intent of a written post can be difficult. In the example cited above, the comment made on the photo of the muddy soccer player (i.e., "OMG! You're disgusting!") could certainly be a joke, but it could also be intended to hurt the person who posted the picture. The only person who truly knows the intent of a posted comment is the person doing the posting. In contrast, the intent of traditional bullying is more obvious based on verbal intonation, body language, and facial expression and usually multiple bystanders witness the bullying and can attest to the harmful intent. However, with cyberbullying there is no vocal intonation, facial expressions, or body language, and bystanders (i.e., those who view the mean posts) may have to guess the perpetrator's intentions. Follow-up comments are particularly illuminating to see if the string of messages is negative or jovial. It is in this back-and-forth messaging that the tone and background of the original post is often explained ("You're disgusting!"—followed by "Just kiddin':–)" versus "Even more disgusting than you usually are"). It is also in these follow-up comments where bystanders might pile-on or stand up for the victim. In all instances, as is the case with traditional bullying, the perception of the victim is paramount. So, even if a child claims he/she did not intend certain comments to be harmful and meant them as a joke, if the victim feels hurt and perceives the comments to be bullying, then cyberbullying is taking place.

In summary, while repetition, power imbalance, and intent to harm are defining features of cyberbullying, nuances of the cyberbullying dynamic can complicate the identification of these features. In Chap. 1, we provided a comprehensive definition of traditional bullying: *Unwanted behavior* that occurs between a more *powerful* perpetrator(s) and weaker victim and *usually* occurs *repeatedly* over time; the behavior is *intended to harm* the victim and does *cause harm* to the victim, bystanders, and/or culture and climate within the enviornment where the bullying occurs. Given the complexities of cyberbullying discussed above we define cyberbullying as the use of electronic means (e.g., e-mail, instant messaging, chat rooms, websites, gaming sites, cellular phones) to purposefully harm a victim through text, photographs, or videos that serve to threaten, humiliate, insult, intimidate, or exclude the victim; this behavior may happen once or repeatedly.

5.2.2 *Cyberbullying Roles*

Like traditional bullying, there are three central roles in cyberbullying dynamics: the cyberbully (i.e., the perpetrator who sends the hurtful, electronic information), the cybervictim (i.e., the victim who is harmed by the cyberbullying behavior), and the cyberbully-victim (i.e., the adolescent who vacillates between cyberbullying others and being cyberbullied). Research suggests that females are significantly more likely to be cybervictims, while males are significantly more likely to be cyberbullies and both are equally likely to be cyberbully-victims. It does not appear that age impacts the likelihood of being a cybervictim, cyberbully, or cyberbully-victim (Bayraktar, Machackova, Dedkova, Cerna, & Sevcikova, 2015).

Bystanders are also present in the cyberbullying dynamic and are those youth who witness the cyberbullying by reading the mean messages or viewing the negative posts. Just like with traditional bullying, bystanders of cyberbullying can behave in three general ways: prosocial cyber-bystander, negative cyber-bystander, or passive cyber-bystander. These bystanders can either take action through electronic means, or take action in the real world (i.e., not online). Prosocial cyber-bystanders intervene in the cyberbullying by sticking up for the victim by writing a nice comment to counteract a nasty post or by directly confronting the perpetrator and writing an admonishment for being mean. If the prosocial cyber-bystander knows who the perpetrator is, he/she might choose to confront the perpetrator in person rather than through electronic means or a prosocial cyber-bystander might decide to get a parent or teacher involved. Negative cyber-bystanders join in the cyberbullying by sending or posting additional mean messages and supporting the perpetrator's cyberbullying. If negative cyber-bystanders know who the perpetrator is, they might also encourage the perpetrator to continue the cyberbullying. Follow-up messages and comments after the original post can be just as toxic as the original cyberbullying. This makes negative cyber-bystanders especially toxic because they keep the traumatic episode going and might forward the materials to others, recruiting more and more negative cyber-bystanders. Passive cyber-bystanders read or view the negative cyberbullying messages or pictures without taking any action. Bystanders are often even more ubiquitous in episodes of cyberbullying than in traditional bullying because a single e-mail or text message can be forwarded to hundreds of people with the click of a button and social media sites can be viewed by countless individuals. However, unlike traditional bullying, it can be difficult to ascertain who the bystanders of cyberbullying are as it is not possible to track who views certain social media pages. Within the online context, the number of "likes" becomes a crude but critical calculation for the victim's self-esteem.

5.2.3 Methods and Forms of Cyberbullying

It is important to distinguish between the actual behaviors that constitute cyberbullying and the methods by which cyberbullying occurs (e.g., e-mail, cell phone, social media). Nancy Willard (2007), attorney and Director of the Center for Safe and Responsible Internet Use established eight cyberbullying behaviors: flaming, harassment, denigration, impersonation, outing, trickery, exclusion, and cyberstalking; cyberbullying research experts added two more: happy slapping and sexting (Kowalski et al., 2012).

1. ***Flaming***. Online fights, usually in a "public" online setting such as a chat room, using angry and vulgar language; both parties mutually insult each other.
2. ***Harassment***. Repeatedly sending mean, harmful, and insulting messages. Harassment differs from flaming in three ways: usually harassment occurs through individual communication channels (e.g., text message, e-mail) as opposed to public areas such as chat rooms; harassment lasts longer than flaming; and harassment is usually one sided with at least one perpetrator targeting a single victim.
3. ***Denigration***. Disrespecting someone online by posting gossip or rumors to damage his/her reputation or social relationships. The information is often untrue, such as digitally altering a photo to portray the victim in a sexualized or harmful way. "Slam books" are an example of denigration; slam books refer to websites where classmates write mean and nasty comments about specific students. Web-based slam books evolved from teenagers carrying actual notebooks to circulate for others to make cruel remarks about targeted youth. This phenomenon dates back to the 1920s but has garnered much more power when communicated on the Internet.

4. ***Impersonation***. The perpetrator gains access to the victim's account and then poses as the victim and sends mean and harmful information to others in order to damage the victim's friendships and reputation. This is an example of cyberbullying-by-proxy (Aftab, 2011; as cited in Kowalski et al., 2012). This form of cyberbullying harms the people who receive mean messages but also harms the person who is impersonated. The person being impersonated may not actually exist. It is simple to create fake accounts on the Internet and exploit others by pretending to be someone else. In one 2007 poll of 511 web users, 55% of respondents said they regularly or always use fake Web identities. Just 12% of people said they always use their real identity (Macmanus, 2007). Indeed, in an online phenomenon called "sockpuppetry," a puppet master creates fake online identities that he uses to reinforce his point of view and attack his enemies (i.e., cyberbullies can create fake negative bystanders to reinforce them in an online fight; Seife, 2014).
5. ***Outing***. Exposing someone's secrets or private and embarrassing information or photos online. For example, forwarding a private e-mail to other people without the permission of the person who wrote the e-mail.
6. ***Trickery***. Tricking someone into revealing their secrets and/or embarrassing and private information and then sharing it online.
7. ***Exclusion***. Purposefully excluding someone from an online group. For example, unfriending someone on Facebook or ignoring them in a chat room or while playing a video game; given our innate human desire to belong and feel part of the group, exclusion can be particularly devastating.
8. ***Cyberstalking***. Repetitive and intense harassment, denigration, and threatening that fosters significant fear. One study found that 88% of respondents spied on their ex partners through Facebook or Instagram. In "catfishing," someone steals another person's online photos and information to create a fake identity and stalk others (Smith, 2015). In an extreme example, a tech-savvy cyberbully may hack into the victim's computer and use their webcam to watch them.
9. ***Happy slapping and hopping***. Perpetrators will slap and/or physically assault someone while a friend videotapes the event; the video is then posted online and/or sent around online to humiliate the victim. In 2010, two teenagers from a happy slapping gang in south London killed Ekram Haque as he waited outside a mosque with his granddaughter. The video remains easily available on YouTube. In happy slapping, teenagers commonly assault elderly victims, making the videos as entertainment.
10. ***Sexting***. Sending or posting nude or partially nude pictures or videos via electronic means. Sometimes, after the breakup of a relationship, these photos or videos are then spread around school as means of cyberbullying.

There are various avenues that adolescents use to carry out these forms of cyberbullying. Kowalski et al. (2012) created a list of the nine most common methods:

1. ***Instant messaging***. Also referred to as "IMing," this is an online chat between two people in real time. Nasty and hurtful messages can be sent (i.e., *harassment*), but perpetrators can also engage in *impersonation* by creating a screen name similar to the name of their intended victim and then sending harmful messages to others pretending they are the victim.
2. ***Electronic mail***. E-mail is a common method for cyberbullying due to the large reach: one message can be sent to hundreds of people with the click of a button. This is a quick and easy way to engage in *denigration*, *outing* and/or *happy slapping*. In addition, e-mail is a convenient method for engaging in *cyberstalking*. Further, fake e-mail accounts can be set up so that the origin of the e-mail cannot be traced to a specific sender.
3. ***Text messaging***. Text messaging through cell phones is another quick way to cyberbully others in a variety of ways such as *denigration*, *outing*, *happy slapping*, *cyberstalking*, and/or *sexting*. Similar to e-mail, one text can be forwarded to many people.
4. ***Bash boards***. An online bulletin board where people can post any information about people. This is a common avenue for *denigration* and *outing*. It is the cyber evolution of slam books.
5. ***Social networking site***. Social networking sites such as Facebook, MySpace, Twitter, and LinkedIn allow users to post profiles and update their followers on every aspect of their lives. This allows perpetrators to post harmful comments in response to updates or photos.
6. ***Chat rooms***. Chat rooms are public, online spaces where people can talk to each other in real time. People may assume fake identities and can lie about their age and gender. Chat rooms are an ideal place for *flaming* to take place.
7. ***Blogs***. These are online journals that youth often use to damage each other's reputation through *denigration* or *outing*.
8. ***Websites***. Youth commonly create websites in order to post harmful information and/or pictures about classmates or to create polls intended to harm peers, such as voting for the most unpopular girl in the class.
9. ***Internet gaming***. Players of online games often harass each other anonymously through gaming sites (e.g., *harassment*) or block other players from participating (i.e., *exclusion*). The side chat and comments made while playing multiplayer online games can be filled with hate speech and denigrating comments. Players have few social norms to filter what they say when they are killing zombies or fighting wars.

Understanding both the methods (e.g., flaming, exclusion) and means (e.g., e-mail, bash rooms, blogs) through which cyberbullying takes place is vital in order for parents and school personnel to properly monitor online activity and use of electronics. These various methods and forms of cyberbullying are incredibly harmful to both perpetrators and victims.

5.3 Psychosocial and Mental Health Impacts of Cyberbullying Engagement

The negative impact of traditional bullying was discussed in Chap. 3 and it is certainly clear that victims suffer from multiple negative outcomes such as poor mental health, disrupted peer relationships, and negative perceptions of school. These effects are often ongoing and impact victims into adulthood. It follows that involvement in cyberbullying would also negatively impact victims. However, given the unique features of cyberbullying (e.g., it can occur 24 h per day, the perpetrator can be anonymous) it is important to fully understand how this devastating experience impacts cybervictims and cyberbully-victims; in addition, researchers have also begun to examine outcomes of cyberbullies as well.

Given that research on cyberbullying is still in its nascence, the first population-based study on cyberbullying was conducted in Finland in 2010. A sample of 2215 Finnish youth ages 13–16 reported on their cyberbullying involvement in the past 6 months (Sourander et al., 2010). Findings indicated that outcomes for cybervictims, cyberbully-victims, and cyberbullies were similar to outcomes for traditional victims, bully-victims, and bullies. About 23% of cyber victims reported they had felt afraid for their safety, indicating possible trauma and also highlighting that the constant, ongoing nature of cyberbullying means youth cannot feel safe at home, as perpetrators can continue to send texts and e-mails even after the school day has ended. While the end of the school day might mean a respite from traditional bullying, cyberbullying follows kids everywhere they go. In addition, pure cybervictimization status was associated with sleeping problems, headaches, stomach aches, and peer problems. Cyberbullying perpetration status was associated with hyperactivity, conduct problems, low prosocial behavior, frequent smoking and alcohol use, headaches, and not feeling safe at school. Cyberbully-victim status was significantly associated with all of the aforementioned risk factors, indicating this group is most at risk, followed, by cybervictims, then cyberbullies (Sourander et al., 2010), which is similar for involvement in traditional bullying.

These findings were replicated in one of the few longitudinal studies of cyberbullying. A sample of 2480 youth participating in the Olympic regeneration in East London study was surveyed at baseline and 1 year later. Compared to youth not involved in cyberbullying, cybervictims and cyberbully-victims were 1.68 and 1.52 (respectively) times more likely to report social anxiety at the 1 year follow-up while being a cyberbully at baseline was not significantly associated with social anxiety at follow-up (Fahy et al., 2016). Further, cybervictims and cyberbully-victims were almost twice as likely compared to non-involved youth to report depressive symptoms at follow-up (Fahy et al., 2016). Another study of 677 Hawaiian youth confirmed these findings and cyberbullying victimization increased the likelihood of depression by almost two times, suicide attempts 3.2 times for females and 4.5 times for males, and increased the likelihood of binge drinking and marijuana use by about 2.5 times (Goebert, Else, Matsu, Chung-Do, & Chang, 2011). These findings suggest that cybervictimization is associated with increased depression and anxiety, perhaps resulting in increased suicide attempts and indicating that cybervictimization erodes mental health functioning in a similar way as traditional bullying victimization.

When it comes to self-esteem, cyberbullies seem to have the best outcomes relative to cybervictims and cyberbully-victims. In one study cyberbullies had significantly higher self-esteem compared to cybervictims; cyberbully-victims also had higher self-esteem but the difference did not reach statistical significance. Cybervictims reported significantly lower self-control and offline aggression compared to both cyberbullies and cyberbully-victims, who did not differ significantly from each other. Cybervictims also had significantly higher secure parental attachment and significantly lower peer rejection compared to cyberbully-victims. Cyberbullies had parental attachment scores quite similar to cybervictims and peer rejection scores in-between cybervictims and cyberbully-victims (Bayraktar et al., 2015).

A meta-analysis of 131 studies of cyberbullying distilled a number of outcomes related to cybervictimization and cyberbullying, in support of the aforementioned findings. For example, cybervictims had poor mental health outcomes and reported high levels of stress ($r = 0.34$), suicidal ideation ($r = 0.27$), depression ($r = 0.24$), anxiety ($r = 0.24$), loneliness ($r = 0.24$), somatic symptoms ($r = 0.19$), conduct and emotional problems ($r = 0.19$ and $r = 0.18$, respectively), and drug and alcohol use ($r = 0.15$) as well as decreased life satisfaction ($r = -0.21$) and self-esteem ($r = -0.17$). Cyberbullies also reported increased depression ($r = 0.15$), anxiety ($r = 0.16$), loneliness ($r = 0.09$), and drug and alcohol use ($r = 0.27$), but to a lesser degree (except for substance use) than cybervictims. Further, cyberbullies also reported decreased life satisfaction ($r = -0.11$) and self-esteem ($r = -0.10$) but again to a lesser degree than cybervictims (Kowalski et al., 2014).

Taken together, findings indicate that any form of participation in cyberbullying is associated with and causes poor mental health outcomes. Cybervictims and cyberbully-victims have worse mental health outcomes while cyberbullies suffer from poorer outcomes in terms of substance use. Of the three groups, cyberbullies fare the best: they have the highest level of self-esteem and appear to avoid suffering from the high levels of depression and anxiety that plague cybervictims and cyberbully-victims. In terms of mental health, cybervictims and cyberbully-victims both had negative outcomes, but cyberbully-victims seem to fare slightly worse, which is similar to traditional bullying.

5.4 The Relationship Between Traditional Bullying and Cyberbullying

Traditional bullying and cyberbullying are closely related, but distinct behaviors. Both involve humiliating a victim and stripping him/her of power in the presence of others, who are either physically present in the case of traditional bullying or virtually present in the case of cyberbullying. However, traditional bullying is typically conducted face-to-face and youth engaged in cyberbullying may never actually see the pain they cause their victims. While these forms of bullying are distinct, there is considerable crossover between them. Youth who are involved in traditional bullying as a perpetrator, a victim and/or both are at increased risk for involvement in cyberbullying as a perpetrator, a victim, and/or both. For example, being a traditional bullying perpetrator was moderately positively related to being a cyberbully perpetrator ($r = 0.45$; Kowalski et al., 2014; Li, 2007). Victims of traditional bullying had significantly higher rates of cybervictimization (Burton, Florell, & Wygant, 2013). Youth who are traditionally bullied are often also cyberbullied and in one sample of 3488 students in Singapore found that 31% reported experiencing both forms of bullying (Chew, 2010). Although both traditional and cyberbullying victimization are harmful, a meta-analysis of 34 studies found that cyberbullying victimization was more strongly related to suicidal ideation (OR = 3.12) compared to traditional bullying victimization (OR = 2.16; van Geel, Vedder, & Tanilon, 2014). This highlights the terrible consequences of the bullying dynamic, leaving victims at double and triple the risk for suicidal ideation in order to end their suffering.

In summary, while traditional bullying and cyberbullying are distinct behaviors, there is substantial overlap between them. This suggests that youth involved in one form of bullying as either a victim or perpetrator, might also be involved in the other form of bullying. Because traditional bullying is much less covert than cyberbullying, this finding suggests that all perpetrators and victims of traditional bullying should be screened for cyberbullying involvement. This "screening" could be as simple as having school personnel and/or parents check in with youth involved in traditional bullying and question them about possible cyberbullying involvement. The more aware adults are of the presence of cyberbullying the more they can take action to intervene. The research results linking both forms of bullying to poor behavioral, mental health, and academic outcomes underscores the toxicity of the bullying dynamic, regardless of how the victimization occurs.

5.5 Conclusions

Cyberbullying is the use of electronic means to purposely cause harm to a victim. Given the widespread adolescent access to smartphones, cellphones, tablets, and computers cyberbullying has become an increasingly common phenomenon. The defining features of traditional bullying (power imbalance, repetition, and intent to harm) are also vital components to cyberbullying; however, nuances of the cyberbullying dynamic complicate these defining features. Involvement in cyberbullying as a cybervictim or a cyberbully-victim results in negative mental health outcomes such as increased depression and anxiety while cyberbullying perpetration is associated with increased substance use. Cyberbullying is often very difficult to detect and adults might be totally unaware that it is occurring. Knowing the harm it can cause highlights the importance of parents and caregivers strictly monitoring adolescent behavior online. Parents and caregivers should also be sure to keep an open dialogue with adolescents about their online activities and should educate them about proper online etiquette. One of the biggest ways to prevent cyberbullying (and traditional bullying) is for parents to foster empathy in their children and help them understand how damaging and hurtful it is to read negative posts or messages about yourself. Further, schools should provide students with education about the negative impact of cyberbullying and should teach students proper online etiquette. Online resources combating cyberbullying have proliferated (i.e., http://www.pacer.org/bullying/resources/cyberbullying/ or https://tylerclementi.org/bullying-stories/) and may be helpful in these educational efforts.

References

Aboujaoude, E., Savage, M. W., Starcevic, V., & Salame, W. O. (2015). Cyberbullying: Review of an old problem gone viral. *Journal of Adolescent Health, 57*, 1018.

Aftab, P. (2011). http://www.wiredsafety.net

Bayraktar, F., Machackova, H., Dedkova, L., Cerna, A., & Sevcikova, A. (2015). Cyberbullying: The discriminant factors among cyberbullies, cybervictims, and cyberbully-victims in a Czech adolescent sample. *Journal of Interpersonal Violence, 30*(18), 3192–3216.

Burton, K. A., Florell, D., & Wygant, D. B. (2013). The role of peer attachment and normative believes about aggression on traditional bullying and cyberbullying. *Psychology in the Schools, 50*(2), 103–115.

Centers for Disease Prevention and Control. (2016a). *High school youth risk behavior surveillance-United States*. Atlanta, GA: Author. Retrieved from https://nccd.cdc.gov/youthonline/App/Default.aspx

Centers for Disease Prevention and Control. (2016b). *Middle school youth risk behavior surveillance-United States*. Atlanta, GA: Author. Retrieved from https://nccd.cdc.gov/youthonline/App/Default.aspx

Chew, C. (2010). Prevalence of cyber bullying in Singapore. In E. Ng & K. Rigby (Eds.), *Breaking the silence: Bullying in Singapore* (pp. 65–84). Singapore: Armour Publishing.

Evans, C. B. R., & Smokowski, P. R. (2016). Understanding weaknesses in bullying research: How school personnel can help strengthen bullying research and practice. *Children and Youth Services Review, 69*, 143–150.

Fahy, A. E., Stansfield, S. A., Smuk, M., Smith, N. R., Cummins, S., & Cark, C. (2016). Longitudinal associations between cyberbullying involvement and adolescent mental health. *Journal of Adolescent Health, 59*, 502–509.

Forbes. (2018). *Donald Trump's 10 most offensive tweets*. Jersey City, NJ: Author. Retrieved from https://www.forbes.com/pictures/flji45elmm/7-lightweight/#435dc286e162

Gladden, R. M., Vivolo-Kantor, A. M., Hamburger, M. E., & Lumpkin, C. D. (2014). *Bullying surveillance among youths: Uniform definitions for public health and recommended data elements, Version 1.0*. Atlanta, GA: National Center for Injury Prevention and Control, Centers for Disease Control and Prevention and U.S. Department of Education.

Goebert, D., Else, I., Matsu, C., Chung-Do, J., & Chang, J. Y. (2011). The impact of cyberbullying on substance use and mental health in a multiethnic sample. *Maternal Child Health Journal, 15*, 1282–1286.

Huang, Y. Y., & Chou, C. (2010). An analysis of multiple factors of cyberbullying among junior high school students in Taiwan. *Computers in Human Behavior, 26*, 1581–1590.

Kowalski, R. M., Giumetti, G. W., Schroeder, A. N., & Lattanner, M. R. (2014). Bullying in the digital age: A critical review and meta-analysis of cyberbullying research among youth. *Psychological Bulletin, 140*, 1073–1137.

Kowalski, R. M., Limber, S. P., & Agatston, P. W. (2012). *Cyberbullying: Bullying in the digital age*. Malden, MA: Wiley-Blackwell.

Langos, C. (2012). Cyberbullying: The challenge to define. *Cyberpsychology, Behavior, and Social Networking, 15*(6), 285–289.

Lenhart, A. (2015). *Teen, social media and technology overview 2015*. Washington, DC: Pew Research Center. Retrieved from http://www.pewinternet.org/2015/04/09/teens-social-media-technology-2015/

Li, Q. (2007). New bottle but old wine: A research of cyberbullying in schools. *Computers in Human Behavior, 23*(4), 1777–1791.

Macmanus, R. (January 31, 2007). *55% Of people regularly or always fake their web identity*. Readwrite. Retrieved from https://readwrite.com/2007/01/31/ake_web_identity_poll_results/

Megan Meier Foundation. (n.d.). *Megan's story*. Saint Charles, MO: Author. Retrieved from https://www.meganmeierfoundation.org/megans-story.html

Olweus, D. (1993). *Bullying at school: What we know and what we can do*. Malden, MA: Blackwell.

Popovic-Citic, B., Djuric, S., & Cvetkovic, V. (2011). The prevalence of cyberbullying among adolescents: A case study of middle schools in Serbia. *School Psychology International, 32*(4), 412–424.

Raskaukas, J., & Stoltz, A. D. (2007). Involvement in traditional and electronic bullying among adolescents. *Developmental Psychology, 43*(3), 564–575.

Roberts-Pittman, B., Slavens, J., & Balch, B. V. (2012). The basics of cyberbullying. *School Administrator, 69*(4), 32–37.

Romer, D. (2010). Adolescent risk taking, impulsivity, and brain development: Implications for development. *Developmental Psychobiology, 52*(3), 263–276.

Salkowitz, R. (January 17, 2017). *Trump's 20 million Twitter followers get smarter under the microscope*. Jersey City, NJ: Forbes. Retrieved from https://www.forbes.com/sites/robsalkowitz/2017/01/17/trumps-20-million-twitter-followers-get-smaller-under-the-microscope/#55c114874407

Seife, C. (July 29, 2014). *The weird reasons why people make up false identities on the internet*. Wired. Retrieved from https://www.wired.com/2014/07/virtual-unreality-the-online-sockpuppets-that-trick-us-all/

Slonje, R., & Smith, P. K. (2008). Cyberbullying: Another main type of bullying? *Scandinavian Journal of Psychology, 49*, 147–154.

Smith, P. (July 4, 2015). *Chilling stories of fake online identities and why people create them*. New York, NY: Buzzfeed. Retrieved from https://www.buzzfeed.com/patricksmith/this-is-why-people-create-false-identities-on-the-internet?utm_term=.bn248G5dRl#.va5wjGbV61

Sourander, A., Klomek, A. B., Ikonen, M., Lindroos, J., Luntamo, T., Koskelainen, M., … Helenius, H. (2010). Psychosocial risk factors associated with cyberbullying among adolescents. *General Psychiatry, 67*(7), 720–728.

Spears, B. A., Taddeo, C. M., Daly, A. L., Stretton, A., & Karklins, L. T. (2015). Cyberbullying, help-seeking and mental health in young Australians: Implications for public health. *International Journal of Public Health, 60*, 219–226.

Steinhauer, J. (November 26, 2008). Verdict in MySpace suicide case. *The New York Times*. Retrieved from http://www.nytimes.com/2008/11/27/us/27myspace.html

Suler, J. (2004). The online disinhibition effect. *Cyberpsychology & Behavior, 7*(3), 321–326.

Sumter, S. R., Valkenburg, P. M., Baumgartner, S. E., Peter, J., & van der Hof, S. (2015). Development and validation of the multidimensional offline and online peer victimization scale. *Computers in Human Behavior, 46*, 114–122.

Van Geel, M., Vedder, P., & Tanilon, J. (2014). Relationship between peer victimization, cyberbullying, and suicide in children and adolescents: A meta-analysis. *Journal of American Medical Association Pediatrics, 168*(5), 435–442.

Vandebosch, H., & van Cleemput, K. (2008). Defining cyberbullying: A qualitative research into the perceptions of youngsters. *CyberPsychology & Behavior, 11*, 499–503.

Willard, N. (2007). *Educators guide to cyberbullying and cyberthreats*. Retrieved from https://education.ohio.gov/getattachment/Topics/Other-Resources/School-Safety/Safe-and-Supportive-Learning/Anti-Harassment-Intimidation-and-Bullying-Resource/Educator-s-Guide-Cyber-Safety.pdf.aspx

Chapter 6
Playground Politics at Home: Child Maltreatment and Sibling Violence

6.1 Introduction

Each year, thousands of children and adolescents are exposed to the harmful impact of child maltreatment at the hands of their parents or caregivers. An even higher number of youth are victims of sibling abuse or bullying, a widespread phenomenon that has received minimal research attention. Both forms of violence have devastating consequences for the development of young victims. Further, both forms of violence are rarely, if ever, understood through the lens of bullying. The current chapter provides an overview of the definitions, prevalence rates, and economic costs of child maltreatment and sibling abuse or bullying. Then a discussion of bullying dynamics is applied to these forms of violence. Discussing these common forms of violence through the definitional framework of bullying provides researchers, practitioners, policy makers, and survivors a nuanced way of understanding violence in the home.

6.2 Child Maltreatment

6.2.1 Overview: Definition, Prevalence Rates, Demographics, and Cost

Horrific stories of child maltreatment dominate the media. A 12-year-old boy was locked in a bathroom for one and possibly 2 years, with a blanket and little else; when the boy was rescued he weighed 30 lb (Larmier, 2017). A 14-year-old girl weighting 48 lb with completely eroded teeth was rescued from her home where she was routinely locked in her room and limited to half a Dixie cup of water per day (Clarridge & Krishnan, 2008). The media is replete with other egregious stories of young babies, toddlers, children, and teenagers hit and beaten; some of this abuse

© Springer Nature Switzerland AG 2019

P. R. Smokowski, C. B. R. Evans, *Bullying and Victimization Across the Lifespan*, https://doi.org/10.1007/978-3-030-20293-4_6

proved fatal. However, there are thousands of maltreated children each year whose stories do not make the headlines, but these youths are, nevertheless, seriously traumatized by the maltreatment that they endure. To fully understand the problem of child maltreatment, it is important to start with some basic information such as the definition and scope of the problem.

Child maltreatment is abuse and/or neglect inflicted upon youth under the age of 18 and includes all forms of physical and emotional mistreatment including sexual abuse, neglect, negligence, and exploitation (World Health Organization, 2016). This chapter focuses specifically on child maltreatment occurring within the home where the parent(s) and/or caregiver(s) are the perpetrators and children under 18 are the victims. Unfortunately, a significant number of US youth endure this mistreatment every year.

In 2014, about 3.2 million children were the subjects of at least one report to Child Protective Services and of those reports, an estimated 702,000 were substantiated; 75% were cases of neglect, 17% physical abuse, and 8% sexual abuse (U.S. Department of Health & Human Services, 2016). In 2015, an estimated 1670 children died from abuse and neglect, which is almost five children per day (U.S. Department of Health & Human Services, 2017). The Fourth National Incidence Study of Child Abuse and Neglect found that one in every 58 children in the USA experiences maltreatment (Sedlak et al., 2010). It is important to note that rates of maltreatment vary widely across studies depending upon the method of research used including the definition of maltreatment, the type of maltreatment studied, the coverage and quality of the statistics, and the coverage and quality of the surveys requesting self-reports from victims and parents or caregivers (World Health Organization, 2016). Indeed, other national studies have found higher rates of maltreatment.

Using a nationally representative sample of 4549 youth ages 0–17, the National Survey of Children's Exposure to Violence found that 18.6% of respondents reported some form of maltreatment over their lifetime and for youth ages 14–17, 32.1% reported lifetime maltreatment (Finkelhor, Turner, Ormrod, & Hamby, 2009). Another study using a nationally representative sample found that 12.3% of youth ages 12–17 had experienced physical abuse (Hawkins et al., 2010). The National Longitudinal Study of Adolescent Health surveyed 15,197 young adults and 28.4% reported childhood maltreatment in the form of physical assault, 11.8% physical neglect, and 4.5% contact sexual abuse (Hussey, Chang, & Kotch, 2006). Further, the World Health Organization (2016) found that 25% of adults reported childhood maltreatment and 20% of women and almost 8% of men specifically reported sexual abuse. These findings indicate that up to one quarter of US youth under 18 suffer from childhood maltreatment and the ensuing devastating physical and emotional consequences (to be discussed later). While child maltreatment knows no boundaries, there are specific demographic factors that put youth at increased risk.

The vast majority of child maltreatment cases are comprised of three racial/ethnic groups: White (44%), Hispanic/Latino (23%), and African American (21%; U.S. Department of Health & Human Services, 2016). While children under three are at the highest risk for maltreatment and comprised over one quarter (27%) of maltreatment cases in 2014, preadolescents and adolescents are also a vulnerable group and youth ages 10–18 comprised 31% of maltreatment cases (U.S. Department of Health & Human Services, 2016). Socioeconomic status (SES), including income, educational attainment, occupational prestige, and perceptions of social status and class, has been linked to child maltreatment (American Psychological Association, 2017). Indeed, a low SES is a risk factor for child maltreatment and increased income significantly decreased the risk for child maltreatment (Cancian, Slack, & Yang, 2010). This finding may be due to the chronic stress that low-income parents struggle with as they single parent, juggle multiple jobs, and cope with meeting basic family needs. Under this stress, parents may become impatient, use extreme discipline techniques, and/or lack capacity to provide adequate supervision to their children (Administration for Children Youth and Families, 2016).

Finally, it is important to consider the economic cost of childhood maltreatment. In 2010 dollars, the lifetime cost of nonfatal child maltreatment per victim was estimated to be $210,012 and fatal cases cost about $1,258,800 per death. In 2008, it was estimated that nonfatal and fatal cases of child maltreatment cost the USA $124 billion; $83.5 billion in lost productivity, $25 billion in health care costs, $14.5 billion for special education, $4.5 billion for child welfare, and $3.5 billion in criminal justice expenses (Fang, Brown, Florence, & Mercy, 2012). In addition to the significant economic cost to society, child maltreatment has an incalculable cost in human suffering and serious negative consequences for victims.

6.2.2 Negative Consequences of Child Maltreatment

The negative consequences of child maltreatment are both immediate (i.e., in childhood when the maltreatment is occurring) and enduring (i.e., lasting into adulthood). For example, as a direct result of physical abuse, youth can suffer from bruises, cuts, broken bones, head trauma, or hemorrhages (Child Welfare Information Gateway, 2013) and neglected youth were at an increased risk for obesity and had a body mass index that grew significantly faster compared to their non-neglected counterparts (Shin & Miller, 2012).

Child maltreatment has been found to actually alter brain structure and function. For example, compared to non-maltreated youth, those who suffered from childhood maltreatment had significantly smaller hippocampal and amygdala volume (Chaney et al., 2014; Gorka, Hanson, Radtke, & Hairi, 2014; Hanson et al., 2015). The hippocampus is responsible for storing and processing long term memories and emotional responses and the amygdala is responsible for the memory of emotions (especially fear) and controls the way we react to events (The Brain Made Simple, n.d.). These brain changes in the hippocampus and amygdala were evident both in childhood (Hanson et al., 2015) and in adulthood (Chaney et al., 2014; Gorka et al., 2014) indicating that maltreatment has an immediate and enduring negative impact on the brain structure and function. Perhaps as a result of these brain changes, compared to non-maltreated youth, maltreated children have lower IQ's and deficits in language and academic achievement (see DeBellis & Zisk, 2014 for a review). Further, youth exposed to interpersonal trauma, such as maltreatment, display dysregulation of affect (e.g., flat, numbed, or inappropriate affect) and behavior (e.g., withdrawal, aggression, substance use); disturbances of attention and consciousness (e.g., dissociation, difficulty concentrating or planning); disturbances of attribution (e.g., difficulty understanding responsibility for personal behavior and behavior of others); and interpersonal difficulties (e.g., poor social skills, disrupted attachment styles; See D'Andrea, Ford, Stolbach, Spinazzola, & van der Kolk, 2012 for a review).

Child maltreatment is a serious form of trauma that can result in a persistent fear response for children and seriously impacts their view of social interactions. Trauma, such as maltreatment, results in the chronic activation of the brain pathways involved in the fear response. This chronic activation can create enduring "memories" that impact how the child perceives and responds to his/her environment (U.S. Department of Health and Human Services, 2001). This means that maltreated youth are on high alert for threatening situations and might interpret innocuous situations as potentially dangerous; in other words, they live in a state of hyperarousal and are constantly on high alert. For example, if someone accidently bumps into a child who has been maltreated, he/she might interpret that accidental bump as an aggressive act intended to cause harm and might respond either with an intensely aggressive action (e.g., yelling or shoving back) or completely retreat in fear. While functioning in this state of high alert and hyperarousal might serve an adaptive function while living in a hostile and abusive environment, it is then translated into every life situation, even when the environment is no longer dangerous (U.S. Department of Health and Human Services, 2001), which can cause serious problems in navigating social relationships as illustrated in the example above.

Child maltreatment can also seriously damage the ability of children to form healthy and functional attachments to other people. Forming an attachment refers to the ability to establish an emotional and physical bond to another person that provides the feeling of stability and security that is necessary in order to take risks that lead to growth and development (Bowlby, 1980; Developmental Psychology, 2017). The attachment relationship between a child and caregiver becomes a template of sorts for later attachments. Thus, a dysfunctional attachment pattern with a parent/caregiver, such as the pattern that might arise from maltreatment, can then be replicated in later relationships (Bowlby, 1980; Developmental Psychology, 2017). Child maltreatment not only makes a mutual and positive attachment relationship with the parent/caregiver difficult, but can also damage a child's ability to form future, healthy attachments. This means that maltreated youth might have difficulty establishing and maintaining functional and healthy social relationships in childhood, adolescence, and adulthood.

Child development researchers have extensively studied infant attachment for 50 years (Bowlby, 1969). Upon a child's birth, every parent's role is to provide food, safety, and a nurturing attachment relationship or bond with the infant; this is called a secure base that provides the foundation for all other learning to occur. An enormous amount of brain development and learning occurs during the first 3 years of life (Thompson, 2001), setting the stage for all other growth across the life span. Attachment theory asserts that disturbances in the early bond between caregiver and infant profoundly impact the developmental processes of the child. In a famous experiment, Dr. Harry Harlow (1962) separated baby rhesus monkeys from their biological mothers and let them choose either a wire mesh mother that provided milk or a cloth mother that provided no milk. Each infant became attached to its particular mother, recognizing its unique face and preferring it above all others. The infant monkeys overwhelmingly preferred the cloth mothers, showing that attachment was not primarily about hunger or thirst and could not be reduced to nursing. Love was emotional rather than physiological and cuddling kept normal development on track, even with cloth mothers. Conversely, infant monkeys with wire mothers became withdrawn, unresponsive, and clearly showed sign of depression and failure to thrive. These wire mother infants had physiological problems, such as diarrhea, which indicated they were under stress. In later experiments, Harlow reared young monkeys in isolation to simulate social deprivation. After 6 months of isolation, monkeys became severely psychologically disturbed, with autistic clutching and rocking and emotional shock. After 12 months, their social functioning was entirely obliterated. These findings paralleled later research findings with human infants in overcrowded orphanages.

Following this classic research, Ainsworth (1964; Ainsworth & Bell, 1970) designed a process for studying mother–infant attachment in humans called the Strange Situation. Mothers and 12–18-month-old toddlers were placed in a room with a stranger. The mother would leave for a short time, usually causing the child to become upset. Researchers would closely document the infant's behavior when the mother returned. Table 6.1 summarizes this attachment research and its connection to maltreatment and bullying. These researchers identified three main attachment styles:

1. **Secure (type B)**—The caregiver was sensitive, responsive to infant's stress, emotionally warm and supportive, protective, and provided the appropriate level of stimulation with a synchrony between the caregiver and the infant. The child was distressed at separation but consolable at the reunion with the caregiver. Later in development, secure children were less likely to experience psychopathology, more socially competent, and demonstrated better academic and cognitive performance.
2. **Insecure avoidant (type A)**—The caregiver was unresponsive, unaffectionate, rejecting, intrusive, and provided excessive stimulation. During the Strange Situation, the child hides distress at separation and reunion, inhibits expression of affect, and is slow to return to pre-separation physiological state. Later in development, insecure-avoidant children are less socially competent, more likely to be rejected by teachers, to victimize others, act compulsively and, have inhibited emotionality such as little empathy. In short, they are at high risk for becoming bullies.
3. **Insecure resistant (type C)**—These caregivers are inconsistently available, unpredictable in parenting, intermittent reinforcement (i.e., sometimes positive sometimes negative in their responses), under involved, and unresponsive. In the

Table 6.1 Attachment styles, maltreatment, and bullying

	Secure attachment	Resistant attachment	Avoidant attachment	Disorganized attachment
Caregiver characteristics	Sensitive; responsive to infant's stress; emotionally warm and supportive; protective; provides appropriate level of stimulation; achieves interactional synchrony with the infant.	Inconsistently available; unpredictable parenting; intermittent reinforcement; under-involved; unresponsive.	Unresponsive; unaffectionate; rejecting; intrusive; provides excessive stimulation.	Unresponsive to infant cues; maltreatment; frightened or frightening behavior; unresolved childhood experiences—possibly violence or abuse; withdrawal and/or hostile intrusive.
Separation anxiety	Distressed when the mother leaves.	The infant shows signs of intense distress when the mother leaves.	The infant shows no sign of distress when the mother leaves.	Inconsistent, a mix of Avoidant and Resistant.
Stranger anxiety	Avoidant of stranger when alone, but friendly when the mother present.	The infant avoids the stranger—shows fear of the stranger.	The infant is okay with the stranger and plays normally when the stranger is present.	Inconsistent, a mix of Avoidant and Resistant.
Reunion behavior	Positive and happy when the mother returns.	The child approaches the mother but resists contact, may even push her away.	The infant shows little interest when mother returns.	Inconsistent, a mix of Avoidant and Resistant.
Assessment	Will use the mother as a safe base to explore their environment.	The infant cries more and explores less than the other two types.	The mother and the stranger are able to comfort the infant equally well.	No discernible pattern.
Child later in development	Less likely to experience psychopathology; more socially competent; better academic and cognitive performance.	More likely to be victims; pampered by teachers; coercive strategies because environment is unpredictable; anxious and clingy in relationships.	Less socially competent; more likely to be rejected by teachers; more likely to victimize others; inhibited in expressing emotions, compulsive.	Aggression; Problems at school; Especially vulnerable to stress or adversity.

(continued)

Table 6.1 (continued)

	Secure attachment	Resistant attachment	Avoidant attachment	Disorganized attachment
Potential connection to child temperament	Easy temperament; eats and sleeps regularly, accepts new experiences.	Slow to warm-up temperament.	Difficult temperament.	Difficult temperament.
Connection to maltreatment	No consistent relationship.	Risk for emotional abuse, sexual abuse, neglect.	Risk for physical abuse, physical neglect, emotional neglect.	Risk for physical abuse, emotional abuse, physical neglect, emotional neglect.
Connection to bullying	Bystanders.	Risk for becoming victims.	Risk for becoming bullies.	Risk for becoming bullies or bully-victims.

Note: Belsky and Rovine (1987), McLeod (2016)

Strange Situation, the child expresses affect, is highly vigilant against abandonment, is difficult to console, and shows mixed emotions at reunion with the mother. Later in development, these children are anxious, pampered by teachers, and more likely to be victims of bullying.

4. **Disorganized** (meaning infant's responses to separation and reunion are inconsistent; may be combination of Types A and C). The caregiver is unresponsive to infant cues, may have a history of maltreatment, frightened or frightening behavior, unresolved childhood experiences—Possibly violence or abuse with withdrawal and/or hostile intrusive parenting. The young child in the Strange Situation displays no consistent response to separation, no consistent strategy to defend self or seek help from environment, and is slow to return to pre-separation physiological state. Later in development, these children show aggression, problems at school, and are especially vulnerable to stress or adversity.

The attachment research summarized above is important because it shifted the focus of early child development research to maternal sensitivity, nurturance, and love. Conversely, the profound negative implications of caregiver deprivation and social isolation on child development were uncovered. In many instances of child maltreatment, caregivers are insensitive to the child's physical, emotional, and social needs. The deprivation from this abuse has both short and long-term effects on the developing child.

In addition to the immediate negative effects of childhood maltreatment, adolescents and adults maltreated in childhood are at an increased risk for negative outcomes. For example, adults abused and neglected as children were at an increased risk for diabetes, vision problems, malnutrition, and lung disease (Widom, Czaja, Bentley, & Johnson, 2012). Maltreatment also increases the likelihood of substance use and those with a history of child abuse and neglect were 1.5 times more likely to report past year illegal drug use in middle adulthood, reported use of a larger number of drugs, and more substance-use-related problems compared to their non-maltreated counterparts (Widom, Marmorstein, & White, 2006). Research suggests that maltreatment is also associated with at least a 25% increased risk of violent delinquency, teenage pregnancy, symptoms of mental illness, and low academic achievement (Kelley, Thornberry, & Smith, 1997). Indeed, child maltreatment negatively impacts adolescent and adult criminality and increased the likelihood of juvenile arrest by 59%, adult arrest by 28%, and engagement by violent crime by 30% (Widom & Maxfield, 2001). Further, maltreatment negatively impacts mental and emotional health. For example, one study found that 80% of young adults maltreated before the age of 18 met the criteria for at least one psychiatric disorder by the age of 21. Compared to their non-maltreated counterparts, those who had been maltreated had increased depressive symptomology, anxiety, psychiatric disorders, emotional-behavioral problems, suicidal ideation, and suicide attempts (Silverman, Reinherz, & Giaconia, 1996).

Taken together, these findings illustrate the devastating short- and long-term consequences of child maltreatment. Victims are at risk for poor mental (e.g., depression) and physical (e.g., lung disease) health outcomes; decreased academic functioning (e.g., low IQ); and behavioral (e.g., criminal behavior) and social (e.g., poor social skills) problems. These negative outcomes are due in part to the altered brain structure caused by maltreatment. Although these issues often begin in childhood when the maltreatment is occurring, they endure into adulthood. To better understand why child maltreatment is so devastating we propose examining this detrimental interaction through the framework of bullying.

6.2.3 *Child Maltreatment Through the Bullying Framework*

The three essential definitional elements of bullying behavior as outlined in Chap. 1 are repetition, power imbalance, and intent to harm. Each of these elements is present in situations of child maltreatment. However, despite this, child maltreatment is not typically defined as a form of bullying and is not understood through these definitional components. We argue that the presence of the repetition, power imbalance, and intent to harm present in maltreatment dynamics suggests that this dysfunctional social interaction can be understood as a form of bullying. We are not suggesting renaming child maltreatment as "bullying in the home," we are simply offering a new and innovative way of examining and understanding the dynamics present in childhood maltreatment.

6.2.3.1 Repetition

Child maltreatment is almost always repeated; it is rare for a parent or caregiver to engage in an isolated act of maltreatment. An example of an isolated act would be a parent slapping his/her child one time and then never engaging in physical abuse again or refusing to take a child to the doctor on one occasion when the child was sick and needed medical attention. While it is possible these behaviors could occur in isolation and then never be repeated, it is more common that these behaviors are indicative of an overall pattern of behavior that is repeated over time. The saying, "the past is the best predictor of the future" comes to mind. Indeed, prospective studies of abuse indicated that the best predictor of whether abuse will be repeated in the future is whether or not abuse has occurred in the past (Honomichl & Brooks, 2009). Researchers studying the repetition of maltreatment use the term "recurrence" or "re-abuse" and define recurrence or re-abuse as maltreatment that occurs after an initial report of abuse or neglect has been made (see Honomichl & Brooks, 2009 for a review). In this regard, researchers do not assess if the maltreatment was ongoing and repeated prior to the initial report, they examine if any maltreatment occurred following an initial report to Child Protective Services (CPS) or other agencies.

Researchers have established a variety of factors that impact whether maltreatment reoccurs after an initial report is made. However, it is likely that these same factors would impact whether maltreatment was repeated, that is, whether the parent or the caregiver engaged in ongoing abusive and/or neglectful behavior over time. For example, timing of past abuse is a major predictor of re-abuse; that is, children are at risk for further maltreatment directly after an episode of maltreatment and this elevated risk can endure for up to a 2-year time period. In one study of abused children admitted to a hospital-based child abuse assessment unit, the greatest risk of re-abuse occurred in the 2 years following discharge and then risk for re-abuse decreased (Levy, Markovic, Chaudhry, Ahart, & Torres, 1995). A systematic review of 16 studies confirmed that youth maltreated in the past were about six times more likely than non-maltreated youth to experience recurrent maltreatment and the risk for recurrence was highest within 30 days of the last maltreatment episode (Hindley, Ramchandani, & Jones, 2006). Further, the likelihood of re-abuse increases after each maltreatment episode (Fluke, Yuan, & Edwards, 1999) and the referral rate to CPS increased as the number of prior referrals increased (English, Marshall, Brummel, & Orme, 1999), again confirming that past maltreatment was associated with future maltreatment. Taken together, these findings suggest that maltreatment begets maltreatment and that youth are at the highest risk for being revictimized right after an episode of maltreatment. This means that as maltreatment continues over time, the likelihood that it will continue steadily increases. Indeed, it is likely that maltreatment begins with less intense incidents that build in severity over time until the behavior potentially comes to the attention of CPS agencies and intervention occurs.

Certain child characteristics such as age, gender, and disability status are also risk factors for re-abuse or the repetition of child maltreatment. For example, research consistently shows that younger children are more likely to experience re-abuse compared to older children and in general, girls are more at risk for recurrence of abuse compared to boys, but this is not a consistent finding. Finally, children with special needs are at an increased for re-abuse (See Honomichl & Brooks, 2009 for a review). For example, children with a disability were 1.5 times more likely compared to children without a disability to experience re-abuse (Fluke, Shusterman, Hollinshead, & Yuan, 2008).

There are also a variety of parent factors that put youth at risk for re-abuse including parental substance use, poor parent mental health, poor parenting skills, and a parental history of child maltreatment. And family factors such as domestic violence and conflict, an increasing number of children, and low financial well-being are also associated with an increased risk of re-abuse (See Honomichl & Brooks, 2009 for a review). Community factors including high levels of mobility within neighborhoods results in an increased risk for re-abuse. Unstable neighborhoods likely lack support and contribute to increased parent and family stress, leading to an increased risk for re-abuse (See Honomichl & Brooks, 2009 for a review).

Not only are maltreatment incidents repeated over time, but types of maltreatment also overlap and co-occur. In the Adverse Childhood Experiences (ACE) studies (Substance Abuse and Mental Health Services Administration, n.d.), 26% of adults reported one ACE, almost 40% of the Kaiser sample reported two or more ACEs (i.e., multiple experiences of emotional, physical, sexual abuse, emotional neglect, physical neglect, domestic violence, substance use by parent, mental illness in parent, divorce, and having an incarcerated family member) and 12.5% experienced four or more. Cumulative effects of ACEs, rather than the individual effects of each, had profoundly negative effects on adult health and well-being. A person's cumulative ACEs score has a strong, dose–response relationship to numerous health, social, and behavioral problems throughout their life span. As shown in Fig. 6.1, individuals who experienced four or more ACEs during childhood had far greater health risks in adulthood; 14 times the risk of suicide attempts, 11 times the risk for intravenous drug use, 4.5 times the risk for depression, four times the risk for early sexual intercourse (before age 15), three times the risk for smoking and lung disease, and two times the risk for liver disease in adulthood (often linked to overuse of alcohol; National Institute on Alcohol Abuse and Alcoholism, n.d.). Adverse child experiences, as shown in Fig. 6.1, are thought to trigger a cascade of problems that build across the life span. Specifically, adverse childhood experiences, such as abuse and neglect, lead to disrupted early neurodevelopment, which leads to social, emotional, and cognitive impairment in childhood, which leads to adoption of health risk behaviors in adolescence and adulthood, followed by disease, disability, and social problems that ultimately end in early death. Indeed, Dr. Robert Block, the former president of the American Academy of Pediatrics, said, "Adverse Childhood Experiences are the single greatest unaddressed public health threat facing our nation today." The problematic pyramid in Fig. 6.1 could be sliced in two based on the bullying dynamic; on one side bullies with ACEs take out their early pain by inflicting harm on others while, on the other side, victims with ACEs often experience revictimization at different points in the life span.

The repeated nature of child maltreatment is one reason this experience is so traumatic. Like bullying, maltreatment usually happens over and over, continually exposing youth to physical and emotional humiliation and harm. However, one central element that differentiates bullying and maltreatment is that parents or caregivers are the perpetrators of maltreatment. These adult figures are supposed to protect and nurture their offspring. Children and adolescents rely on their parents or caregivers for love, nurturance, and basic needs (e.g., food, water, clothing, education,

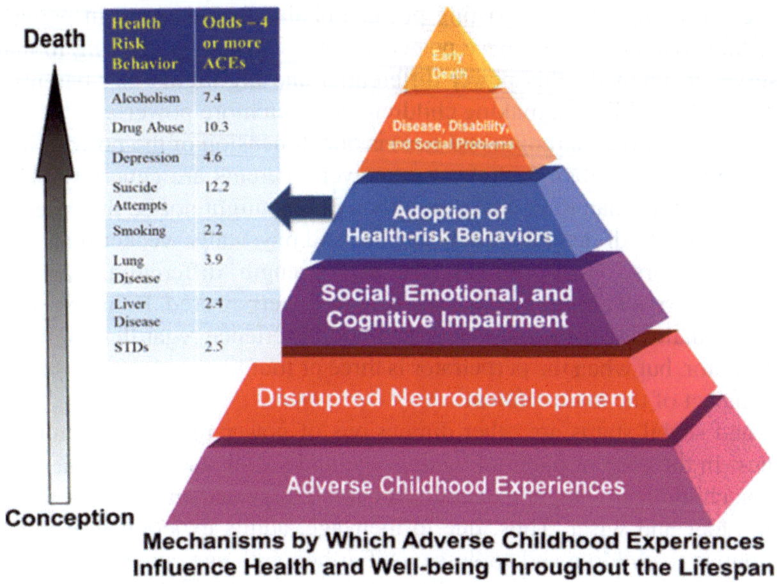

Fig. 6.1 Adverse childhood experiences and health consequences

medical care). When the person who is supposed to love you unconditionally, continually physically and/or emotionally abuses and/or neglects you, your trust in social relationships is eroded. While being maltreated even once is traumatic, it is the repeated nature of maltreatment that can physically, psychologically, and emotionally damage youth in both the short and long term. The repeated nature of maltreatment is a central reason this form of violence is so harmful to young victims. Further, the repetition of child maltreatment incidents directly connects this form of violence to bullying, suggesting that child maltreatment can be understood through the framework of bullying.

6.2.3.2 Power Imbalance

There are clear power differentials within families. Most notably, children are subordinate to parents (Miller-Perrin & Perrin, 2007) and, as the adults in the family, parents have the majority of the power. Children are expected to follow parents' directions, rules, and requests. Unlike the ambiguity of the power imbalance in bullying dynamics discussed in Chap. 1, the power imbalance in parent–child relationships is very clear-cut: parents are physically stronger until later in adolescence, in charge, control finances, and have the power inherent in their role. As discussed in Chap. 1, the power imbalance in a bullying dynamic can be ambiguous until one person begins to bully another. It could appear that two youth are on an equal playing field in terms of power, but the very act of aggression gives the perpetrator power over the victim and creates a power imbalance (if one was not already in existence) or strengthens an existing power imbalance. However, in parent–child relationships, parents already have power over the child and engaging in maltreatment serves to intensify this power differential and highlights that parents are in control over their children, making children feel even more powerless.

Physical power (i.e., strength and size) is one dimension of the power imbalance between children and their parents or caregivers. Parents are generally physically larger and stronger than their children; although this might not be the case for adolescents, young children are certainly smaller and physically weaker than their parents or caregivers. This physical size and strength differential can be very intimidating to small children who can easily feel overpowered. Being physically or emotionally maltreated is a scary and traumatic experience regardless of the size of the perpetrator, but when the perpetrator is three or four times your size, this intensifies the impact of the maltreatment.

Age and social status are other dimensions of power relevant in maltreatment dynamics. In the case of parental figures, age and social status are somewhat synonymous; children are taught that adults are to be respected and listened to because they are older and wiser. Thus, due to their age, adults experience higher social status relative to children and adolescents. Further, with age comes privileges such as driving or access to money that children lack. Age and social status gives parents or caregivers additional power over youth, making it easy for caregiving adults to exploit their power by engaging in maltreatment. Indeed, even the most common forms of parental discipline, such as "time-out" or taking away privileges, can be seen as demonstration of power and authority. Maltreatment occurs when that inherent power and authority is used to abuse the child.

It is common for researchers to discuss interpersonal violence and domestic violence through the lens of power imbalance. However, the child maltreatment literature does not generally address the power imbalance inherent in this dynamic. This is an oversight because the power imbalance inherent in parent– or caregiver–child relationships is one factor that allows maltreatment to continue; children are powerless to stop it. Just like victims in a bullying situation, victims of child maltreatment lack the power to end their victimization.

6.2.3.3 Intent to Harm

As discussed in Chap. 1, the element of intent to harm is fairly straight forward in bullying dynamics; the perpetrator intends to harm the victim and uses physical, relational, and/or verbal bullying tactics to inflict this harm. Intent to harm is more complex in child maltreatment dynamics because there are a myriad of reasons that parents or caregivers engage in maltreatment. Certainly, inflicting harm upon their child might be one reason, but there are many other reasons that adults maltreat their children. For example, the Administration for Children Youth and Families (2016) note a number of reasons that child maltreatment occurs: (1) Immature parents—young parents often lack the experience for rearing children and are unprepared for the responsibility and therefore do not know proper ways of disciplining children;

(2) Unrealistic expectations—parents or caregivers might lack knowledge about normal child development and therefore not understand normative behavior leading to frustration and ultimately abusive discipline; (3) Stress—poverty, unstable housing, divorce, or unemployment cause stress which can result in maltreatment; (4) Parental substance use—substance use impairs parents' ability to adequately care for their children; (5) Intergenerational trauma—past maltreatment or trauma impacts how parents interact with their own children and past abuse increases the likelihood of engaging in maltreatment; and (6) Isolation—a lack of a supportive partner, community, or family makes parenting more difficult and increases the likelihood of maltreatment. Thus, the reason parents or caregivers engage in maltreatment is not necessarily to harm their children. Let us take an extreme example: Sean Cole, a 29-year-old Alabama father with an 11-year-old son diagnosed with autism, had his girlfriend rape and sodomize the boy because he feared his son was gay. Cole, who had previously been arrested for domestic violence, thought he would straighten out the boy. The young victim asked police, "Why is my dad doing this to me?" and later said, "Dad said to tell no one. I failed him. I just told you [i.e., the police interviewer]." This disturbing example underscores that, however misguided they are, parents may have a justification for their abusive behavior that may or may not place the harm in context.

Similarly, consider how deeply ingrained the notion "spare the rod and spoil the child" is in our culture. Violence is commonly justified as discipline; take the common and controversial practice of spanking as an example. UNICEF (2014) reports that 80% of children worldwide are spanked or physically punished by their parents. Ostensibly spanking is a punishment to reduce misbehavior and has the support of many cultural and religious groups (e.g., "spare the rod" comes from the Bible). The terms "corporal punishment," "physical punishment," and "spanking" are largely synonymous and can be defined as non-injurious, open-hand hitting with the intention of modifying child behavior; spanking is defined as hitting a child on their buttocks or extremities using an open hand (Gershoff & Grogan-Kaylor, 2016). Researchers have conducted hundreds of studies to examine if this physical punishment is effective. Syntheses of research results showed that spanking and other physical punishments are largely ineffective and harmful (Gershoff, 2002) and are linked with children's cognitive, emotional, and behavioral problems (Ferguson, 2013; Paolucci & Violato, 2004).

Gershoff and Grogan-Kaylor (2016) analyzed 111 studies representing 160,927 children; 99% of studies (102 out of 111) indicated an association between spanking and a detrimental child outcome. In childhood, parental use of spanking was associated with low moral internalization, aggression, antisocial behavior, externalizing behavior problems, internalizing behavior problems, mental health problems, negative parent–child relationships, impaired cognitive ability, low self-esteem, and risk of physical abuse from parents. In adulthood, prior experiences of parental use of spanking were significantly associated with adult antisocial behavior, adult mental health problems, and with positive attitudes about spanking. These researchers also showed that the effects for spanking were quite similar to effects from physical abuse. This strongly conclusive scientific research underscores how even socially sanctioned bullying in the home, such as spanking, is toxic to victims and serves as a precursor to seriously detrimental consequences in adulthood.

As cited above, severe stress, not the desire to harm, is often the catalyst of child maltreatment. However, regardless of whether or not parents or caregivers intend to cause harm by engaging in maltreatment, this behavior without a doubt *does* cause harm. Which begs the questions: is it the perpetrator's intent to harm or the victim's perception of harm that is most salient in identifying bullying? In child maltreatment dynamics, harm is inflicted regardless of the parent's or the caregiver's intent, suggesting that the perception of the victim is paramount.

Taken together, the definition of bullying accurately describes child maltreatment dynamics. Repetition, power imbalance, and harm are present illustrating that child maltreatment can be understood as a form of bullying. Using the definition of bullying to understand child maltreatment dynamics is an innovative addition to violence literature and highlights the commonalities between bullying and child maltreatment. Moreover, the discussion above provides evidence that maltreatment may form the foundation for the bullying dynamic in childhood and throughout the life span. In the never-ending debate between nature and nurture, bullies are made in adverse environments; there is no gene that turns on bullying. What is the recipe for creating a bully? The answer would arguably be to place an infant with vast natural potential in an environment characterized by multiple adversities (i.e., emotional, physical, or sexual abuse, emotional or physical neglect, domestic violence, substance abuse, mental illness, parent separation/divorce or incarceration) add insensitive, inconsistent, unresponsive caregiving with coercive physical punishment, like spanking, and the result is likely to be a child that is insecurely attached to others, has neurological damage, a hyperactive biological stress response system, low social skills, and a tendency to compulsively lash out when feeling threatened (which is most of the time). That recipe, or some variation of it, happens to one in every 58 children in the USA. Some of these maltreated children cope with their suffering by anxiously withdrawing; others cope by lashing out with aggression. As discussed in previous chapters, anxious withdrawn children are targets for victimization on the playground and aggressive children with low empathy are perpetrators on the playground. Early adverse childhood experiences set the stage for the playground politics that dominate middle school. Then, place these same wounded children in college, in marriages, in workplaces, and in retirement homes and it is clear why a life span approach is needed to fully understand bullying perpetration and victimization.

6.3 Sibling Violence and Bullying

> "Mommmmmmmm Louis hit me. Mom, he did it again. He won't stay on his side of the car. Mom! He keeps poking me and hitting me!"
>
> "Stuart called me an idiot! Mom, he won't stop calling me mean names, make him stop!"

"DAD! Katy took the book I was reading and won't give it back. She hid it somewhere and I can't find it!"

Just about every parent or caregiver who has more than one child has likely heard complaints similar to these. While siblings can get along beautifully and play quietly together or engage in supportive conversations, arguments and disagreements are common and normative. However, there is a fine line between developmentally appropriate fighting and sibling bullying. With parent inattention, small daily conflicts can escalate.

David and Sterling were playing feed the dolphin with Sterling catching peanuts in her mouth as David tossed them from the top bunk bed. He quietly switched from peanuts to pieces of chalk. After Sterling successfully ate a piece of chalk, she chased David around the house threatening him with a fork.

In her book titled Girl In The Water: A True Story of Sibling Abuse, Nancy Kilgore describes how her older sister, Sherry, strangled her into unconsciousness and smashed a piggybank over her head, among other horrible acts. As the family grew larger, Sherry was put in charge of Nancy so that her mother could tend to the babies.

And finally, in the Forgiveness Project, Clare describes how her older brother began physically and sexually assaulting her when she was seven. Her parents were going through a divorce and left the children alone a lot. As discussed below, sibling sexual abuse is more common than parent–child sexual abuse (The Forgiveness Project, 2018).

In the above examples, Louis hitting his sibling a few times or Stuart calling his sibling a mean name once or twice is one thing, but engaging in these behaviors multiple times per day, day after day, is a different story. Suddenly, Louis's sibling might be beaten up on a daily basis while Stuart's sibling might be emotionally and psychologically scarred from constant verbal harassment. Further, if Katy constantly terrorized her sibling by stealing and hiding possessions, this could move quickly from normative sibling pestering to a serious case of sibling bullying if she engaged in this behavior repeatedly over time.

Out of all of the forms of violence across the life span, sibling violence is arguably the most ignored. Indeed, it is often passed off as normative ("boys will be boys") and tolerated by society. Parents often daydream about having a second or third child so the first child can have a best friend. When inevitable conflicts happen between siblings, there are so many squabbles that beleaguered parents have to choose their battles, ignoring many harmful incidents. These inattentive parents are reflecting deeply ingrained societal attitudes. Consider the archetypal biblical story of Cain and Abel that has been discussed in pulpits for hundreds of years.

Cain and Abel are the first two sons of Adam and Eve in the biblical Book of Genesis; Cain, the firstborn, was a farmer, and his brother Abel was a shepherd. After the brothers made sacrifices to God, Abel's sacrifice was favored by God more than Cain's. Consequently, Cain murdered Abel, God punished Cain to a life of wandering; he built a city and fathered the line of descendants beginning with Enoch.

If God was a parent who played favorites and gave out ineffective punishment, what are mere human parents supposed to do? We do not mean to delve into biblical scholarship; however, churchgoing families hear this story of sibling homicide at least once a year as they attend services. The topic of sibling conflict has deep roots in cultural discourse, yet this has led to a normalization of violence between brothers or sisters. Because a certain level of sibling discord is socially ignored, identifying and addressing sibling violence and bullying is often quite difficult. In the following sections we provide an overview of sibling violence and argue that it in fact should be referred to as sibling bullying. We also discuss the negative associated consequences of sibling violence and then apply the bullying framework to sibling violence.

6.3.1 Overview: Definition, Prevalence Rates, and Demographic Risk Factors

Despite the fact that sibling violence is the most common form of family violence, it is under studied (Button & Gealt, 2010; Eriksen & Jensen, 2006). Further, there is disagreement in the literature as to how to refer to sibling violence: should it be called sibling violence or sibling abuse or sibling bullying? Difficulties in naming and describing this phenomenon hinder researchers' ability to study it and also makes cross-study comparisons difficult because it is unclear if researchers are studying the same construct. According to the CDC, bullying only occurs between non-siblings (Gladden, Vivolo-Kantor, Hamburger, & Lumpkin, 2014), which suggests that sibling violence should not be referred to as bullying. However, we disagree. In this section of the book we will argue that sibling violence should indeed be considered bullying and referred to as such; a number of violence researchers agree with this assessment and define ongoing sibling violence as bullying (e.g., Hoetger, Hazen, & Brank, 2015; Menesini, Camodeca, & Nocentini, 2010; Skinner & Kowalski, 2013; Tanrikulu & Campbell, 2015; Wolke, Tippett, & Dantchev, 2015). However, other researchers refer to this behavior as sibling violence or abuse (e.g., Caffaro, n.d.; Button & Gealt, 2010; Kiselica & Morrill-Richards, 2007). We will refer to sibling bullying, however, when citing others' research, we will use the nomenclature used in the study. For example, Hoetger et al. (2015) refer to sibling bullying, while Button and Gealt (2010) refer to either sibling violence or sibling abuse; thus we follow suit when discussing each of their findings.

Regardless of whether the term sibling violence, abuse, or bullying is used, this phenomenon is difficult and complicated to define and identify because a certain level of sibling conflict and discord is unfortunately normative. Routine sibling conflict is generally a mutual disagreement, whereas sibling abuse occurs when one sibling is consistently the aggressor and the other sibling is consistently victimized (Kiselica & Morrill-Richards, 2007). Sibling abuse is a repeated pattern of verbal and physical aggression where the aggressor intends to inflict harm and is motivated by the desire for power and control (Caffaro, n.d.); this definition has many similarities to the definition of bullying discussed in Chap. 1. Like child maltreatment and peer bullying, sibling abuse comes in various forms including psychological abuse (e.g., ridicule, intimidation, provocation), physical abuse (e.g., purposefully inflicting physical harm by shoving, hitting, slapping, biting), and sexual abuse (e.g., unwanted sexual interactions; Kiselica & Morrill-Richards, 2007). A large number of youth are at risk for these forms of sibling violence.

The vast majority (78%) of US children live with a sibling (Kreider & Ellis, 2011), indicating a significant number of youth are at risk for engagement in sibling conflict that could turn into sibling bullying. It is difficult to gauge the prevalence of sibling violence given limited research in this area, however, small-scale studies confirm that sibling bullying is a widespread phenomenon. In a sample of 336 middle school youth, 30% reported they were commonly bullied by their siblings (Duncan, 1999). And in a study of 455 youth grades 5 through 12, about 32% reported sibling bullying, a rate more than three times higher than the percentage reporting peer bullying (in that study 10%; Tanrikulu & Campbell, 2015).

These rates are confirmed by nationally representative studies. One group of researchers assessed prevalence rates with a nationally representative sample of 1705 youth ages 1 month to 17 years from the National Survey of Children's Exposure to Violence survey. Findings indicated that 37.6% of youth from two child families experienced as least one incident of sibling victimization in the past year, with an average of 1.3 incidents over the course of the year. About 32% of the sample reported physical assault and 4% reported physical assault with a weapon or resulting injury (Tucker, Finkelhor, Shattuck, & Turner, 2013). A second group of researchers examined data from the National Incident-Based Reporting System from 2000 to 2005 and found that during this period there were 33,066 reports of sibling violence (Krienert & Walsh, 2011). Males were the offender in 73% of the cases and the majority of incidents resulted in minor injury (52%) and 3% of cases resulted in major injury. Weapons were common and were present 85% of the time and personal weapons (hands and feet) were used in 69% of incidents. The majority of incidents were simple assault (80%; no weapon and no severe injury to the victim), 15% were aggravated assaults (weapon and serious victim injury), and 5% were intimidation (Krienert & Walsh, 2011). In a third large scale study of 8122 eighth and 11th graders, 42% reported sibling violence (Button & Gealt, 2010). These studies confirm that sibling violence is widespread and impacts a significant number of youth; however, certain demographic factors put youth at increased risk for sibling bullying.

For example, younger children are at higher risk for engaging in physical sibling violence (Eriksen & Jensen, 2006) and are more often victimized (Tippett & Wolke, 2015). Indeed, as the age of the victim increased, the number of acts of physical violence he/she experienced decreased (Eriksen & Jensen, 2006). Research indicates that boys are more likely compared to girls to engage in sibling violence (Eriksen & Jensen, 2006) and bullying (Menesini et al., 2010), while girls are more likely to be victims (Button & Gealt, 2010). Having an older brother is a risk factor associated with increased sibling bullying for both boys and girls (Menesini et al., 2010). Low levels of empathy and sibling relationships fraught with conflict were significantly associated with increased sibling bullying perpetration for both boys and girls (Menesini et al., 2010). Further, individual characteristics such as trait anger (i.e., becoming easily angered across a variety of situations) and moral disengagement increased the likelihood of bullying ones sibling (Tanrikulu & Campbell, 2015).

Parental relationship and behavior also had a significant impact on sibling bullying and increased parental consideration of separation or divorce was significantly associated with increased sibling violence (Eriksen & Jensen, 2006). Further, parent-to-child violence (Button & Gealt, 2010; Eriksen & Jensen, 2006), mother engaging in physical punishment, and the father losing his temper were also significantly associated with increased sibling violence (Eriksen & Jensen, 2006). Indeed, negative sibling interactions are four times more frequent in abusive and neglectful families (see Kiselica & Morrill-Richards, 2007 for a review). Youth who experienced child maltreatment had four times the risk of experiencing sibling abuse compared to their non-maltreated counterparts and those who witnessed adult domestic violence had two times the risk of experiencing sibling violence (Button & Gealt, 2010). These findings highlight the impact of family climate on children's behavior; parents considering separation or divorce likely argue frequently which might result in a hostile family climate, leading to increased sibling discord. Similarly, if parents model physical punishment, abuse, and yelling as acceptable behaviors, children will pick up on this and might reenact these behaviors with their siblings. Social learning theory, which has several decades of social science research behind it, holds that children learn through watching and imitating role models. In this case, the role modeling comes from parents exhibiting violence against each other or against children. That behavior becomes imprinted in the child's mind as an acceptable response to social situations. These children then replicate this aggression in bullying others—their siblings, other children, dating partners, spouses, and work colleagues.

Because physical sibling bullying is so common, it is important to note that we have no data on relational bullying among siblings, which may be even more prevalent. Relational bullying would be spreading rumors or nasty information about one's sibling in order to undermine their relationships. Excluding them from social groups or poisoning their friendships would also fall into this category. Siblings often know each other's deepest secrets and are in a powerful position to humiliate each other with sensitive information. We hypothesize that this sibling behavior is very common, but research needs to be conducted in this area.

6.3.2 Negative Consequences of Sibling Violence, Abuse, and Bullying

Victims of sibling violence and bullying reported a multitude of negative outcomes. For example, a study of 8122 eighth and 11th graders found that sibling violence was associated with a significantly increased likelihood of using tobacco, alcohol, or marijuana and engaging in delinquency and aggression (Button & Gealt, 2010).

This is illustrated in Clare's case from the Forgiveness Project who was physically and sexually assaulted by her brother.

> At the time the abuse began happening my parents were going through a divorce and my brother and I were left alone a lot. My mom had gone back to school in the evening and was dating regularly on Friday and Saturday nights. During this time I was also introduced to cigarettes, drugs and alcohol. By the time I was nine years old I was addicted to cigarettes, and was lying to my mom regularly about my whereabouts so that I could smoke, drink and get high. I stopped participating in extra-curricular events and went from being a top-achieving student to not caring about school. I felt alienated from my peers and anytime I felt uncomfortable socially I simply dropped out, or left, or went somewhere else mentally. This became a habitual pattern for me which I still struggle with as an adult (The Forgiveness Project, 2018).

Being punched or kicked by a sibling increased the odds of using substances by 31.4%, and being threatened with a weapon during a sibling fight increased the odds of substance use by 52.6%. Sibling verbal abuse and/or sibling shoving, pushing, or slapping increased the odds of delinquency by 39.0% and being threatened with a weapon increased the odds of delinquency by 119.2% (Button & Gealt, 2010). Other researchers found that victims of sibling bullying suffered from depression, insecurity, and low self-esteem even later in life (See Hoffman & Edwards, 2004 for a review). Indeed, victims of sibling bullying were about twice as likely to suffer from depression, anxiety, and self-harm compared to their counter parts who did not endure sibling bullying (Bowes, Wolke, Joinson, Lereya, & Lewis, 2014). These findings were corroborated in a nationally representative probability sample of 3599 youth ages 0–17, which found that experiencing one or more forms of mild or severe sibling aggression was significantly associated with worse mental health outcomes (e.g., anxiety, depression; Tucker, Finkelhor, Turner, & Shattuck, 2013). Being a victim of sibling abuse can also put youth at increased risk for other forms of violence such as dating violence (Simonelli, Mullis, Elliot, & Pierce, 2002). Most alarming, sibling bullying and victimization were significantly associated with peer bullying and victimization suggesting that exposure to sibling bullying might prime or train children to take on their sibling role (i.e., the perpetrator or the victim) in the larger peer group (Menesini et al., 2010; Tucker, Finkelhor, Turner, & Shattuck, 2014). Once again applying Social Learning Theory, we can think of sibling relationship dynamics as a form of social training for peer relationships whereby siblings replicate their role from their sibling dynamic in peer social dynamics. Indeed, every one unit standard deviation increase in the sibling victimization scale increased the odds of being a victim of peer bullying at school by 69% and every one unit standard deviation increase in the sibling perpetration scale increased the odds of being a bully perpetrator at school by 163% (Tippett & Wolke, 2015). This research establishes a clear link between sibling bullying and peer bullying, highlighting the critical importance of examining these phenomena using an integrated, life span approach. Indeed, the maltreatment discussion above established that aggressive parents likely serve as mentors or role models for bullying while sibling relationships may be the training labs where children become good at victimizing others.

6.3.3 *Sibling Violence Through the Bullying Framework*

Although sibling violence occurs in the home and therefore lacks the mob mentality often present with school bullying, there are similarities between sibling and peer bullying in terms of form (i.e., physical, verbal, or relational), intention (e.g., the perpetrator intentionally seeks to harm the victim), repetition (i.e., the behavior is repeated over time), and power imbalance (i.e., the perpetrator is stronger and more powerful than the victim; Menesini et al., 2010). Researchers who label sibling violence as sibling abuse agree that intent and severity of the act (i.e., duration, intensity) are paramount, but also focus on perception (Morrill-Richards & Leierer, 2010). Perception refers to whether one of the siblings in the dyad considers the behavior to be abusive, which would indicate that behavior beyond routine sibling disagreement is occurring (Morrill & Bachman, 2013). These similarities between peer and sibling bullying contradict the CDC and suggest that ongoing violence between siblings can and should be defined as bullying. Establishing that sibling violence is in fact a form of bullying means that researchers who focus on sibling violence can benefit from the past research on peer bullying, which includes well-established interventions, measurement tools, and definitions (Hoetger et al., 2015). Using this existing research could help in the creation of new and innovative interventions aimed at specifically reducing sibling bullying.

6.3.3.1 Repetition

Repetition is a vital element that distinguishes routine sibling disagreement from sibling bullying. It is considered normal in some households for siblings to verbally argue and/or to hit or shove each other once in a while. However, these "normal" disagreements become bullying when they happen over and over again. To continue labeling this ongoing violence as "normal" and "sibling rivalry" trivializes it; it should be referred to as bullying. This is not to say that we should rush to label all sibling conflicts as bullying. However, if sibling conflicts occur day after day and one sibling is consistently victimized by the other, this conflict should be labeled as bullying. Parents need to be constantly vigilant about repetition and when it crosses the line into abusive territory. Let us take a simple example.

> Pablo, in 4th grade, and Albert, in 3rd grade, are brothers who have to walk to school together every day. Their mother bought Albert a new winter coat that was brown and textured. When Pablo would see Albert put on the coat, he would loudly start singing "Fuzzy Wuzzy was a bear. Fuzzy Wuzzy had no hair. Fuzzy Wuzzy wasn't fuzzie was he?" This irritated Albert, especially as Pablo did it every day over and over. Then Pablo told the kids at school that Albert wanted to be called Fuzzy Wuzzy because of his new coat. It quickly caught on. Their mother did not intervene until Albert came home in a snowstorm without his coat, which he threw away on the playground, and refused to go back to school.

Repetition often comes with escalation if the behavior is effective (i.e., in this example, it effectively irritated Jaime). An attentive parent could stop this kind of small behavior before it explodes into sibling bullying. Unfortunately, many parents do not give these behaviors appropriate attention until a crisis happens.

6.3.3.2 Power Imbalance

Power imbalance plays an important role in sibling bullying and there are actually many more forms of power imbalance in the sibling dynamic as compared to power imbalance in peer bullying discussed in Chap. 1. There is often an easily identifiable power imbalance between siblings where older siblings hold the power over younger siblings. However, physical size also creates a power imbalance and age and physical size might not always align. It is possible, but not the norm, that a younger sibling could be physically larger than the older sibling and might therefore hold the power in the relationship. Gender is another potential area of power imbalance where male siblings might hold power over female siblings. Disability status is also an important potential dimension of power in sibling relationships; if one sibling suffers from an intellectual or physical disability he/she might feel or actually be less powerful than his/her non-disabled sibling(s). Yet this needs to be looked at closely because a disabled sibling may also hold the power if parents pay more attention to that child and give him or her more latitude for poor behavior. Sibling physical appearance, personality, and skills and abilities might also serve to create a power imbalance. A handsome, athletic, academically oriented older brother might make a chubby, clumsy, dyslexic younger sister feel very powerless. In this example, appearance, athletic and academic ability, gender, and age accumulate to give the older brother power over his younger sister. However, similar to peer bullying as discussed in Chap. 1, forms of power might not align and therefore it depends on how power is perceived. For example, if a younger female sibling is physically larger than her older brother, who has the power? Does the older brother have more power because he is older and is a male? Or does physical size give the younger sister the power? The answer depends upon how the two individuals view their dynamic. If the brother feels unable to protect himself from his sister's aggression due to her physical size, then physical size is the determinant of power. However, if the brother uses his age and gender to bully his sister and she feels intimidated by him, then gender and age become the determinants of power.

It is also important to consider family dynamics. There is an inescapable power imbalance between older and younger siblings based on age and development; older siblings are always going to be more developed physically and cognitively until late adolescence, unless there is some type of disability. In large families, some older children may be invested with power by parents to be "in charge" of younger siblings. This may make the older sibling responsible and perhaps "parentified" or "adultified" (Burton, 2007); however, it also raises the risk for abuse of that power. Perhaps one sibling is favored by the parents, which provides him/her with power over the other children in the family. It is also possible that one child is disliked by the parents and is therefore treated as a second-class citizen of sorts, which strips him/her of power and makes him/her an easy target for sibling bullying. Further, blended families in which all siblings are not fully biologically related present even more complexity, with power coming from being a biological child versus a step-child. For example, in a family with one adopted daughter and one biological daughter, the adopted daughter could feel less powerful or important than the biological daughter by virtue of being adopted. Conversely, in an effort to "even the playing field" the parents might actually consciously or subconsciously favor the adopted daughter to make sure she does not feel left out, thus leaving the biological daughter feeling less powerful. Half-siblings pose another interesting power imbalance dynamic. If a divorced mother with a son remarries and has a second son with her new husband, the first son has one biological parent and one step-parent, while the second son has two biological parents. If the father favors his biological son, this could create a power dynamic whereby although younger, the second son has the power by virtue of being his father's favorite. These varied situations create a power imbalance between siblings that can be exacerbated if one sibling consistently victimizes the other. Clearly, a variety of power imbalances exist within families and specifically between siblings, and these power imbalances play a significant role in the bullying dynamic.

Evolutionary psychology, discussed in relation to peer bullying in Chap. 2, suggests that there is always a scramble for resources that results in power imbalances, perpetration, and victimization. In sibling bullying, the ultimate scramble is likely for parent attention, acceptance, and love. Children who receive their parent's acceptance either overtly (i.e., "Your brother is just teasing you. Don't be so sensitive") or covertly (i.e., through a smile or glance, by the parent NOT intervening) have substantially magnified power within the family. Indeed, in families with permissive parenting styles (Baumrind, 1978), certain dominant children may wield more power than their parents because those parents set few boundaries. In these situations, sibling victimization would go unchecked because the parent has little authority.

6.3.3.3 Intent to Harm

The intent of the perpetrator in sibling bullying dynamics could be twofold. First, it is possible that the intent of the bullying behavior is to gain access to limited resources such as parental time and affection, physical space, or objects such as toys or clothing. This is the evolutionary perspective mentioned above and in Chap. 2 (i.e., survival of the fittest in the family). However, it is also possible that the bullying behavior is simply to cause harm and to hurt the victimized sibling (Morrill & Bachman, 2013). Although intent to harm is a hallmark of peer bullying behavior, we argue that it is less salient in the sibling bullying dynamic. Even if the intent of the bullying behavior is to gain access to resources, the behavior is still harmful and results in negative consequences for the victimized sibling. Therefore, as long as sibling violence is repeated and there is a power imbalance, this behavior is bullying because, regardless of the intent, the victim is harmed. Without a doubt, harm is also caused by sibling bullying.

Taken together, repetition, power imbalance, and harm are present in sibling bullying dynamics. While it is completely accurate to label ongoing sibling conflict as sibling violence or sibling abuse, we feel that labeling this behavior as sibling bullying and understanding this behavior through the definitional framework of bullying has powerful and important consequences. First, it allows sibling violence researchers to use preexisting and well-established research on peer bullying to inform additional and much needed research on sibling bullying and to begin to create some prevention and intervention programs. Second, using the term sibling bullying highlights the severity of harmful sibling relationship dynamics and the fact that this type of sibling conflict is not normative and needs immediate intervention.

6.4 Conclusions

Although child maltreatment and sibling violence are distinct forms of family violence, the definitional framework of bullying can be used to understand each form of familial violence. Repetition, power imbalance, and intent to harm are present in child maltreatment dynamics, highlighting that researchers can view this form of violence through a bullying lens. We are not proposing renaming child maltreatment as "bullying in the home" or "parent–child bullying," we are simply presenting a new and innovative means of understanding this harmful dynamic. However, we do suggest replacing the terms sibling violence and sibling abuse with sibling bullying. Repetition, power imbalance, and harm are inherent in sibling bullying dynamics. The only elements that distinguish peer bullying from sibling bullying is location (i.e., home versus school) and the fact that siblings are biologically related or share a home. Relabeling sibling violence and sibling abuse as bullying would enable researchers of peer bullying and sibling bullying to join forces and create more comprehensive intervention and prevention programs.

The prevalence rates for adverse child experiences (67% in the Kaiser studies; Substance Abuse and Mental Health Services Administration, n.d.), like maltreatment (11% emotional abuse, 28% physical abuse, 21% sexual abuse, and 25% emotional or physical neglect) and sibling violence (conservative estimates of 30% of youth with siblings) are shockingly high and in line with rates for peer bullying (approximately 20–30%). Along with similar prevalence rates, the consequences of adverse childhood experiences, such as maltreatment, and sibling violence are in line with the negative effects of peer bullying victimization (i.e., short-term depression, loss of self-esteem, PTSD symptoms, neurodevelopmental damage, adult depression, substance use, suicidal behavior). This leads us to emphasize the importance of understanding the overall bullying dynamic, which gets reflected in different contexts (i.e., the infant's nursery, the playroom with siblings, the playground at school with peers, with dating partners, in marriages, and workplaces). Child maltreatment is the earliest and most intense form of childhood bullying because of the enormous power difference between parents and children. Maltreatment has profound negative consequences for children across the life span. Considering the inherent role of parents as mentors and role models, maltreatment experiences prime some children to behave in aggressive, coercive ways with their siblings and peers (i.e., to become bullies) and others to withdraw inward (i.e., a major risk factor for sibling and peer victimization). With 80% of children worldwide experiencing spanking and other forms of physical punishment (UNICEF, 2014), it is clear that we are socializing our children to the use of power, control, and coercion from the very beginning of the life span.

Meanwhile, sibling violence is the most common, and most ignored, form of abuse in our society. Sibling groups can serve as training laboratories for bullies and victims to test out their strategies before bringing these behaviors to the playground. Parents, who are often overwhelmed and see the need to choose their battles, often do not intervene until a crisis occurs and the damage is done. These bullying dynamics in the home when children are young and vulnerable set the stage for bullying behaviors to be generalized to many different contexts across the life span.

References

Administration for Children Youth and Families. (2016). *Building community building home: 2016/2017 prevention resource guide*. Washington, DC: Author. Retrieved from https://www.childwelfare.gov/pubPDFs/guide_2017.pdf

Ainsworth, M. D. (1964). Patterns of attachment behavior shown by the infant in interaction with his mother. *Merrill-Palmer Quarterly of Behavior and Development, 10*, 51–58.

Ainsworth, M. D. S., & Bell, S. M. (1970). Attachment, exploration, and separation: Illustrated by the behavior of one-year-olds in a strange situation. *Child Development, 41*, 49–67.

American Psychological Association. (2017). *Children, youth, families and socioeconomic status*. Washington, DC: Author. Retrieved from http://www.apa.org/pi/ses/resources/publications/children-families.aspx

Baumrind, D. (1978). Parental disciplinary patterns and social competence in children. *Youth & Society, 9*(3), 239–276.

Belsky, J., & Rovine, M. (1987). Temperament and attachment security in the strange situation: An empirical rapprochement. *Child Development, 58*(3), 787–795.

Bowes, L., Wolke, D., Joinson, C., Lereya, S. T., & Lewis, G. (2014). Sibling bullying and risk of depression, anxiety, and self-harm: A prospective cohort study. *Pediatrics, 134*, 1–8.

Bowlby, J. (1969). *Attachment: Attachment and loss* (Vol. 1). New York, NY: Basic Books.

Bowlby, J. (1980). *Loss: Sadness and depression* (Vol. III). New York, NY: Basic Books.

Burton, L. (2007). Child adultification in economically disadvantaged families: A conceptual model. *Family Relations, 56*(4), 329–345.

Button, D. M., & Gealt, R. (2010). High risk behaviors among victims of sibling violence. *Journal of Family Violence, 25*, 131–140.

Caffaro, J. (n.d.). *Sibling violence*. Alexandria, VA: American Association for Marriage and Family Therapy. Retrieved from https://www.aamft.org/iMIS15/AAMFT/Content/Consumer_Updates/Sibling_Violence.aspx

Cancian, M., Slack, K. S., & Yang, M. Y. (2010). *The effect of family income on risk of child maltreatment*. Institute for Research on Poverty Discussion Paper no. 1385-10. Madison, WI: Institute for Research on Poverty. Retrieved from https://www.irp.wisc.edu/publications/dps/pdfs/dp138510.pdf

Chaney, A., Carballedo, A., Amico, F., Fagan, A., Skokauskas, N., Meaney, J., & Frodl, T. (2014). Effect of childhood maltreatment on brain structure in adult patients with major depressive disorder and healthy participants. *Journal of Psychiatry and Neuroscience, 39*(1), 50–59.

Child Welfare Information Gateway. (2013). *Long-term consequences of child abuse and neglect.* Washington, DC: Author. Retrieved from https://www.childwelfare.gov/pubPDFs/long_term_consequences.pdf

Clarridge, C. & Krishnan, S. (October 13, 2008). Carnation couple charged in "worse case" child abuse of teen daughter. *The Seattle Times*. Retrieved from https://www.seattletimes.com/seattle-news/carnation-couple-charged-in-worst-case-child-abuse-of-teen-daughter/

D'Andrea, W., Ford, J., Stolbach, B., Spinazzola, J., & van der Kolk, B. A. (2012). Understanding interpersonal trauma in children: Why we need a developmentally appropriate trauma diagnosis. *American Journal of Orthopsychiatry, 82*(2), 187–200.

DeBellis, M., & Zisk, A. (2014). The biological effects of childhood trauma. *Child & Adolescent Psychiatric Clinics of North America, 23*(2), 185–222.

Duncan, R. D. (1999). Peer and sibling aggression: An investigation of intra- and extra- familial bullying. *Journal of Interpersonal Violence, 14*(8), 871–886.

English, D. J., Marshall, D. B., Brummel, S., & Orme, M. (1999). Characteristics of repeated referrals to child protective services in Washington state. *Child Maltreatment, 4*(4), 297–307.

Eriksen, S., & Jensen, V. (2006). All in the family? Family environment factors in sibling violence. *Journal of Family Violence, 21*, 497–507.

Fang, X., Brown, D. S., Florence, C. S., & Mercy, J. A. (2012). The economic burden of child maltreatment in the United States and implications for prevention. *Child Abuse & Neglect, 36*(2), 156–165.

Ferguson, C. J. (2013). Spanking, corporal punishment and negative long-term outcomes: A meta-analytic review of longitudinal studies. *Clinical Psychology Review, 33*, 196–208.

Finkelhor, D., Turner, H., Ormrod, R., & Hamby, S. (2009). Violence, abuse, and crime exposure in a national sample of children and youth. *Pediatrics, 124*, 1411–1423.

Fluke, J. D., Shusterman, G. R., Hollinshead, D. M., & Yuan, Y. Y. T. (2008). Longitudinal analysis of repeated child abuse reporting and victimization: Multistate analysis of associated factors. *Child Maltreatment, 13*(1), 76.

Fluke, J. D., Yuan, Y. T., & Edwards, M. (1999). Recurrence of maltreatment: An application of the national child abuse and neglect data system (NCANDS). *Child Abuse & Neglect, 23*(7), 633–650.

Gershoff, E. T. (2002). Corporal punishment by parents and associated child behaviors and experiences: A meta-analytic and theoretical review. *Psychological Bulletin, 128*(4), 539–579.

Gershoff, E. T., & Grogan-Kaylor, A. (2016). Spanking and child outcomes: Old controversies and new meta-analyses. *Journal of Family Psychology, 30*(4), 453–469.

Gladden, R. M., Vivolo-Kantor, A. M., Hamburger, M. E., & Lumpkin, C. D. (2014). *Bullying surveillance among youths: Uniform definitions for public health and recommended data elements, Version 1.0*. Atlanta, GA: National Center for Injury Prevention and Control, Centers for Disease Control and Prevention and U.S. Department of Education.

Gorka, A. X., Hanson, J. L., Radtke, S. R., & Hairi, A. R. (2014). Reduced hippocampal and medial prefrontal gray matter mediate the association between reported childhood maltreatment and trait anxiety in adulthood and predict sensitivity to future life stress. *Biology of Mood & Anxiety Disorders, 4*(12), 1–10.

Hanson, J. L., Nacewicz, B. M., Sutterer, M. J., Cayo, A. A., Schaefer, S. M., Rudolph, K. D., … Davidson, R. J. (2015). Behavioral problems after early life stress: Contribution of the hippocampus and amygdala. *Biological Psychiatry, 77*, 314–323.

Harlow, H. F. (1962). Development of affection in primates. In E. L. Bliss (Ed.), *Roots of behavior* (pp. 157–166). New York, NY: Harper.

Hawkins, A. O., Danielson, C. K., Ruggiero, K. J., de Arellano, M. A., Hanson, R., Smith, D., … Kilpatrick, D. G. (2010). Ethnic/racial differences in the prevalence of injurious spanking and other child physical abuse in a national survey of adolescents. *Child Maltreatment, 15*, 242–249.

Hindley, N., Ramchandani, P., & Jones, D. (2006). Risk factors for recurrence of maltreatment: A systematic review. *British Medical Journal, 91*(9), 744.

Hoetger, L. A., Hazen, K. P., & Brank, E. M. (2015). All in the family: A retrospective study comparing sibling bullying and peer bullying. *Journal of Family Violence, 30*, 103–111.

Hoffman, K. L., & Edwards, J. N. (2004). An integrated theoretical model of sibling violence and abuse. *Journal of Family Violence, 19*(3), 185–200.

Honomichl, R. D., & Brooks, S. (2009). *Predicting and minimizing the recurrence of maltreatment: Literature review*. Davis, CA: Northern California Training Academy. Retrieved from http://www.childsworld.ca.gov/res/pdf/LR-PredictingRecurrence.pdf

Hussey, J., Chang, J., & Kotch, J. (2006). Child maltreatment in the United States: Prevalence, risk factors, and adolescent health consequences. *Pediatrics, 118*, 933–942.

Kelley, B. T., Thornberry, T. P., & Smith, C. A. (1997). *In the wake of childhood maltreatment. Juvenile Justice Bulletin*. Washington, DC: U.S. Department of Justice, office of Justice Programs, Office of Juvenile Justice and Delinquency prevention. Retrieved from https://www.ncjrs.gov/pdffiles1/165257.pdf

Kiselica, M. S., & Morrill-Richards, M. (2007). Sibling maltreatment: The forgotten abuse. *Journal of Counseling & Development, 85*, 148–160.

Kreider, R. M., & Ellis, R. (2011). *Living arrangements of children: 2009. Current population reports*. Washington, DC: U.S. Census Bureau.

Krienert, J. L., & Walsh, J. A. (2011). My brother's keeper: A contemporary examination of reported sibling violence using national level data, 2000-2005. *Journal of Family Violence, 26*, 331–342.

Larmier, S. (January 13, 2017). The 'heinous' case of a child whose mother allegedly kept him locked in a bathroom for months. *Washington Post*. Retrieved from https://www.washingtonpost.com/news/true-crime/wp/2017/01/13/mother-arrested-in-heinous-case-of-child-who-was-allegedly-kept-locked-in-a-bathroom/?utm_term=.42745ec209f6

Levy, H. B., Markovic, J., Chaudhry, U., Ahart, S., & Torres, H. (1995). Reabuse rates in a sample of children followed for 5 years after discharge from a child abuse inpatient assessment program. *Child Abuse and Neglect, 19*(11), 1363–1377.

McLeod, S. (2016). *Mary Ainsworth*. Simply Psychology. Retrieved from https://www.simplypsychology.org/mary-ainsworth.html

Menesini, E., Camodeca, M., & Nocentini, A. (2010). Bullying among siblings: The role of personality and relational variables. *British Journal of Developmental Psychology, 28*, 921–939.

Miller-Perrin, C. L., & Perrin, R. (2007). *Child maltreatment: An introduction* (2nd ed.). Thousand Oaks, CA: Sage Publications.

Morrill, M., & Bachman, C. (2013). Confronting the gender myth: An exploration of variance in male versus female experience with sibling abuse. *Journal of Interpersonal Violence, 28*(8), 1693–1708.

Morrill-Richards, M., & Leierer, S. (2010). The relationship between sibling maltreatment and college students' sense of well-being. *Journal of College Counseling, 12*, 17–30.

National Institute on Alcohol Abuse and Alcoholism. (n.d.). *Alcohol's effects on the body*. Bethesda, MD: Author. Retrieved from https://www.niaaa.nih.gov/alcohol-health/alcohols-effects-body

Paolucci, E. O., & Violato, C. (2004). A meta-analysis of the published research on the affective, cognitive, and behavioral effects of corporal punishment. *The Journal of Psychology, 138*, 197–221.

Psychologist World. (2017). *Developmental Psychology. Attachment theory*. South Yorkshire: Author. Retrieved from https://www.psychologistworld.com/developmental/attachment-theory.php

Sedlak, A. J., Mettenburg, J., Basena, M., Petta, I., McPherson, K., Greene, A., & Li, S. (2010). *Fourth national incidence study of child abuse and neglect (NIS–4): Report to congress.*

Washington, DC: U.S. Department of Health and Human Services, Administration for Children and Families.
Shin, S. H., & Miller, D. P. (2012). A longitudinal examination of childhood maltreatment and adolescent obesity: Results from the National Longitudinal Study of Adolescent Health (AddHealth) Study. *Child Abuse & Neglect, 36*(2), 84–94.
Silverman, A. B., Reinherz, H. Z., & Giaconia, R. M. (1996). The long-term sequelae of child and adolescent abuse: A longitudinal community study. *Child Abuse & Neglect, 20*(8), 709–723.
Simonelli, C. J., Mullis, T., Elliot, A. N., & Pierce, T. W. (2002). Abuse by siblings and subsequent experiences of violence within the dating relationship. *Journal of Interpersonal Violence, 17*(2), 103–121.
Skinner, J. A., & Kowalski, R. M. (2013). Profiles of sibling bullying. *Journal of Interpersonal Violence, 28*(8), 1726–1736.
Substance Abuse and Mental Health Services Administration. (n.d.). *Adverse childhood experiences*. Rockville, MD: Author. Retrieved from https://www.samhsa.gov/capt/practicing-effective-prevention/prevention-behavioral-health/adverse-childhood-experiences
Tanrikulu, I., & Campbell, M. A. (2015). Sibling bullying perpetration: Associations with gender, grade, peer perpetration, trait anger, and moral disengagement. *Journal of Interpersonal Violence, 30*(6), 1010–1024.
The Brain Made Simple. (n.d.). *Hippocampus and amygdala*. Retrieved from http://brainmadesimple.com/
The Forgiveness Project. (2018). *Clare's story of childhood abuse*. London: Author. Retrieved from http://theforgivenessproject.com/visitor/clares-story-of-childhood-abuse/
Thompson, R. A. (2001). Development in the first years of life. *Caring for Infants and Toddlers, 11*(1), 21–33.
Tippett, N., & Wolke, D. (2015). Aggression between siblings: Associations with the home environment and peer bullying. *Aggressive Behavior, 41*, 14024.
Tucker, C. J., Finkelhor, D., Shattuck, A. M., & Turner, H. (2013). Prevalence and correlates of sibling victimization types. *Child Abuse & Neglect, 37*, 213–223.
Tucker, C. J., Finkelhor, D., Turner, H., & Shattuck, A. (2013). Association of sibling aggression with child and adolescent mental health. *Pediatrics, 132*(1), 79–84.
Tucker, C. J., Finkelhor, D., Turner, H., & Shattuck, A. M. (2014). Sibling and peer victimization in childhood and adolescence. *Child Abuse & Neglect, 38*, 1599–1606.
U.S. Department of Health & Human Services, Administration for Children and Families, Administration on Children, Youth and Families, Children's Bureau. (2001). *Understanding the effects of maltreatment on early brain development*. Retrieved from https://www.childwelfare.gov/pubPDFs/earlybrain.pdf
U.S. Department of Health & Human Services, Administration for Children and Families, Administration on Children, Youth and Families, Children's Bureau. (2016). *Child maltreatment 2014*. Retrieved from http://www.acf.hhs.gov/programs/cb/research-data-technology/statistics-research/child-maltreatment
U.S. Department of Health & Human Services, Administration for Children and Families, Administration on Children, Youth and Families, Children's Bureau. (2017). *Child maltreatment 2015*. Retrieved from http://www.acf.hhs.gov/programs/cb/research-data-technology/statistics-research/child-maltreatment
UNICEF. (2014). *Hidden in plain sight: A statistical analysis of violence against children*. New York, NY: UNICEF.
Widom, C. S., Czaja, S. J., Bentley, T., & Johnson, M. S. (2012). A prospective investigation of physical health outcomes in abused and neglected children: New findings from a 30-year follow-up. *American Journal of Public Health, 102*(6), 1135–1144.
Widom, C. S., Marmorstein, N., & White, H. (2006). Childhood victimization and illicit drug use in middle adulthood. *Psychology of Addictive Behavior, 20*(4), 394–403.

Widom, C. S., & Maxfield, M. G. (2001). *An update on the "Cycle of violence"*. Washington, DC: U.S. Department of Justice, Office of Justice Programs, National Institute of Justice. Retrieved from https://www.ncjrs.gov/pdffiles1/nij/184894.pdf

Wolke, D., Tippett, N., & Dantchev, S. (2015). Bullying in the family: Sibling bullying. *Lancet Psychiatry, 2*, 917–929.

World Health Organization. (2016). *Child maltreatment: Fact sheet.* Geneva: WHO. Retrieved from http://www.who.int/mediacentre/factsheets/fs150/en/

Chapter 7
Bullying in Young Adulthood: College Hazing as a Form of Bullying

7.1 Dying to be Accepted

In 2002 students Kristin High and Kenitha Saafir were pledging Alpha Kappa Alpha at California State University at Los Angeles and were forced to engage in hours of exercise and then walk backwards into the ocean. Saafir, who could not swim, was swept out to sea by a wave, and High swum after her in an attempt to save her. Both girls drowned.

In 2005, Chico State University Student Mathew Carrington joined Chi Tau fraternity and was forced to do calisthenics in the basement of the fraternity house while freezing water was dumped on him and fans blew cold air. He was not allowed to use the bathroom and had to ask permission to wet himself. This torture lasted for 5 h at which point he was forced to chug a gallon of water. Carrington died of water intoxication and hypothermia.

In 2008, 19-year-old Harrison was pledging a college fraternity. One night during "hell week," Harrison and another pledge were told to dress in light clothing and were taken to a field 20 miles from their college campus. They were instructed to run the "gauntlet" from one end of the field to another where they had to touch the "sacred rock." Unbeknownst to the two sophomore pledges, fraternity brothers dressed in dark clothing came out of nowhere and tackled them as they ran the length of the field. Some of the brothers were football players and weighed 220 lb. Harrison was hit multiple times and ended up hitting his head on the frozen field and ultimately died.

In 2017, Maxwell Gruver was pledging Phi Delta Theta House at Louisiana State when he was forced to participate in a hazing ritual called "Bible Study." Pledges were forced to drink alcohol if they answered questions about the fraternity incorrectly. Gruver died with a blood alcohol level of 0.495.

Even when hazing rituals do not result in death, they often cross a line and turn into serious bullying. For example, consider the following:

© Springer Nature Switzerland AG 2019

P. R. Smokowski, C. B. R. Evans, *Bullying and Victimization Across the Lifespan*, https://doi.org/10.1007/978-3-030-20293-4_7

In 2008, fraternity pledge Kit was forced to stand with his nose against a concrete wall during rush. If he or the other pledges moved, their heads were slammed into the wall. The pledges were also forced to clean the floor with their fingernails and drink "pitch black water."

In 2010, a student pledging Rutgers University Sigma Gamma Rho Sorority was hospitalized after being beaten with paddles.

In 2012, pledges at Binghamton University were forced into freezing showers while reciting the Greek alphabet. They were fed pills to make them vomit on each other and were forced to hold hot hookah coals in their hands.

Not all hazing is bullying. Sometimes hazing can be good natured and fun. For example, sending fraternity or sorority pledges on an innocuous scavenger hunt around the college where the goal is to collect specific objects or take pictures of certain landmarks; the goal is not to break the law, be humiliated, or put the pledges in harm's way. The goal is simply to provide a fun and entertaining team building activity. Sometimes new members of sports teams might be tasked with carrying the bag of balls or taking sweaty uniforms to the laundry to be washed. Again, the goal is not to cause harm or humiliation, it is to give newcomers responsibility that veteran team members do not want to deal with. However, when misguided or taken to the extreme, which hazing often is, this rite of passage becomes a vicious and life-threatening form of bullying. In the following chapter, we will focus on hazing rituals that cross the line from fun and carefree group bonding activities to become emotional and physical experiences of bullying.

7.2 Introduction

News stories (see Chap. 1 and above) of fraternity pledges, like Tim Piazza who was forced to drink until he blacked out, fell down a flight of stairs, and died, or marching band members, like Robert Champion who was physically beaten to death on a bus, remind the world that bullying does not stop with high school graduation. Indeed, hazing, which we argue in this chapter is a form of bullying, is all too common in young adulthood and usually occurs on college campuses, but also happens in the military and other organizations such as the Boy Scouts or middle and high school sports teams. While hazing stories that end in death capture the attention of the news networks and make horrifyingly captivating headlines, hazing does not usually end in death, but most certainly causes physical and emotional scars that can result in enduring emotional trauma. For example, sorority, fraternity, military, and athletic team hazing stories include newcomers being beaten with paddles, drinking strange and unidentified substances, being used as a human trash can and having garbage dumped on them, being told to drink alcohol until they pass out, being doused with boiling water, staying awake all night without being allowed to use the bathroom, and being verbally and physically abused (e.g., called stupid; hit; or punched). Although it may seem that hazing is distinct from bullying because pledges, freshman, or newcomers to groups, clubs, organizations, or teams "willingly" engage in these activities, hazing is a brutal form of bullying. One of the hallmarks of hazing is intense humiliation, which is also a component of bullying that we touched on in Chap. 3. In this chapter, we will first discuss hazing in general by defining this egregious behavior and discussing the definition in regard to state anti-hazing laws. We will also provide prevalence rates and talk about the consequences of hazing and then apply the three definitional components of bullying (repetition, power imbalance, intent to harm) to help understand how the bullying dynamic is infused in hazing.

7.3 Overview of Hazing

7.3.1 A Brief History of Hazing

There is evidence that hazing has roots in ancient Greece and medieval Europe. In 1495, Leipzig University banned hazing of freshmen by other students.

> Statute Forbidding Any One to Annoy or Unduly Injure the Freshmen. Each and every one attached to this university is forbidden to offend with insult, torment, harass, drench with water or urine, throw on or defile with dust or any filth, mock by whistling, cry at them with a terrifying voice, or dare to molest in any way whatsoever physically or severely, any, who are called freshmen, in the market, streets, courts, colleges and living houses, or any place whatsoever, and particularly in the present college, when they have entered in order to matriculate or are leaving after matriculation.

The practice was imported to America during the colonial period. Joseph Webb, a Harvard student, was expelled for hazing in 1684. After the Civil War in the 1860s, hazing grew in popularity. According to John Hechinger's (2017) book titled *True Gentlemen: The Broken Pledge of America's Fraternities*, "… returning soldiers brought military-style hazing to college campuses ... the pledge period soon grew to weeks or months, devolving into the orgy of abuse so familiar today… Early hazers doled out beatings, force-fed vile substance, and staged kidnappings" (Hechinger, 2017, pp. 51–52). In 1873, a Kappa Alpha Society pledge at Cornell was taken to the countryside, blindfolded, and left to find his way back in the dark. He fell off a cliff and died, marking the first high profile hazing death in America. By the early 1900s, Stanford fraternity members submerged naked pledges in water until they nearly drowned (similar to the controversial torture practice of waterboarding) a practice called "tubbing" (Hechinger, 2017, p. 52). After Reginald Stringfellow died from the tubbing ritual in 1925, the practice was banned at the University of Utah. Delta Kappa Epsilon (DKE) at Yale and Dartmouth branded its pledges with triangles on their lower backs. In 1967, George W. Bush was associated with one of these incidents and dismissed the injury as "only a cigarette burn" when the fraternity was fined for the behavior. The term "Hell Week" and movies such as Animal House, Frat House, Fraternity Row, and the Hazing have sensationalized hazing rituals, ingraining them into popular culture.

7.3.2 Definition

The best place to begin the discussion of hazing is with a definition. What exactly is hazing? The word likely brings to mind news stories of horrific deaths caused by excessive alcohol consumption or physical beatings likely involving college fraternities, sororities, sports teams, or marching bands. These images suggest that hazing involves humiliation and harm as a way to inculcate new members into a group. Indeed, the Merriam-Webster Dictionary (n.d.) defines hazing as "An initiation process involving harassment." A website dedicated to hazing (Hazingprevention.org, 2015a) defines hazing as "… any action taken or any situation created intentionally that causes embarrassment, harassment or ridicule, and risks emotional and/or physical harm to members of a group or team, whether new or not, regardless of the person's willingness to participate." In the USA, these activities are called hazing, in the UK "initiation ceremonies," in Australia "bastardisation," and in South Asia "ragging." A comprehensive, multi-university investigation of hazing practices conducted by Alfred University (Hoover, 1999) defined hazing as,

> Any activity expected of someone joining a group that humiliates, degrades, abuses or endangers, regardless of the person's willingness to participate. This does not include activities such as rookies carrying the balls, team parties with community games, or going out with your teammates, unless an atmosphere of humiliation, degradation, abuse or danger arises.

These definitions confirm that hazing causes humiliation and is a form of harmful abuse inflicted upon newcomers to a team or group.

Currently, 44 states have anti-hazing laws and each state defines hazing slightly differently; however, there are commonalities across the laws that reinforce the above definitions (Hazingprevention.org, 2015b). All 44 state laws confirm that hazing causes harm by either directly stating that the person being hazed is physically and/or emotionally harmed and/or humiliated or by providing examples of hazing that make it clear that harm and/or humiliation would result. The vast majority of state laws (42) refer directly to the fact that hazing involves some sort of initiation (i.e., into a group, club, team, organization), while two state laws (Maine, South Carolina) fail to mention initiation as a hallmark of hazing; however, the South Carolina law states that hazing is performed by a "superior" student who has authority over the "subordinate" student who is being hazed, which implies that the student getting hazed is new. Almost all the state laws (39) define hazing as occurring in some sort of educational institution while five state laws (Indiana, Kansas, Mississippi, New York, and North Dakota) mention initiation into any sort of organization and do not specify that the organization is connected to an educational institution. Thirty-five state laws note that hazing is a willful or intentional act and 24 state laws provide examples of specific forms of hazing. For example, the Texas state law provides a comprehensive array of forms of hazing:

> (A) Any type of physical brutality, such as whipping, beating, striking, branding, electronic shocking, placing of a harmful substance on the body, or similar activity; (B) any type of physical activity, such as sleep deprivation, exposure to the elements, confinement in a

small space, calisthenics, or other activity that subjects the student to an unreasonable risk of harm or that adversely affects the mental or physical health or safety of the student; (C) any activity involving consumption of a food, liquid, alcoholic beverage, liquor, drug, or other substance that subjects the student to an unreasonable risk of harm or that adversely affects the mental or physical health or safety of the student; (D) any activity that intimidates or threatens the student with ostracism, that subjects the student to extreme mental stress, shame, or humiliation, that adversely affects the mental health or dignity of the student or discourages the student from entering or remaining registered in an educational institution, or that may reasonably be expected to cause a student to leave the organization or the institution rather than submit to acts described in this subdivision; and (E) any activity that induces, causes, or requires the student to perform a duty or task that involves a violation of the Penal Code.

Taking these definitions and state laws into account, we will define hazing according to the first part of the definition by the study conducted by Alfred University (Hoover, 1999) and define hazing as: "Any activity expected of someone joining a group that humiliates, degrades, abuses or endangers, regardless of the person's willingness to participate." Unfortunately, hazing begins in middle school, continues through high school, and peaks in college and an alarming number of US youth are negatively impacted by engagement in this harmful practice.

7.3.3 Prevalence of Hazing in the United States

Research on hazing remains minimal and few studies of prevalence rates have been conducted. Although hazing commonly occurs on college campuses, one research team surveyed 1541 high school juniors and seniors from a random national sample of 20,000 US high school students. Overall, 48% of students belonging to a group reported being hazed and based on these findings, it was estimated that 1.5 million high school students are subjected to hazing each year (Hoover & Pollard, 2000). Findings indicated that 43% of students belonging to groups reported being hazed by humiliation (e.g., being yelled, cursed, or sworn at; embarrassing themselves publicly; eating or drinking disgusting things; depriving themselves of food, sleep or cleanliness), 23% were hazed by substance abuse (e.g., drinking alcohol; smoking cigarettes or cigars; using illegal drugs), and 22% were hazed in a dangerous way (e.g., stealing, cheating, or committing a crime; beating up others or picking a fight with someone; inflicting self-pain by branding or satanic rite; being physically abused or beaten).

Another group of researchers surveyed 1105 middle and high school student-athletes in grades 6 through 12 in three middle-class school districts in the suburbs of New York City. Athletes were asked about hazing activities they were forced to engage in (i.e., wearing embarrassing clothing; undressing; acting as a slave or maid; exercising too much; cutting or shaving hair; drinking alcohol; eating something unusual; doing a scavenger hunt) and actions done to them (e.g., being punched, beaten, or paddled; being yelled, screamed, or cursed at; being called names; being ignored; being tied or taped up; being confined in a locker or car trunk; being abandoned somewhere; being kidnapped). Results indicated that 17.4% of surveyed youth had experienced some form of hazing mentioned above (Gershel, Katz-Sidlow, Small, & Zandieh, 2003). This study confirmed that hazing begins early, with 13.3% of sixth grade students reporting engagement in hazing. These findings suggest that while we commonly consider hazing to be a college problem, youth as young as sixth grade are being victimized by this brutal practice and additional research and interventions for middle- and high-school hazing are warranted.

However, the vast majority of hazing occurs in college and this age group is the focus of the current chapter. In a large-scale study of hazing in college athletes, 224 colleges and universities across the country submitted the names and addresses of 61,258 student athletes. A random sample of 10,000 athletes were taken from this list and of those 2027 participated in the study. Almost half (45%) of participants stated that they knew of, had heard of, or suspected that hazing occurred on their campus (Hoover, 1999). When students were questioned about specific forms of hazing activities, 65% reported engagement in at least one "questionable" initiation activity (i.e., being yelled, cursed, or sworn at; being forced to wear embarrassing clothing; being tattooed, pierced, shaved, or branded; engaging in calisthenics not related to the sport; associating with specific people, not others; being a personal servant; being deprived of food, sleep, or hygiene; consuming disgusting concoctions), 51% reported an alcohol related initiation activity (i.e., consuming alcohol on a recruitment visit; participating in a drinking contest), and 21% reported engagement in "unacceptable" hazing activities (i.e., making prank calls or harassing others; destroying or stealing property; engaging in or simulating sexual acts; being tied up, taped, or confined in a small space; being paddled, whipped, beaten, kicked, or beating others; being kidnapped or transported and abandoned). More alarming, 17% of respondents were deeply immersed in a culture of hazing and participated in or were subjected to five or more hazing behaviors (Hoover, 1999). When these results were projected onto the national population of college athletes, over a quarter of a million athletes are hazed each year. These findings were confirmed in a more recent national survey.

In the most comprehensive study of hazing to date, researchers examined hazing in a sample of 11,482 undergraduate students ages 18–25 across a wide range of student clubs, organizations, and teams in a national sample of 53 diverse colleges and universities (Allan & Madden, 2012). Almost half of the sample (48%) belonged to one group or team and 15% belonged to two groups of teams. Findings indicated the widespread nature of hazing across groups and teams on US college campuses ranging from 74% of varsity athletic team members to 20% of Honor Society members; in total, 55% of students involved in clubs and teams reported being hazed. Certain hazing practices including alcohol consumption, humiliation, isolation, sleep-deprivation, and sex acts were common across student groups (Allan & Madden, 2012). See Table 7.1.

Although limited, the existing literature on the prevalence of hazing indicates it is a serious problem in middle school, high school, and college. Nationally, almost half (48%) of high school juniors and seniors are involved in hazing (Hoover & Pollard, 2000). However, this rate dropped to 17.4% when students in middle and

Table 7.1 Percentage of group members who experienced different hazing behavior

Group	% Experienced at least 1 hazing behavior	% Hazed by drinking games	% Hazed by sleep deprivation	% Hazed by engaging in a sexual act
Varsity athletic team	74	54	16	16
Social fraternity or sorority	73	53	17	10
Club sports	64	41	10	7
Performing arts organization	56	23	17	5
Service fraternity or sorority	50	26	10	3
Intramural team	49	28	7	9
Recreation Club	42	20	9	4
Other group	30	N/A	10	2
Academic Club	28	10	7	1
Honor society	20	5	6	1

early high school were included (Gershel et al., 2003), perhaps indicating that rates of hazing are lower in younger age groups and increase over time. Rates of hazing on college sports teams ranged from 21% (unacceptable hazing activities) to 65% (questionable hazing activities; Hoover, 1999). When a multitude of collegiate clubs and teams were assessed, 55% of student members reported being hazed (Allan & Madden, 2012). This means that over half of college students involved in a team, club, or organization are hazed each year. These numbers paint an alarming picture and indicate that beginning in middle school and continuing through college, children, adolescents, and young adults are at risk for engagement in hazing activities and the ensuing negative consequences.

7.3.4 Negative Consequences Associated with Hazing

The most obvious negative consequence of hazing is physical injury and possible death. Deaths are often related to excessive alcohol consumption and injuries that occur while the person is so drunk he or she blacks out. Afraid of getting in trouble, group or team members fail to call 911 and let victims of hazing perish when medical attention could be life-saving. Hazing expert Hank Newer has closely tracked hazing related deaths and found that from 1961 to 2017 at least one hazing death per year occurred on a North American college campus, and many years multiple deaths occurred (Nuwer, 2018). However, even in less severe cases of hazing, when death does not occur, long lasting physical and emotional scars may ensue.

Hazing has serious psychological consequences. For example, Post Traumatic Stress Disorder and suicide have both resulted from hazing (Maxwell, 2018; Sussberg, 2003). In addition, depression and poor self-esteem can result from hazing (Finkel, 2002). Finkel (2002) summarized the most common forms of hazing and the ensuing negative consequences (see Table 7.2). As illustrated in Table 7.2, hazing results in a multitude of physical injuries ranging in severity from first degree burns to organ failure or hypoxic brain damage as well as psychological consequences including depression, PTSD, and low self-esteem.

Despite these horrific consequences, victims of hazing are often reticent to disclose the true source of their injuries and can thus be difficult to identify. There are several guidelines that emergency room staff can rely upon to accurately identify victims of hazing: (1) Gender—males are more likely to engage in hazing compared to females; (2) Race—there were three times as many hazing incidents involving Caucasian students compared to African American students; (3) Time of year—hazing most often

Table 7.2 Overview of hazing practices and negative consequences

Hazing practices	Mechanism	Negative consequences
Alcohol, binge drinking	Acute alcohol intoxication	Aspiration, alcoholic coma, hematemesis, injuries associated with concomitant hazing practices
Beating/paddling/whipping/striking	Blunt trauma	Intracranial, intrathoracic, intra-abdominal, and extremity injuries
Blood pinning[a]	Penetrating trauma to chest	Superficial chest trauma, pain, bleeding
Branding/tattooing/cigarette burning/burning	Burns	1st, 2nd, third degree burns; oropharyngeal and esophageal burns
Calisthenics	Heat-related	Syncope, vomiting, end-organ damage including seizure and coma
	Cardiac	Ischemia in people with underlying heart disease
Confinement in a restricted area	Heat-related	Syncope, vomiting, end organ damage
	Hypoxia	Multiorgan system failure, hypoxic brain damage
Consumption of nonfood substances	Toxicity to gastrointestinal tract	Gastrointestinal disease
Drowning, near drowning	Hypoxia	Multiorgan system failure, hypoxic brain damage
Falls	Blunt trauma	Spinal cord/c-spine; intracranial, intrathoracic, intra-abdominal, and extremity injury
Immersion in noxious substances	Heat- or cold-related	Burns, cold exposure, dermatitis
Psychological abuse	Verbal humiliation, coercion into performing demeaning acts, forced sleep deprivation	Depression, post-traumatic stress, poor self-esteem
Sexual assaults	Blunt trauma to mouth, vagina, or anus	Anal, oral, or vaginal trauma; human immune-deficiency virus, hepatitis C, and other sexually transmitted diseases; unwanted pregnancy

[a]Note: Most commonly seen in military hazing; involves a senior officer inserting the sharp points of ceremonial wings into the subcutaneous tissue of the initiate (Finkel, 2002)

occurs in February, March, April, September, and October (Finkel, 2002). In summary, hazing results in serious physical and psychological consequences, yet it is an enduring tradition, which begs the question, "What causes hazing?"

7.3.5 Causes of Hazing

If hazing has such horrendous consequences, why does it occur? There are various reasons groups justify hazing: (1) hazers think that "breaking people down and building them back up" (Maxwell, 2018, p. 50) provides some sort of benefit to victims by toughening them up for life; (2) hazing is seen as a test of loyalty and if the victim performs well, he/she will be a trustworthy and contributing member of the group; (3) hazing serves to bond people together, creating unity and cohesion (Maxwell, 2018). Existing group members often justify hazing based on one or all of these premises.

Other researchers contend that three main macro theories best explain why hazing occurs. According to solidarity macro theory, hazing occurs as a way to foster solidarity among group members; individuals being hazed increase their liking for a group as a means of justifying the horrendous hazing acts in which they engage (see Cimino, 2011 for a review). Thus, one reason hazing occurs is because existing group members want to ensure that new, incoming members are devoted to the group and that there is a feeling of unity and camaraderie. However, research with athletes suggests that the more hazing individuals endured, the less cohesive they perceived the sports team to be in sports related tasks. Conversely, the more appropriate team building activities there were, the more cohesive athletes perceived their team to be (Van Raalte, Cornelius, Linder, & Brewer, 2007). And a second study of 154 college athletes in the UK found that there was no relationship between hazing and team cohesion, again suggesting that using hazing to increase team cohesion is an ineffective practice (Lafferty, Wakefield, & Brown, 2017). So, although students might perceive hazing as an effective means of creating team unity, research suggests it does not impact team cohesion and can actually erode team cohesion.

A second applicable theory is the dominance macro theory, which posits that hazing occurs because the existing group members want to maintain their power and dominance over incoming members (see Cimino, 2011 for a review). Groups often have well established social hierarchies and adding new members introduces the possibility that the current social hierarchy could be altered. Thus, existing group members could use hazing as a way of reminding incoming group members who is in charge. If existing group members feel threatened by incoming members and worry that their social status might be usurped, hazing could be a means of keeping new members in a subordinate position.

The famous Stanford prison experiments by Zimbardo (Haney, Banks, & Zimbardo, 1973; McLeod, 2017) provide evidence for dominance theory. Twenty-one undergraduate, male students were randomly assigned to either play the role of guard or prisoner in a simulated prison created in the basement of Stanford's psychology department. Prisoners underwent a de-individuation process where they were given numbers instead of names, wore prison clothing, stocking caps on their heads, and chains around their ankles. Guards were given whistles and billy clubs (power symbols, although violence was not allowed) and mirrored sunglasses to prevent eye contact. Within a very short amount of time, guards were asserting their authority and started to act in an abusive way towards some prisoners (e.g., giving pointless and boring tasks, physical punishment such as doing push-ups with other prisoners sitting on their backs). Guards put down a rebellion with a fire extinguisher and gave special privileges, like eating, to "good prisoners." Prisoners quickly became dehumanized, submissive, and dependent; some deteriorated psychologically with uncontrollably sobbing, delusions, and rages. The experiment had to be terminated early and ignited many ethical questions. This research showed that participants conformed with social roles; those with authority became more sadistic in the prison setting and those without power decompensated into neurotic dependency. Results are highly relevant for bullying in general and hazing in particular where the power differential is manipulated to keep newcomers subordinate while veteran group members hardly realize how sadistic they become during the indoctrination. For those in power, deindividuation is a state when you become so immersed in the norms of the group that you lose your sense of identity and personal responsibility. You may feel that you are upholding the group tradition that you lived through years ago. For the victims, learned helplessness may prompt submitting to the abuse when you feel that whatever you do has little effect and you give up responding.

Finally, the commitment macro theory views hazing as a means of testing newcomers commitment; those who are truly committed to the group will not be deterred by having to endure hazing (see Cimino, 2011 for a review). Conversely, newcomers whose commitment is lukewarm, might balk at being asked to engage in humiliating and/or dangerous acts and decide to forgo joining the group. In this regard, hazing is used to weed out noncommitted individuals and is a means of ensuring the best and most dedicated (or at least most submissive) members are added to the group.

It is also important to consider why new group members endure hazing. Social belonging is a basic and fundamental human need (Baumeister & Leary, 1995) and individuals often alter their behavior in order to conform to group norms, avoiding ostracism and social isolation. Thus, the egregious nature of hazing rituals is overshadowed by the biological need for acceptance and belonging. A seminal study that demonstrated this need for group acceptance was Asch's (1951) line length discrimination study. In this study, seven confederates and one subject were presented with a line and were told to select the line of the same length from three comparison lines. The confederates answered before the subject and in some cases purposefully selected a comparison line that was clearly not the same length as the original line. When an incorrect line was selected by all confederates, one third of the subjects, overwhelmed by the desire to be accepted by the group, went along with the group and endorsed the incorrect selection. This study highlights that the powerful desire for acceptance and belonging caused individuals to alter their behavior to conform to group norms. Thus, new group members might quietly endure harsh hazing practices in order to feel the social acceptance inherent in group membership. They are told the abuse is part of conforming to group norms.

Indeed, it appears that human beings are biologically wired for conformity. In one study using fMRI machines, 24 females were asked to rate the attractiveness of 222 faces. After providing a rating, each subject was presented with the "average European rating" (i.e., the group rating) of attractiveness, which was altered to either coincide with or differ from the subjects rating. When the group rating differed from the subject's rating, indicating a lack of conformity with the group, a neuronal response occurred in areas of the brain that signal error processing and detection. Behavior deviating from the group norm was processed by the brain as problematic (Klucharev, Hytonen, Rijpkema, Smidts, & Fernandez, 2009), suggesting that the human brain is wired to enhance and promote group conformity, and fires a warning signal when individual behavior conflicts with the group. Thus, even if victims of hazing feel hesitant about participating, they may refrain from speaking up because no one else in their group is protesting. The aforementioned research highlights the importance of group belonging and hazing is likely viewed as a mechanism for obtaining this coveted and biologically necessary commodity.

7.4 Hazing as a Form of Bullying

Before applying the definitional framework of bullying to hazing, there are important differences between hazing and bullying that we must highlight. Bullying is typically used to target one individual who is socially excluded through the bullying; this social exclusion could go on endlessly and victims of bullying often see no hope of social acceptance by the peer(s) bullying them. Hazing, on the other hand, is often directed at a small group of individuals and is used as means to obtain social inclusion (Hazingprevention.org, 2015c). Thus, the end points of bullying and hazing are quite different: bullying results in ongoing social exclusion, while hazing begins as an experience of social exclusion, but ultimately results in acceptance and group membership (if initiates survive the ritual). Chapter 4 discusses the innate human desire to belong to a group; thus, it is possible that because hazing is a means of acquiring group belonging, it is less harmful than bullying because it is time limited and a desired outcome is achieved. Conversely, bullying can go on indefinitely and does not ultimately result in social acceptance and group membership but often results in prolonged ostracism. This is not to say that while hazing is occurring it is not damaging, but at least victims of hazing know the abuse is time limited and may result in coveted group membership.

Further, victims of bullying are often bullied alone; they are the only victim bullied by one or more perpetrators, often in front of a crowd. Victims of hazing are typically hazed alongside a cohort of their peers; so, although they are forced to engage in embarrassing, humiliating, and often dangerous acts, they do so alongside other people. In this regard, hazing can be considered a form of "group bullying" (Allan & Madden, 2012) because other people are always present: the peers getting hazed as well as the group members conducting the hazing. Although bullying also often occurs in a group setting (i.e., bystanders are usually present), it can also occur privately such as an upperclassman slamming a freshman into a locker in an empty hallway; however, hazing always occurs in a group setting. The presence of peers who are also being hazed might mitigate the trauma and humiliation that hazing practices often cause (due to the social support of going through the ritual together) but could also serve to further traumatize victims who feel even more self-conscious and embarrassed that they were forced to engage in hazing behaviors in front of others. Further, the audience of existing group members watching the hazing could also exacerbate the humiliation felt by the incoming members and fellow initiates may pressure each other to press further into the humiliation than if each newcomer were hazed alone.

Despite these distinctive features of hazing that seem to render it separate from bullying, we argue below that the definitional framework of bullying can actually be quite useful in understanding the hazing dynamic. Like the bullying dynamic, repetition is often but not always present in hazing; however, a power imbalance is a fundamental element of all hazing situations. Finally, intent to harm may or may not be present in hazing situations, but regardless of the intent, hazing victims are often harmed both physically and psychologically. Although two of the three definitional features of bullying are inconsistently present in hazing dynamics, we maintain that the bullying definitional framework is useful for better understanding hazing. Indeed, other researchers confirm that hazing is a form of bullying (Allan & Madden, 2012; Srabstein et al., 2008).

7.4.1 Repetition

The duration of hazing varies and it may or may not be repeated over time. For example, hazing practices might extend over a period of days or weeks (Allan & Madden, 2012), such as "Hell Week" at fraternities and sororities where pledges are often required to live at the fraternity or sorority house for an entire week while they endure multiple hazing incidents day after day. However, hazing might also be limited to a single event such as a "rookie initiation night" for a sports team (Allan & Madden, 2012, p. 1). While bullying is almost always repeated over time and repetition is a seemingly vital component necessary to define bullying, as mentioned in Chap. 1, there are certain one-time events that are so egregious they constitute bullying. Thus, while hazing might be a one-time event, we argue that hazing practices are often so horrendous that even a one-time hazing event can be considered a form of bullying.

Regardless of whether hazing occurs over one evening or over an entire week, newcomers are likely forced to engage in multiple hazing practices during the allotted hazing period. Thus, even in one evening, initiates can be subjected to multiple, dangerous and humiliating practices that can put them in harm's way and can result in the serious negative outcomes discussed in Table 7.2. And hazing that lasts over an extended period of time, such as "Hell Week," certainly increases victims' risk for harm and trauma as multiple hazing rituals are forced on initiates during this time period. However, as we mentioned above, unlike bullying, hazing is time limited. So, even though hazing practices can be repeated over time, new group members enduring the hazing know (or at least hope) that the hazing will not continue indefinitely.

7.4.2 Power Imbalance

As discussed in Chap. 1, power imbalance is fundamental to bullying, but can often be difficult to establish. The very act of bullying creates a power imbalance so it can be difficult to know if the power imbalance was created by the bullying or if the bullying exacerbated an existing power imbalance. Further, there are many dimensions of power (e.g., race, age, gender, socioeconomic status) and a power imbalance exists only if the victim views the perpetrator's sources of power as more salient than his/her sources of power.

An imbalance of power is central to the hazing dynamic; existing group members have more power than the newcomers simply by virtue of the fact that they are already members of the group. The senior group members wield their power over new initiates and demand that they engage in hazing as a way to gain access to group membership. The existing members of the group have power for a few reasons. First, they are veteran members of the group and have a nuanced understanding of the group dynamics, group culture and climate, and group social hierarchy; thus, they are able to seamlessly navigate the group social structure and use their knowledge of the group dynamics to control the newcomers. It is likely that existing group members have already endured the hazing rituals and are thus viewed as being in charge by the incoming group members. Incoming members desperately want to be liked and accepted by veteran group members and will do almost anything to gain this acceptance.

Second, the veteran group members are likely older and more experienced than the incoming group members; this is especially true for freshman athletes or pledges to fraternities or sororities who look up to the older, veteran group members. This age discrepancy gives veteran members additional power over the new, incoming members. As discussed in Chap. 6 for sibling violence, age is a form of power and gives current group members additional power and prestige over the incoming group members.

Finally, the existing group members have something the incoming members desperately want: group membership. The incoming members are in a vulnerable position where the fear of rejection motivates them to do almost anything to gain group acceptance. This gives the current group members great power over the initiates because they can say, "If you don't drink this alcohol or accept this physical punishment then you can't be in our group," and the incoming group members have absolutely no recourse to fight against this injustice if they want to pursue group membership.

It is important to note that once the hazing is over, the power imbalance inherent in the hazing dynamic may or may not be greatly diminished. Although veteran group members continue to maintain status due to their tenure in the group, once hazing ends, the newcomers become group members, and the playing field might be slightly evened. Conversely, just as in bullying dynamics, the power imbalance can endure endlessly and victims might never feel equal to their perpetrators. Senior group members may continue to abuse junior group members in less intense ways, which may be a reason why junior group members adopt the same hazing behavior once they become the seniors. Turning the abuse on others may finally be therapeutic (i.e., similar to bully-victims); however, this keeps the hazing cycle going.

7.4.3 Intent to Harm

As discussed in Chap. 1, regardless of the perpetrators' intentions, bullying undoubtedly causes harm to the victim. Further, only the perpetrator knows his/her true intentions; thus, harm is in the eyes of the victim: if the victim feels harmed, then harm is present and the victim will likely define his/her experience as bullying. Conversely, if the victim interprets teasing as a joke and does not view it as harmful, then he/she might not label the experience as bullying. The same can be said of hazing; regardless of the existing group members' intent, if newcomers feel that the hazing practice is harmful to them, then harm is present. Even if the intent of the hazing was meant to be lighthearted and fun, if victims of the hazing feel embarrassed, humiliated, or suffer negative physical or psychological consequences, then harm is present. However, it is possible that victims are so desperate to be accepted into the group that they are in denial about the harm the hazing causes them. Similarly, drinking until you black out may be perceived as wild, perhaps normative, college fun. Yet this can take a tragic turn when these poor decisions are made. Thus, it is conceivable that only a third party (i.e., someone external to the group) is cognizant of the harm the hazing practices are causing.

While the victim's interpretation of hazing practices is paramount, it is also important to consider the perpetrator's intent (i.e., the existing group members who enforce the hazing). It is possible that existing group members blindly follow past group protocol and enforce hazing practices that they themselves engaged in and reason "I survived these hazing rituals so they really can't be that bad." If this is the case, the existing group members are not even stopping to consider the potential harm they might cause initiates and simply force them to engage in hazing rituals because it is a historical legacy, what happened to them when they were new. These cognitions are identical to the rationalizations that propagate intergenerational patterns of child maltreatment (i.e., "My father whipped me and I turned out okay. So, this discipline is good enough for my child"). However, it is also conceivable that existing group members do want to harm initiates as a way to test their loyalty to the group. In line with commitment macro theory discussed above (see Cimino, 2011 for a review), existing group members may purposefully choose harmful hazing practices as a way of testing incoming members' dedication to the group. Indeed, the harder it is to secure group membership, the higher the status of the group appears. If new members are willing to put up with harmful, abusive, and humiliating hazing practices, existing members might see this as their true dedication to the group. New members who lack dedication to the group would be unwilling to endure harmful hazing practices and might drop out of the initiation. In this regard, harming incoming members through egregious hazing practices is a means of ensuring dedicated and loyal (as well as disempowered and obedient) newcomers are admitted to the group.

7.5 Conclusions

Hazing is defined as "Any activity expected of someone joining a group that humiliates, degrades, abuses or endangers, regardless of the person's willingness to participate." Over half of college students who belong to a team, club, or organization have engaged in hazing, indicating that each year hundreds of thousands of college students are at risk for the physical, emotional, and psychological negative outcomes associated with hazing. Although some hazing practices are fun and harmless group bonding activities, many hazing rituals cross a line and should be viewed as a form of bullying. Despite the distinct characteristics of bullying and hazing (e.g., hazing ultimately results in group acceptance while bullying has no foreseeable end and results in ongoing social isolation), the three definitional components of bullying can be applied to the hazing dynamic. Hazing is often ongoing, there is a power imbalance, and harm is often caused. Taken together, this chapter highlights how the bullying dynamic does not end in high school but continues into young adulthood on college campuses.

References

Allan, E., & Madden, M. (2012). The nature and extent of college student hazing. *International Journal of Adolescent Medicine and Health, 24*(1), 1–8.

Asch, S. (1951). Effects of group pressure upon the modification and distortion of judgments. In H. Guetzkow (Ed.), *Groups, leadership and men research in human relations* (pp. 177–190). Pittsburgh, OH: Carnegie Press.

Baumeister, R. F., & Leary, M. R. (1995). The need to belong: Desire for interpersonal attachments as a fundamental human motivation. *Psychological Bulletin, 117*(3), 497–529.

Cimino, A. (2011). The evolution of hazing: Motivational mechanisms and abuse of newcomers. *Journal of Cognition and Culture, 11*, 241–267.

Finkel, M. A. (2002). Traumatic injuries caused by hazing practices. *American Journal of Emergency Medicine, 20*, 228–233.

Gershel, J. C., Katz-Sidlow, R. J., Small, E., & Zandieh, S. (2003). Hazing of suburban middle school and high school athletes. *Journal of Adolescent Health, 32*, 333, 335.

Haney, C., Banks, W. C., & Zimbardo, P. G. (1973). A study of prisoners and guards in a simulated prison. *Naval Research Review, 30*, 4–17.

Hazing. (n.d.). In *Merriam-Webster's collegiate dictionary*. Retrieved from https://www.merriam-webster.com/dictionary/hazing

Hazingprevention.org. (2015a). *What hazing looks like*. Retrieved from www.hazingpreveint.org/home/facts-what-hazing-looks-like/

Hazingprevention.org. (2015b). *Hazing law-Interactive state map*. Retrieved from https://hazing-prevention.org/home/hazing/statelaws/

Hazingprevention.org. (2015c). *Hazing and bullying*. Retrieved from https://hazingprevention.org/home/hazing/hazing-and-bullying/

Hechinger, J. (2017). *True gentlemen: The broken pledge of America's fraternities*. New York, NY: Hachette Book Group.

Hoover, N. C. (1999). *National survey: Initiation rites and athletics for NCAA sports teams*. Retrieved from http://www.alfred.edu/sports_hazing

Hoover, N. C., & Pollard, N. J. (2000). *Initiation rites in American high schools: A national survey*. Alfred, NY: Alfred University.

Klucharev, V., Hytonen, K., Rijpkema, M., Smidts, A., & Fernandez, G. (2009). Reinforcement learning signal predicts social conformity. *Neuron, 61*, 140–151.

Lafferty, M. E., Wakefield, C., & Brown, H. (2017). We do it for the team-student athletes' initiation practices and their impact on group cohesion. *International Journal of Sport and Exercise Psychology, 15*(4), 438–446.

Maxwell, T. (2018). The hidden harm of hazing for victims and hazers. In H. Nuwer (Ed.), *Hazing: Destroying young lives* (pp. 50–56). Bloomington, IN: Indiana University Press.

McLeod, S. A. (2017). *Zimbardo - Stanford Prison Experiment*. Retrieved from www.simplypsychology.org/zimbardo.html

Nuwer, H. (2018). Introduction: The perils of hazing, a few thoughts on forty years of writing about hazing. In H. Nuwer (Ed.), *Hazing: Destroying young lives* (pp. 1–4). Bloomington, IN: Indiana University Press.

Srabstein, J., Joshi, P., Due, P., Wright, J., Leventhal, B., Merrick, J., … Riibner, K. (2008). Prevention of public health risks linked to bullying: A need for a whole community approach. *International Journal of Adolescent Medicine and Health, 20*(2), 185–199.

Sussberg, J. A. (2003). Shattered dreams: Hazing in college athletics. *Cardoza Law Review, 24*, 1421–1491.

Van Raalte, J. L., Cornelius, A. E., Linder, D. E., & Brewer, B. W. (2007). The relationship between hazing and team cohesion. *Journal of Sport Behavior, 30*(4), 491–507.

Chapter 8
Bullying in Intimate Partner Relationships: Teen Dating Violence and Adult Intimate Partner Violence as Forms of Bullying

8.1 Introduction

Teen dating violence (TDV) and adult intimate partner violence (IPV) share many similarities. The abuser often starts out sweet and charming by doling out compliments, giving presents, and writing thoughtful love notes. This behavior lulls the victim into a false sense of security, strengthening the bond and attachment between the victim and perpetrator, often making the victim fall deeply "in love." Gradually, this loving behavior is replaced with abusive behavior, which often times begins as verbal abuse that escalates into physical and/or sexual abuse that increases in severity over time. Like the fable of the frog and the boiling water in which a frog dropped into a pot of boiling water will jump out, but a frog put in tepid water that is gradually heated to a boil will not perceive danger and will be cooked to death, the escalation of abuse gradually entraps the victim in a coercive cycle of abuse. It is important to consider the developmental course of intimate relationships. The romantic love that marks the early stages of many intimate relationships often comes with high levels of personal disclosure and shared vulnerability. There may not be any particular power imbalance in these early encounters that are characterized by sharing and caring. However, if romance gives way to stress and conflict in the intimate relationship later on, fighting between partners can become abusive and evolve into bullying. We discuss these dynamics in more detail below.

While TDV and IPV are closely aligned, we have opted to first discuss them separately because TDV is a specific form of IPV that occurs when the victim is under the age of 18 and IPV generally refers to adults. Both TDV and IPV result in serious, long-term negative consequences for the victim. Further, although both of these forms of violence are not usually considered to be forms of bullying, both include repetition and power imbalance and can include intent to harm, highlighting the fact that the bullying definitional framework is a useful way of understanding the nuances of TDV and IPV. Following an overview of TDV and IPV, the bullying definitional framework is applied to both forms of violence.

© Springer Nature Switzerland AG 2019

P. R. Smokowski, C. B. R. Evans, *Bullying and Victimization Across the Lifespan*, https://doi.org/10.1007/978-3-030-20293-4_8

8.2 Teen Dating Violence

8.2.1 Overview: Definition, Prevalence Rates, Demographics

"I need to speak to that fucking whore right there … Bitch, get your fucking stupid ass out here now." Crystal Sanchez was a junior in high school when her boyfriend of over 1 year burst into her classroom and shouted these degrading words in front of her classmates. Overwhelmed by shame and humiliation, Crystal left the classroom where her boyfriend spit in her face, yanked her necklace off her neck and threw it in a trash can, and hurled her up against a locker where he threatened her. The abuse Crystal experienced did not begin with this horrific incident. In fact, Crystal and her boyfriend happily dated for almost a year before he began saying he disliked her shirts and that her skirts were too short; controlling and jealous behavior Crystal mistook for adoration. Her boyfriends' behavior gradually intensified to name-calling, insults, unfounded accusations, humiliation, degradation, isolation, and physical assault (Sanchez, 2017).

The trajectory of the TDV that Kimberly Segovia experienced was similar. Kimberly's abuse began when her boyfriend started asking things like: "Why are you dressed like that? You look like a slut." One day Kimberly's boyfriend became enraged because she was wearing a strapless dress and he slapped her across the face. Soon, he began to isolate her from her friends and family, and often dragged her away at gunpoint. One-night Kimberly awoke to her boyfriend pointing a gun to her head; he pulled the trigger, but thankfully it was not loaded. After that terrifying incident, she was too scared to break up with him, believing that her boyfriend would follow through on his threats to kill her and her family (Nguyen, 2017).

Most broadly, teen dating violence (TDV) is defined as "… a pattern of abusive behavior used to control another person" that involves coercion and power assertion (Offenhauer & Buchalter, 2011, p. 3). However, TDV is often defined in a variety of ways, and some researchers limit the definition to only include physical force or threats of force (Offenhauer & Buchalter, 2011). The Centers for Disease Control and Prevention (CDC) defines TDV as a form of physical, psychological/emotional, sexual, or stalking violence between two adolescents in a close relationship. Physical TDV involves one partner being physically abused (e.g., pinched, hit, shoved, slapped, punched, kicked) by the other partner (e.g., Crystal's boyfriend slamming her against a locker); psychological/emotional TDV involves one partner being threatened by the other partner through name calling, shaming, humiliation, or isolation (e.g., Kimberly's boyfriend cutting her off from friends and family); sexual TDV occurs when one partner forces the other partner to engage in a sexual act without consent; and stalking TDV refers to one partner using repeated harassment or threats aimed to scare the other partner. These forms of violence can occur both in person and/or electronically, such as one partner repeatedly texting or posting sexual pictures of his/her partner online or threating to post such pictures (CDC, 2016). For the purposes of this chapter, we will define TDV as any abusive behavior (physical, psychological/emotional, sexual, or stalking) used in person or electronically to control an adolescent dating partner.

TDV is a widespread problem, however, prevalence rates vary because studies define and measure TDV differently and use different periods of time (National Institute of Justice, 2016). The 2015 National Youth Risk Behavior Survey (YRBSS) found that in a national sample of 15,624 high school students, 68.6% reported dating and of those, 9.6% reported physical dating violence and 10.6% reported sexual dating violence, which equates to about one in five adolescents being victims of physical or sexual dating violence. Females were more likely than males to report these two types of TDV (physical—11.7% of females versus 7.4% of males; sexual—15.6% of females versus 5.4% of males). Prevalence rats of physical TDV increased throughout high school from 8.1% in 9th grade to 10.5% in 12th grade, while prevalence rates of sexual dating violence fluctuated over the 4 years of high school increasing from 10.8% in 9th grade to 11.8% in 10th grade then decreasing to 10.3% in 11th grade and 9.2% in 12th grade (Kann et al., 2016).

However, other national samples have found higher rates of TDV. For example, the National Longitudinal Study of Adolescent Health (NLSAH) assessed 7500 adolescents in heterosexual romantic relationship and found that almost one third (29%) of adolescents reported psychological TDV (i.e., being sworn at, insulted, threatened), 12% reported physical TDV (i.e., being pushed, having something thrown at you), and 32% reported experiencing any form of TDV. Interestingly, roughly equal percentages of males and females experienced each form of TDV (Halpern, Oslak, Young, Martin, & Kupper, 2001). A second analysis from the same study examined 117 adolescents in same-sex relationships. Findings indicated that 21% reported psychological TDV, 11% reported physical TDV, and 24% reported any form of TDV (Halpern, Young, Waller, Martin, & Kupper, 2004).

A third study, The National Survey of Adolescents (NSA), surveyed a nationally representative sample ($N = 3614$) of adolescents ages 12–17 and found that 1.6% (2.7% of girls, 0.6% of boys) reported TDV victimization. These findings are markedly lower than previous findings, however, this low percentage still equates to 400,000 US adolescents being victimized by TDV each year (Wolitzky-Taylor et al., 2008). It is not clear why these prevalence rates would be so low compared to other studies. Taken together, findings indicate that somewhere between 1.6% and 30% of adolescent's experience in person TDV. With only one study reflecting the exceptionally low rate, an informed estimate is that between 20% and 30% of teenagers experience some form of psychological or physical TDV (see Table 8.1).

Interestingly, almost as many youths reported being victims of technology based TDV. Technology based TDV refers to Teen Dating Violence that occurs through cellphones (mainly text messaging) or over the internet (e.g., e-mail, websites, instant messaging). A national survey of 615 adolescents ages 13–18 found that more than one in four adolescents (27%) reported that their dating partner had "checked" on them by text 10 or more times per hour and 9% reported being "text checked" by their dating partner more than 50 times an hour (nearly every minute!). In total, almost one third (30%) of adolescents in a relationship reported that they had been texted 10, 20, or 30 times an hour by their partner asking them what they were doing and/or who they are with. Further, one in five adolescents (21%) reported they had gotten ten or more e-mails from their partner per hour and almost one

Table 8.1 Rates of TDV in three national samples

	YRBSS (*N* = 15,624)	NLSAH (*N* = 7500)	NSA (*N* = 3614)
Any TDV	N/A	32.0%	1.6%
Females	N/A	31.0%	2.7%
Males	N/A	32.0%	0.6%
Psychological TDV	N/A	29.0%	N/A
Physical TDV	9.6%	12.0%	N/A
Females	11.7%	29.0%	N/A
Males	7.4%	28.0%	N/A
9th Grade	8.1%	N/A	N/A
10th Grade	9.6%	N/A	N/A
11th Grade	10.1%	N/A	N/A
12th Grade	10.5%	N/A	N/A
Sexual TDV	10.6%	N/A	N/A
Females	15.6%	N/A	N/A
Males	5.4%	N/A	N/A
9th Grade	10.8%	N/A	N/A
10th Grade	11.8%	N/A	N/A
11th Grade	10.3%	N/A	N/A
12th Grade	9.2%	N/A	N/A

quarter (24%) of surveyed youth in a relationship stated that from midnight to 5:00 AM they communicated with their partner via hourly texting. Technology is also frequently used to engage in TDV beyond "text checking." For example, one in five (22%) adolescents have received a text or e-mail asking them to engage in a sexual activity when they did not want to, 19% say their partner used a cellphone or the internet to spread a rumor about them, 18% reported a partner using a networking site (e.g., Facebook) to harass them or put them down, 11% reported that a partner used electronic means to share a private and/or embarrassing picture or video of them, 25% have been called names, harassed, or put down by their partner through cellphones, and 10% reported being threatened physically by a partner via electronic means. These behaviors resulted in 17% of adolescent saying that they are afraid to not respond to their partner via cellphone or e-mail because of what the partner might do (Picard, 2007). Similar to cyberbullying discussed in Chap. 5, youth have no respite from cyber-TDV as the internet and cell phones provide possessive and abusive partners with unfettered access to their dating partner. Technology allows perpetrators to engage in ongoing TDV even when they are not physically with their dating partner, using text messages and e-mails as a means of exerting power and control over the victim (see Table 8.2).

The media typically highlights cases where females are victims of TDV and males are perpetrators; however, this is not accurate. In fact, one meta-analysis found that in general, females engaged in slightly higher rates of more minor physical aggression (i.e., throw something, slap, kick, bite, punch, hit with an object) towards their heterosexual partners compared to males, while males engaged

Table 8.2 Prevalence rates of electronic TDV

Form of electronic TDV	Percentage
Text checking	
10+ per hour	27.0
50+ per hour	9.0
Hourly 12 am–5 am	24.0
E-mail checking	
10+ per hour	21.0
Bullying via text	
Sexual request	22.0
Spread rumor	19.0
Send embarrassing picture	11.0
Called names	25.0
Threatened	10.0

in higher rates of more serious violence (i.e., beat up, choke, strangle; Archer, 2002). Other studies have found that 28–33% of girls reported engaging in physical TDV, compared to 11–20% of males who reported engaging in similar behavior; however, rates of sexual perpetration were higher for males and ranged between 3–37% while rates were 2–24% for females (see Hickman, Jaycox, & Aronoff, 2004 for a review). Despite the fact that TDV perpetration might be fairly equal between males and females it is important to highlight that (1) adolescent female aggression often stems from self-defense, while male aggression stems from the desire for power and control; (2) adolescent males often engage in more serious forms of violence compared to adolescent females; and (3) compared to adolescent males, females reported greater injury, fear, and psychological consequences as a result of TDV victimization (see Edwards, Dardis, & Gidycz, 2011 for a review). Overall, a large number of US youth are involved in both in-person TDV and cyber-TDV, indicating that many adolescents are at risk for the negative consequences associated with TDV.

8.2.2 Negative Consequences of Teen Dating Violence

Similar to the other forms of interpersonal violence we have discussed thus far (school-based bullying—Chap. 3, cyberbullying—Chap. 5, child abuse—Chap. 6, sibling violence—Chap. 6, college hazing—Chap. 7), TDV causes and is associated with a number of negative consequences for victims. TDV is a relatively new field of study and in depth research began in about 2000 (Offenhauer & Buchalter, 2011), yet in the short intervening time period, a number of studies have confirmed the multiple negative outcomes caused by and associated with TDV including increased substance use, poor mental health, poor grades, decreased close social relationships, increased antisocial behavior, and an increased risk for future intimate partner victimization (e.g., Exner-Cortens, Eckenrode, & Rothman, 2013; Foshee, Reyes, Gottredson, Chang, & Ennett, 2013; Roberts, Klein, & Fisher, 2003).

For example, one 2.5-year longitudinal study of 3328 adolescents in grades 8 through 12 found that psychological TDV predicted increased alcohol use and physical TDV predicted increased cigarette use and increased marijuana use (for girls only). In terms of mental health outcomes, psychological TDV predicted increased internalizing symptoms for girls (findings were marginally significant for boys), and physical TDV was marginally predictive of having fewer close friends for boys (Foshee et al., 2013). The National Longitudinal Study of Adolescent Health includes surveys of 5681 youth ages 12–18 and found that TDV significantly predicted worse outcomes 5 years later relative to youth who did not endure TDV. Specifically, females who experienced TDV reported increased episodic drinking, smoking, depression, suicidal ideation, and intimate partner violence and males who were victimized through TDV reported increased antisocial behavior, suicidal ideation, marijuana use, and intimate partner violence victimization (Exner-Cortens et al., 2013). Although these longitudinal studies are of short duration (2.5 and 5 years, respectively), they provide preliminary evidence for the fact that experiencing TDV in adolescence results in poor mental health such as increased depression and suicidal ideation, increased substance use (i.e., alcohol, tobacco, marijuana), and most alarming, increased risk for future intimate partner violence victimization. Taken together, these findings suggest that TDV victimization in adolescence can set the stage for ongoing involvement in future violent relationships as well as a host of other risky behaviors.

Being victimized in an adolescent relationship might prime youth to think that relationships are based on power and control and that abusive behavior is a normal part of intimate relationships. Adolescents are vulnerable and impressionable and early intimate dating relationship experiences can potentially create a template for future relationships. Thus, if an early dating relationship is abusive, youth might actually be drawn to future partners who replicate this early learned pattern of abuse. Indeed, a cognitive template with a victimization narrative may result from the TDV experience, leaving victims to anticipate similar outcomes in future relationships. The depression and self-esteem difficulties that result from the past abuse may also guide future expectations of intimate relationships, creating a self-propagating cycle which would warrant therapeutic intervention. This could especially be true if youth have witnessed domestic violence between their parents or been the victims of child abuse, which could both serve as past traumas that impact the person's world view of abusive interpersonal relationships being normal.

Given the short duration of research on dating violence, more cross-sectional studies (as opposed to longitudinal studies) of associated risk factors have been conducted. The 2009 National Youth Risk Behavior Survey found that 20% of youth who reported getting D's/F's also reported being victims of TDV. The percentage of TDV victimization decreased as grades increased: 12% of those who received mostly C's were victims, 9% of those who received B's, and only 6% of those who received A's were TDV victims. These findings were statistically significant ($p < 0.001$), indicating that youth receiving higher grades were statistically significantly less likely to be victims of TDV compared to youth receiving lower grades (CDC, n.d.). Given the cross-sectional nature of these data it is not possible to ascertain if TDV caused decreased grades or if getting low grades was a risk factor for TDV, but this research indicates that TDV is associated with lower grades. It is also possible that adolescents with higher grades spend less time dating. Another study of 4443 adolescents found that TDV was associated with increased depression for both males and females and increased substance use, antisocial behavior, and suicidal behavior for females only (Roberts et al., 2003). Other studies confirm that TDV was associated with posttraumatic stress disorder, major depressive episodes (Wolitzky-Taylor et al., 2008), suicide attempts, disordered eating, decreased self-esteem (Ackard & Neumark-Sztainer, 2002), illicit substance use (i.e., binge drinking, inhalants, cocaine-girls only), fighting (boys only), multiple sexual partners, and nonuse of condoms (Howard & Wang, 2003a, 2003b). Quite alarmingly, in a sample of 81,247 high school students from Minnesota, 50% of youth reporting both TDV and date rape also reported attempting suicide. Girls who experienced both of these events were over five times more likely and boys were more than six times as likely to attempt or contemplate suicide compared to their non-involved counterparts (Ackard & Neumark-Sztainer, 2002). Taken together, these findings highlight that TDV victimization is connected to a host of long- and short-term negative outcomes. Given the lasting negative impact of TDV, it is vital to understand why this form of violence occurs.

8.2.3 Risk Factors for Teen Dating Violence

When discussing the causes of TDV, researchers refer to the risk factors that increase the likelihood for engaging in TDV perpetration or for being a victim of TDV, however, these risk factors are correlates of TDV and cannot necessarily be considered direct causes (Offenhauer & Buchalter, 2011). For example, one systematic review uncovered 20 articles examining the risk and protective factors for engaging in TDV perpetration. Overall, 19 articles identified 53 risk factors that led to an increased risk of TDV perpetration; however, 7 specific risk factors were found across multiple studies including: depression, general aggression, previous dating violence, engagement in peer violence, having friends who engage in TDV perpetration, race/ethnicity, and parental marital conflict. Only three studies identified a variety of protective factors which were found to prevent TDV which included: high cognitive dissonance about TDV (i.e., a perpetrator realized what he/she was doing was wrong), high empathy, high grade point average, high verbal IQ, positive maternal relationship, and school attachment (Vagi et al., 2013). These findings suggest that prior aggression, violence, and engagement in TDV increased the likelihood of future TDV, which makes sense given that past behavior is the best predictor of future behavior. Further, the lack of findings on significant protective factors (i.e., only three articles identified significant protective factors) is worrisome and indicates a lack of research on protective factors related to TDV.

In general, risk factors for TDV involvement span multiple ecological levels including individual, family, peer, and community levels (Offenhauer & Buchalter,

2011). It is important to note that some of the negative consequences of TDV victimization noted above are also risk factors for TDV victimization; thus, consequences of TDV victimization and causes of TDV victimization become somewhat of a chicken and the egg conundrum. For example, low self-esteem was associated with TDV victimization (Ackard & Neumark-Sztainer, 2002) which means it could be both a cause and a consequence and is thus discussed as both. Low self-esteem could make it difficult for an adolescent to stand up for him/herself and might make him/her believe he/she deserves to be treated badly, which would make him/her a prime target for a TDV perpetrator. However, being victimized by TDV would certainly cause self-esteem to decrease. Thus, it is difficult to sort out if low self-esteem contributed to the initial onset of TDV by making someone a desirable victim, and then victimization caused self-esteem to decrease further or if low self-esteem was the result of enduring TDV. The answer depends on the situation, but it is important to keep in mind that both the causes and consequences of TDV are intertwined. While more longitudinal research is needed to explore pathways of effects, it is critical to note that depression, aggression, peer violence, and parental marital conflict/aggression all cluster into a toxic environment for adolescent development that sets the stage for TDV and various other forms of bullying that we discuss in this book.

There are a myriad of individual factors that put youth at increased risk for engagement in TDV and low socioeconomic status is one of the most prominent risk factors for both TDV victimization and perpetration (Ackard, Neumark-Sztainer, & Hannan, 2003; Foshee et al., 2009; see Offenhauer & Buchalter, 2011 for a review). Other individual factors associated with an increased risk for TDV involvement are mental-health problems such as low self-esteem (TDV victims—Ackard & Neumark-Sztainer, 2002), anxiety, depression (female TDV perpetrators—Chase, Treboux, & O'Leary, 2002), externalizing behavior (male TDV perpetrators—Chase et al., 2002), suicidality (female TDV victims—Howard, Wang, & Yan, 2007) as well as difficulty taking responsibility for ones actions (male TDV perpetrators-Feiiring, Deblinger, Hoch-Espada, & Haworth, 2002). In addition, family factors, such as childhood maltreatment (discussed in Chap. 6) was associated with increased risk for verbal, physical, and sexual dating violence perpetration and victimization (Foshee, Benefield, Ennett, Bauman, & Suchindran, 2004; Foshee, Ennett, Bauman, Benefield, & Suchindran, 2005); maltreated males and those who have witnessed parental conflict are at a particular increased risk for TDV perpetration (Kingsfogel & Grych, 2004; Lavoie et al., 2002). Indeed, witnessing martial violence sets an example for adolescents that interpersonal violence is acceptable, which could serve to justify TDV perpetration (see Offenhauer & Buchalter, 2011 for a review).

The peer group also presents a source of risk for TDV perpetration and early association with antisocial peers increases the likelihood of TDV perpetration (Schnurr, 2009). Interestingly, research indicates that the impact of violent peers on future TDV perpetration is stronger than the impact of familial violence, highlighting the strong influence that adolescent peers have on each other's behavior (Arriaga & Foshee, 2004). Further, Hispanic and African American males engaged in community violence were more likely to report TDV perpetration (Gorman-Smith, Tolan, Sheidow, & Henry, 2003), suggesting an overlap between these two forms of violence, such that engaging in community violence might normalize violent behavior, making it part of youths' everyday lives, including dating relationships. Overall, there are many risk factors in youths' lives across multiple ecological levels that put them at risk for engagement in TDV and paramount among these factors is exposure to multiple forms of bullying, aggression, and violence in the environment. This confirms hypotheses purported by social learning theory that adolescents learn how to be in the world through the behavior that is modeled by others, particularly others who have significance and emotional salience in the adolescent's ecology (i.e., parents, siblings, peers; Bandura, 1977, 1997). Toxic behaviors would be introduced in an adolescent's relationships through observation and imitation of interactions he or she sees from other salient actors. These reflections of perpetration and victimization are consequently linked and disseminated across different parts of a toxic ecology (i.e., parental conflict to TDV, peer aggression to TDV, sibling aggression to TDV).

To better understand the TDV dynamic, we will use the bullying framework. The dynamics delineated in the discussion above clearly show that TDV has the bullying components of intent to harm, repetition over time, and power imbalance. Considering the intensity and turbulence of teenage relationships, adolescent romantic love may be augmented by the novelty of physical and psychological intimacy, leading to high levels of personal disclosure and shared vulnerability. Cultural messages in films and music commonly depict romance as powerful, dramatic, turbulent, stormy, and rough. Sexuality and conflict are both narrated as intensely emotional and necessary for true romance. When adolescent romance fades, however, there are far fewer cultural narratives to help navigate this difficult territory. Sharing and caring transforms to hurt, frustration, jealousy, and despair, often prompting one wounded partner to nurture the intent to harm the other partner in order to get revenge. A TDV bully is born when he or she combines this new intent to harm with a plan to use physical or psychological power over the other partner.

In TDV, there are unique aspects to the power imbalance. In playground politics in middle school, bullies may be stronger physically or have more resources or social status to fuel a power imbalance with the victim. TDV bullies may be physically larger, but the psychological power imbalance may not surface until romance is waning and emotional reinforcement is cut off. In that context, power comes from the ability to hurt one's partner. Physical intimidation, social humiliation in person or online, or damaging the former partner's reputation are all viable strategics to seek revenge, feel empowered, and cover up one's feelings of sensitivity and rejection. Unfortunately, the intent to harm and power imbalance are super charged in TDV because the bully now knows the victims' innermost sensitivities. It is terribly unpleasant to be abused by someone you hate on a middle school playground; however, being abused by someone you loved and trusted, and perhaps lost your virginity to, is a different order of intensity for the resulting pain and suffering.

8.3 Intimate Partner Violence

8.3.1 *Overview: Definition, Prevalence Rates*

Intimate partner violence (IPV) refers to physical violence, sexual violence, stalking, or psychological aggression (e.g., coercive acts) by a current or former intimate partner (i.e., spouse, boy/girlfriend, dating partner, ongoing sexual partner). Physical violence includes the intentional use of physical force (e.g., pushing, shoving, choking, punching, use of weapon) to cause harm. Sexual violence is any sexual act committed without the consent of the victim such as forced penetration, alcohol/drug facilitated penetration, or sexual touching. Stalking is a repeated pattern of unwanted attention that engenders fear for one's safety or the safety of someone else (e.g., family, friend). Finally, psychological aggression is the use of verbal and non-verbal communication to emotionally or mentally harm another person and/or control another person (e.g., humiliating; name calling; limiting access to money, friends, or family; monitoring persons whereabouts; threating violence; Breiding, Basile, Smith, Black, & Mahendra, 2015). A significant number of US adults are victims of IPV.

The National Intimate Partner and Sexual Violence Survey (NISVS) is a national random-digit-dial telephone survey of the US population over age 18. The most recent NISVS was completed in 2011 and included 12,727 full interviews and 1428 partial interviews. Findings indicated that more than one in five women (22.3%) and one in ten men (14.0%) experienced physical IPV over their lifetime and 2.3% of women and 2.1% of men experienced this form of IPV in the last year. An estimated 8.8% of women and 0.5% of men were raped by an intimate partner over their lifetime (0.8% of women were raped in the past year by their intimate partner), and 15.8% of women and 9.5% of men experienced another form of sexual IPV over their lifetime (2.1% of men and women experienced another form of sexual IPV in the past year). In terms of stalking, 9.2% of women and 2.4% of men reported stalking by an intimate partner over their lifetime while 2.5% of women and 0.8% of men reported IPV stalking within the past year (Breiding et al., 2014). In total, about 1.3 million women and 835,000 men experience physical IPV each year in the USA (Tjaden & Thoennes, 2000). While these prevalence rates indicate that a higher percentage of women are the victims of IPV, the above national data highlights the fact that men are also often victimized, indicating that millions of US adults are at risk for the negative outcomes associated with IPV (see Table 8.3).

8.3.2 *Negative Consequences of Intimate Partner Violence*

There is some overlap between the negative consequences of IPV and the negative consequences associated with TDV discussed above (e.g., poor mental and physical health, increased substance use). However, the samples in studies examining the

Table 8.3 Prevalence rates of IPV

	Lifetime	Past 12 months
Physical IPV		
Female	22.3%	2.3%
Male	14.0%	2.1%
Rape IPV		
Female	8.8%	0.8%
Male	0.5%	N/A
Other sexual IPV		
Female	15.8%	2.1%
Male	9.5%	2.1%
Stalking		
Female	9.2%	2.5%
Male	2.4%	0.8%

consequences of IPV are usually adults as opposed to the adolescent samples used in TDV research. Thus, a brief discussion of the negative consequence of IPV will follow.

A serious consequence of IPV is physical injury, ranging from minor injuries to death (Black, 2011). In fact, for women, 2 million injuries and 1300 deaths result from IPV every year (National Center for Injury Prevention and Control, 2003). In addition to physical injury, IPV is associated with an increased risk of negative health outcomes impacting the brain and nervous system (e.g., headaches, seizures, traumatic brain injury), cardiovascular system (e.g., stroke, hypertension, cardiovascular disease), gastrointestinal system (e.g., stomach ulcers, gastric reflux, diarrhea), genitourinary system (e.g., bladder/kidney infections), immune and endocrine system (e.g., chronic pain, inflammation, diabetes), musculoskeletal system (e.g., broken bones, arthritis, functional impairment), and reproductive system (e.g., poor sexual health, chronic pelvic pain). In addition, victims of IPV are at an increased risk for somatic symptoms (e.g., chronic fatigue, chronic pain, fibromyalgia), poor pregnancy outcomes (e.g., neonatal death, preterm delivery, abortion), poor mental health outcomes (e.g., depression, suicidality, posttraumatic stress disorder), health risk behaviors (e.g., heavy drinking, smoking, lack of medical care), and overall poor health (e.g., chronic health conditions, asthma, poor physical health; see Centers for Disease Control and Prevention, 2018 for a review; see Black, 2011 for a review). Both men and women victimized by IPV are almost 1.5–2 times more likely to smoke and/or engage in heavy/binge drinking compared to their counterparts not victimized by IPV (Breiding, Black, & Ryan, 2008). And women victimized by IPV are more likely to engage in other risky behaviors compared to women not victimized by IPV (e.g., substance abuse, suicide attempts, alcoholism; Centers for Disease Control and Prevention, 2018). It appears that there is a dose response relationship between IPV and negative outcomes and the more severe the IPV, the stronger the relationships between IPV and the negative outcomes including high risk sexual behavior (e.g., unprotected sex, multiple sexual partners, trading sex for food or money), substance use (e.g., smoking, drinking, drug use), and unhealthy diet related behaviors (e.g., fasting, overeating, vomiting; Centers for Disease Control and Prevention, 2018). Taken together, victims of IPV are at risk for a host of negative psychological, emotional, physical, and behavioral outcomes.

8.3.3 Risk Factors for Intimate Partner Violence

There are a variety of risk factors that are associated with an increased likelihood of IPV. Similar to the risk factors for TDV, risk factors for IPV span multiple ecological levels including the individual (e.g., prior aggression, age, substance use, poverty, unemployment), family (e.g., witnessed parental IPV, childhood abuse), and social relationships (e.g., social support).

The strongest risk factor for both IPV perpetrators and victims was a record of aggressive delinquency prior to age 15 (Moffitt & Caspi, 1999). This finding suggests that youth who engage in early aggression might become accustomed to behaving violently and witnessing violence and are therefore more likely to engage in later violence in the form of IPV and also to spend time with violent individuals who could victimize them. Early parenthood is also a risk factor for IPV and women who had children by age 21 were twice as likely to be IPV victims compared to non-mothers and men who had children by age 21 were three times more likely than non-fathers to be IPV perpetrators (Moffitt & Caspi, 1999). In general, age is a protective factor for IPV and the risk of IPV decreases with age (see Capaldi, Knoble, Shortt, & Kim, 2012 for a review). While increased substance use is a negative potential consequence of IPV victimization, it is also an associated risk factor for IPV perpetrators. Perpetrators are more likely than victims to engage in substance use and one study found that 80% of males who killed or abused a female partner had an issue with alcohol the year before the incident and two thirds of homicide and attempted homicide offenders used alcohol, drugs, or both during the incident (Sharps, Campbell, Campbell, Gary, & Webster, 2003). Poverty is another individual risk factor for IPV and research suggests that a higher income is correlated with a lower rate of IPV. The stress of poverty is overwhelming, which can negatively impact the perpetrator by decreasing patience and increasing anger and hostility, but poverty might also make the victim dependent upon the perpetrator and make it difficult for the victim to leave (see Carlson, Worden, van Ryn, & Bachman, 2000 for a review). Related to poverty and income, researchers have found that unemployment is associated with increased IPV (see Capaldi et al., 2012 for a review).

There are also family level risk factors for IPV including witnessing IPV between parents and being the victim of child abuse. Both witnessing abuse and being abused increased the risk for IPV perpetration and victimization (see Capaldi et al., 2012 for a review). Childhood exposure to IPV and child abuse normalizes interpersonal violence and puts youth at risk for later IPV involvement. Social relationships can serve as a huge source of support and social support has been found to decrease the risk of IPV victimization and perpetration, so a lack of support can be considered a risk factor (see Capaldi et al., 2012 for a review). Individual, family, and social factors are among the most influential risk factors for IPV.

8.4 Teen Dating Violence and Intimate Partner Violence Through the Bullying Framework

In the following section, we apply the three fundamental definitional components of traditional bullying (repetition, power imbalance, and intent to harm) to TDV and IPV. TDV and IPV share common characteristics with traditional bullying and can be considered severe forms of bullying within intimate partner relationships.

8.4.1 Repetition

By definition, TDV and IPV are considered to be a pattern of abusive behaviors that occur repeatedly over the course of time (Break the Cycle, 2014). Clearly, repetition is a key element in both TDV and IPV and is an important element of partner violence (Hebert, Van Camp, Lavoie, Blais, & Guerrier, 2014). As mentioned in Chap. 6 in regard to child abuse, it is conceivable that an isolated incident of TDV or IPV could occur; however, this is the exception rather than the norm. Generally, TDV and IPV represent a pattern of repeated and ongoing abusive behavior. Indeed, one study found that a third of female IPV victims experienced more than three incidents of violence from the perpetrator of their worst IPV incident. And when IPV was defined as non-sexual threats and force, on average, women experienced about 20 incidents per year; however, this mean was inflated by women with a very high number of incidents and the median number of incidents per year was 4 (Walby & Allen, 2004).

TDV has little data on repetition due to the field being so new. We can extrapolate that most TDV comes from within ongoing relationships, thus meeting the threshold for repetition. A single violent event may be considered assault, but the potential for the repeated occurrence and variable nature of the victimization (physical/psychological/cyber) all make it likely that there is a temporal component that is salient.

Just like the repetition inherent in school bullying dynamics, the repetition of TDV and IPV is part of what makes this form of abuse so devastating for victims. Research indicates that the more severe IPV is, the worse the developmental outcomes (Centers for Disease Control and Prevention, 2018). It is likely that IPV (and TDV) repetition might have a similar dose response relationship and the longer victims endure TDV and IPV over time, the worse consequences the victim suffers. The repeated nature of TDV and IPV means that victims are repeatedly exposed to trauma at the hands of their partner. The more that TDV and IPV are repeated, the harder it is for victims to extricate themselves from the harmful relationship. The repeated violence inherent in TDV and IPV could paralyze victims in fear and prevent them from leaving the relationship. Indeed, few victims of IPV leave. For example, in a large-scale study across ten countries, only between 19% and 51% of women who experienced physical IPV left their partner for at least one night and between 8% and 21% left 2–5 times while the vast majority (between 49% and 81%) reported never leaving (Garcia-Moreno, Jansen, Ellsberg, Heise, & Watts, 2005). These data highlight how few female victims of IPV leave their partners. It is possible that the repeated violence inherent in IPV is so terrifying that victims are unable to leave. Alternately, the fact that violence happens between partners who once shared a loving bond may make it harder to leave a potentially intimate relationship; some victims may not leave because they still care for their abuser.

Further, youth victimized by traditional school-based bullying were more likely to have experienced physical and emotional dating violence than their non-bullied peers (Debnam, Bradshaw, & Waasdorp, 2016). This finding suggests that the repeated nature of school-based bullying might turn some youth into chronic victims who are bullied repeatedly at school and then are victimized repeatedly by dating partners. These adolescents who experience multiple victimizations may be desperate to maintain interpersonal relationships despite the abuse. They may have a deeply ingrained role being the victim that recreates itself in different social situations. Dominant peers may sense this and take advantage—all while the chronically victimized teen is struggling to make some type of connection. The repeated nature of bullying, TDV, and IPV intensifies the negative impact of these harmful forms of violence.

8.4.2 *Power Imbalance*

Similar to school-based bullying discussed in Chap. 1, power imbalance is central to both TDV and IPV. As soon as TDV or IPV begins, the perpetrator has more power than the victim. In some cases, the power differential might not appear until the violence begins when the perpetrator immediately gains power over the victim through use of violence or coercion. However, in other cases, one partner in the relationship might already have more power due to gender (e.g., males often have more social power than females), income (e.g., one partner might have more financial resources than the other), race (e.g., people of color often suffer from racism and discrimination that white people do not endure), or physical size (i.e., one partner might be physically larger and stronger). If the more powerful partner is also the perpetrator, the violence serves to strengthen the existing power imbalance. However, if the less powerful partner engages in violence then the violence becomes a means of equaling the playing field and perhaps even makes the less powerful partner more powerful.

The power differential in TDV and IPV is another reason why victims might not leave—they are afraid of the powerful perpetrator. Perpetrators often threaten victims and/or their loved ones, stating that they will hurt or kill the victim or his/her family/close friends if the victim leaves. The powerful fear that these threats engender keep the victim silently trapped in the abusive relationship. Further, perpetrators might use physical strength, threats, or coercion to subdue victims, perhaps by physically harming the victim if he/she tries to leave or by cutting off the victims' access to financial resources. Empowering victims is one way to help them extricate themselves from a TDV or IPV relationship. As long as victims feel powerless, they will remain in the abusive relationship and the power differential will continue. However, empowering victims is one way of weakening the power differential and helping victims' escape. Thus, it is extremely important for practitioners to be aware of the power differential inherent in TDV and IPV situations so that they can try and empower victims and lessen the power differential.

As mentioned above in the TDV discussion, we believe power imbalance in TDV and IPV is a particularly important aspect of this form of bullying. Any person who has experienced the end of an intimate relationship can attest to the fact that there is more power in being the partner who terminates the relationship (i.e., the "rejecter") rather than the rejected partner. This fear of being rejected may lead the victim to continue with the abuse rather than to leave, being alone may seem like a worse fate. The bully's awareness that the abusive tactics are effective in keeping his or her partner powerless also feeds into and intensifies the imbalance.

8.4.3 *Intent to Harm*

As discussed in Chap. 1, intent to harm is very tricky because only the perpetrator truly knows his/her intent. Further, even if the intent of the perpetrator is not to cause harm, but to gain power or popularity, the victim still endures harm. That is why in Chap. 1 we amended the definition of bullying to state not that harm was intended, but that harm was caused. Without a doubt, victims of TDV and IPV are harmed regardless of the perpetrator's intent. In some cases of TDV and IPV the perpetrator's main goal is to maintain power and control; however, the victim is undoubtedly harmed, as discussed in the consequences section above (Sects. 8.2.2 and 8.3.2). Harm is the means of obtaining power and control. The multiple negative consequences associated with both TDV and IPV discussed above highlight the harm these forms of violence cause and indicate that regardless of the perpetrator's intent, harm is caused.

In most cases, the bully fully intends to cause harm. For TDV and IPV victims, this harm is particularly tragic because it comes from a person who previously was a confidante, companion, or lover. The prior physical and psychological intimacy makes intent to harm immeasurably powerful. The nude photo that was so cute to share while sexting becomes a psychological nuclear bomb when disseminated on Instagram. Personal secrets shared during times when support was needed now become fodder for gossip. There is a bitter sense of deep betrayal when the person you once loved transforms into the one you hate the most. And this explosive intent to harm unfolds either in the presence of peer groups for TDV or in view of family members (i.e., children watching) for IPV, adding shame and humiliation. Unfortunately, the harm caused is often permanent and the consequences severe for victims.

8.5 Conclusions

Both TDV and IPV are harmful forms of interpersonal violence where victims are physically, psychologically, and/or emotionally abused by their intimate partner. The numerous negative consequences of TDV and IPV include poor mental health (e.g., depression, anxiety), poor physical health (e.g., physical injury, chronic pain), increased substance use, and increased involvement in violent relationships. These two related forms of violence are repeated over time, involve a power imbalance where the perpetrator has more power than the victim, and cause harm to the victim. In this regard, TDV and IPV can be understood as severe forms of bullying where the perpetrator uses physical force and coercive techniques to control the victim. Using this framework helps partially explain why victims often remain in an abusive relationship—the repeated violence creates a power differential that leaves victims feeling helpless and unable to leave. There is a faint hope that the intimacy that once characterized the relationship might somehow return. And perhaps being abused but together is better than being alone. Considering the linkages among violence categories that foster polyvictimization experiences over time, it is important to provide victims with therapeutic intervention. Practitioners working with victims of TDV and IPV should focus on empowering victims in order to decrease the power imbalance, changing cognitive narratives concerning victimization so that they do not keep propagating, and providing hope that human relations do not have to consistently be characterized by bullying.

References

Ackard, D. M., & Neumark-Sztainer, D. (2002). Date violence and date rape among adolescents: Associations with disordered eating behaviors and psychological health. *Child Abuse & Neglect, 26*(5), 455–473.

Ackard, D. M., Neumark-Sztainer, D., & Hannan, P. J. (2003). Dating violence among a nationally representative sample of adolescent girls and boys: Associations with behavior and mental health. *Journal of Gender-Specific Medicine, 6*(3), 39–48.

Archer, J. (2002). Sex differences in physically aggressive acts between heterosexual dating partners: A meta-analytic review. *Aggression and Violent Behavior, 7*, 313–351.

Arriaga, X. B., & Foshee, V. A. (2004). Adolescent dating violence: Do adolescents follow in their friends' or their parents' footsteps. *Journal of Interpersonal Violence, 19*(2), 162–184.

Bandura, A. (1977). *Social learning theory*. New York, NY: General Learning Press.

Bandura, A. (1997). *Self-efficacy: The exercise of control*. New York, NY: W.H. Freeman.

Black, M. C. (2011). Intimate partner violence and adverse health consequences: Implications for clinicians. *American Journal of Lifestyle Medicine, 5*, 428–439. https://doi.org/10.1177/1559827611410265

Break the Cycle. (2014). *What is dating abuse?* Retrieved from https://www.breakthecycle.org/learn-about-dating-abuse

Breiding, M. J., Basile, K. C., Smith, S. G., Black, M. C., & Mahendra, R. R. (2015). *Intimate partner violence surveillance: Uniform definitions and recommended data elements, Version 2.0.* Atlanta, GA: National Center for Injury Prevention and Control, Centers for Disease Control and Prevention.

Breiding, M. J., Black, M. C., & Ryan, G. W. (2008). Chronic disease and health risk behaviors associated with intimate partner violence—18 U.S. states/territories, 2005. *Annals of Epidemiology, 18*, 538–544. https://doi.org/10.1016/j.annepidem.2008.02.005

Breiding, M. J., Smith, S. G., Basile, K. C., Walters, M. L., Chen, J., & Merrick, M. T. (2014). Prevalence and characteristics of sexual violence, stalking, and intimate partner violence victimization—National intimate partner and sexual violence survey, United States, 2011. *Morbidity and Mortality Weekly Report, 63*(SS08), 1–18.

Capaldi, D. M., Knoble, N. B., Shortt, J. W., & Kim, H. K. (2012). A systematic review of risk factors for intimate partner violence. *Partner Abuse, 3*(2), 231–280.

Carlson, B. E., Worden, A. P., van Ryn, M., & Bachman, R. (2000). *Violence against women: Synthesis of research for service providers.* Final report to the National Institute of Justice. Washington, DC: U.S. Department of Justice, National Institute of Justice, NCJ 199578.

Centers for Disease Control and Prevention. (2018). *Intimate partner violence: Consequences.* Retrieved from https://www.cdc.gov/violenceprevention/intimatepartnerviolence/consequences.html

Centers for Disease Control and Prevention. (n.d.). *Unintentional injury and violence-related behaviors and academic achievement.* Retrieved from https://www.cdc.gov/healthyyouth/health_and_academics/pdf/unintentional_injury_violence.pdf

Centers for Disease Control and Prevention, National Center for Injury Prevention and Control, Division of Violence Prevention. (2016). *Understanding teen dating violence: Fact sheet.* Retrieved from https://www.cdc.gov/violenceprevention/pdf/teen-dating-violence-factsheet-a.pdf

Chase, K. A., Treboux, D., & O'Leary, K. D. (2002). Characteristics of high-risk adolescents' dating violence. *Journal of Interpersonal Violence, 17*(1), 33–49.

Debnam, K. J., Bradshaw, C. P., & Waasdorp, T. E. (2016). Examining the contemporaneous occurrence of bullying and teen dating violence victimization. *School Psychology Quarterly, 31*(1), 76–90.

Edwards, K. M., Dardis, C. M., & Gidycz, C. A. (2011). The role of victimization experiences in adolescent girls and young women's aggression in dating relationships. In M. A. Paludi (Ed.), *The psychology of violence and victimization: Prevention strategies for families and schools* (Vol. 2, pp. 71–85). Santa Barbara, CA: Praeger.

Exner-Cortens, D., Eckenrode, J., & Rothman, E. (2013). Longitudinal associations between teen dating violence victimization and adverse health outcomes. *Pediatrics, 131*(1), 71–78.

Feiiring, C., Deblinger, E., Hoch-Espada, A., & Haworth, T. (2002). Romantic relationships aggression and attitudes in highs school students: The role of gender, grade, and attachment and emotional styles. *Journal of Youth and Adolescence, 31*(5), 373–385.

Foshee, V. A., Benefield, T., Suchindran, C., Ennett, S. T., Karriker-Jaffe, K. J., Reyes, H. H. M., & Mathias, J. (2009). The development of four types of adolescent dating abuse and selected demographic correlates. *Journal of Research on Adolescence, 19*(3), 380–400.

Foshee, V. A., Benefield, T. S., Ennett, S. T., Bauman, K. E., & Suchindran, C. (2004). Longitudinal predictors of serious physical and sexual dating violence victimization during adolescence. *Preventive Medicine, 39*, 1007–1016.

Foshee, V. A., Ennett, S. T., Bauman, K. E., Benefield, T., & Suchindran, C. (2005). The association between family violence and adolescent dating violence onset: Does it vary by race, socioeconomic status, and family structure? *The Journal of Early Adolescence, 25*(3), 317–344.

Foshee, V. A., Reyes, H. L. M., Gottredson, N. C., Chang, L., & Ennett, S. T. (2013). A longitudinal examination of psychological, behavioral, academic, and relationship consequences of dating abuse victimization among a primarily rural sample of adolescents. *Journal of Adolescent Health, 53*, 723–729.

Garcia-Moreno, C., Jansen, H. A. F. M., Ellsberg, M., Heise, L., & Watts, C. (2005). *WHO multi-country study on women's health and domestic violence against women: Initial results on prevalence, health outcomes and women's responses*. Geneva, Switzerland: World Health Organization.

Gorman-Smith, D., Tolan, P. H., Sheidow, A. J., & Henry, D. B. (2003). Partner violence and street violence among urban adolescents: Do the same family factors relate? *Journal of Research on Adolescence, 11*(3), 273–295.

Halpern, C. T., Oslak, S. G., Young, M. L., Martin, S. L., & Kupper, L. L. (2001). Partner violence among adolescents in opposite-sex romantic relationships: Findings from the National Longitudinal Study of Adolescent Health. *American Journal of Public Health, 91*(10), 1679–1685.

Halpern, C. T., Young, M. L., Waller, M. W., Martin, S. L., & Kupper, L. L. (2004). Prevalence of partner violence in same-sex romantic and sexual relationships in a national sample of adolescents. *Journal of Adolescent Health, 35*(2), 124–131.

Hebert, M., Van Camp, T., Lavoie, F., Blais, M., & Guerrier, M. (2014). Understanding the hesitancy to disclose teen dating violence: Correlates of self-efficacy to deal with teen dating violence. *Temida, 17*(4), 43–64.

Hickman, L. J., Jaycox, L. H., & Aronoff, J. (2004). Dating violence among adolescents: Prevalence, gender distribution, and prevention program effectiveness. *Trauma, Violence, & Abuse, 5*(2), 123–142.

Howard, D. E., & Wang, M. Q. (2003a). Risk profiles of adolescent girls who were victims of dating violence. *Adolescence, 38*(149), 1–14.

Howard, D. E., & Wang, M. Q. (2003b). Psychosocial factors associated with adolescent boys' reports of dating violence. *Adolescence, 38*(151), 519–533.

Howard, D. E., Wang, M. Q., & Yan, F. (2007). Psychosocial factors associated with reports of physical dating violence among U.S. adolescent females. *Adolescence, 42*(166), 311–324.

Kann, L., McManus, T., Harris, W. A., Shanklin, S. I., Flint, K. H., Hawkins, J., … Zaza, S. (2016). Youth risk behavior surveillance—United States, 2015. *Morbidity and Mortality Weekly Report, 65*(6), 1–174.

Kingsfogel, K. M., & Grych, J. H. (2004). Interparental conflict and adolescent dating relationships: Integrating cognitive, emotional, and peer influences. *Journal of Family Psychology, 18*(3), 505–515.

Lavoie, F., Robitaille, L., Hebert, M., Tremblay, R., Vitaro, F., Veina, L., & McDuff, P. (2002). History of family dysfunction and perpetration of dating violence by adolescent boys: A longitudinal study. *Journal of Adolescent Health, 30*(5), 375–383.

Moffitt, T. E., & Caspi, A. (1999). *Finding about partner violence from the Dunedin multidisciplinary health and development study. Research Brief.* Washington, DC: U.S. Department of Justice, National Institute of Justice, NCJ 170018.

National Center for Injury Prevention and Control. (2003). *Costs of intimate partner violence against women in the United States*. Atlanta, GA: Centers for Disease Control and Prevention. Retrieved from http://www.cdc.gov/violenceprevention/pub/IPV_cost.html

National Institute of Justice. (2016). *Prevalence of teen dating violence*. Retrieved from https://www.nij.gov/topics/crime/intimate-partner-violence/teen-dating-violence/pages/prevalence.aspx#note2

Nguyen, B. (2017, February 22). *Teen dating violence: Kim's story. Break the silence against domestic violence*. Retrieved from http://www.breakthesilencedv.org/teen-dating-violence-kims-story/

Offenhauer, P., & Buchalter, A. (2011). *Teen dating violence: A literature review and annotated bibliography*. Washington, DC: U.S. Department of Justice. Retrieved from https://www.ncjrs.gov/pdffiles1/nij/grants/235368.pdf

Picard, P. (2007). *Tech abuse in teen relationships study*. Liz Claiborne Inc. Retrieved from https://www.breakthecycle.org/sites/default/files/pdf/survey-lina-tech-2007.pdf

Roberts, T. A., Klein, J. D., & Fisher, S. (2003). Longitudinal effect of intimate partner abuse on high-risk behavior among adolescents. *Archives of Pediatrics and Adolescent Medicine, 157*, 875–881.

Sanchez, C. (2017, February 8). A story about teen dating violence. *The HuffPost*. Retrieved from https://www.huffingtonpost.com/crystal-sanchez/a-story-about-teen-dating_b_9191604.html

Schnurr, M. P. (2009). *Precursors to adolescents' dating violence perpetration and health romantic relationships*. Graduate Theses and Dissertations, 10369. Retrieved from http://lib.dr.iastate.edu/etd/10369

Sharps, P., Campbell, J. C., Campbell, D., Gary, F., & Webster, C. (2003). Risky mix: Drinking, drug use, and homicide. *NIJ Journal, 250*, 8–13.

Tjaden, P., & Thoennes, N. (2000). *Full report of the prevalence, incidence, and consequences of violence against women*. Washington, DC: U.S. Department of Justice, Office of Justice Programs. Retrieved from https://www.ncjrs.gov/pdffiles1/nij/183781.pdf

Vagi, J. V., Rothman, E. F., Latzman, N. E., Tharp, A. T., Hall, D. M., & Breiding, M. J. (2013). Beyond correlates: A review of risk and protective factors for adolescent dating violence perpetration. *Journal of Youth and Adolescence, 42*, 633–649.

Walby, S., & Allen, J. (2004). *Domestic violence, sexual assault and stalking: Findings from the British crime survey*. Home Office Research Study 276. London, UK: Home Office.

Wolitzky-Taylor, K. B., Ruggiero, K. J., Danielson, C. K., Resnick, H. S., Hanson, R. F., Smith, D. W., … Kilpatrick, D. G. (2008). Prevalence and correlates of dating violence in a national sample of adolescents. *Journal of the American Academy of Child and Adolescent Psychiatry, 47*(7), 755–762.

Chapter 9
Playground Politics, Power, and Privilege in the Workplace: How Bullying and Harassment Impacts Employees

9.1 Introduction

Harvey Weinstein was cofounder of Miramax films and one of the most powerful executive producers in Hollywood. He was also the largest proponent of the infamous "casting couch" (i.e., using his power as a white male to exploit young actresses trying to break into the movie business) and used his power and invulnerability to advance predatory behavior. In 2017, after many years of Mr. Weinstein's misconduct being an open secret, the New York Times and The New Yorker published stories of a 30-year pervasive pattern of Mr. Weinstein's sexual abuse against young actresses and other women starting out in the film industry. More than 80 women have accused Mr. Weinstein of sexual misconduct (13 for sexual assault or harassment and 3 for rape), while he denies any allegations of nonconsensual sex. At least 16 former and current executives and assistants who worked with Weinstein either witnessed or knew of the inappropriate behavior but did nothing for years. Indeed, assistants were tasked with setting up meetings with young actresses who would come to Mr. Weinstein's hotel room to talk about their careers and he would ask them for massages or sex. Actresses who complained or rejected his advances were removed from projects and negative stories were planted about them in the media. Mr. Weinstein hired intelligence firms and private investigators to follow his enemies, victims, and journalists who might expose him to keep them quiet. His lawyers facilitated settlements and threatened victims to remain quiet. However, 2017 seemed to be the year that society would no longer keep silent about workplace harassment and bullying. The Weinstein scandal sparked the #MeToo movement, which triggered many similar allegations against powerful men around the world (the Weinstein effect). The New York Times and The New Yorker won the 2018 Pulitzer Prize for Public Service for their reporting and the #MeToo movement went on to expose misconduct and abuse of power across multiple workplaces.

© Springer Nature Switzerland AG 2019

P. R. Smokowski, C. B. R. Evans, *Bullying and Victimization Across the Lifespan*, https://doi.org/10.1007/978-3-030-20293-4_9

For example, Charlie Rose, a world-famous journalist for the television news programs 60 Minutes, 60 Minutes II, the Charlie Rose Show on PBS, and CBS This Morning, was accused of widespread sexual misconduct by female coworkers from 1986 to 2017. Allegations included making lewd phone calls, walking around naked in the presence of coworkers, and groping breasts, buttocks, or genital areas. His PBS show was canceled, and he was fired from CBS News after investigations reported by the Washington Post published articles based on interviews with 107 current and former CBS News employees. Supervisors knew of his inappropriate behavior and over the course of Mr. Rose's 31-year career sometimes warned new employees to be leery of Mr. Rose, but no disciplinary action was taken.

In April 2018, actor and comedian Bill Cosby was found guilty of three counts of sexual assault. He was found guilty of drugging and assaulting Andrea Constand, a Temple University women's basketball operations director. Cosby, who was on the Temple University Board of Directors for many years, lured Constand to his home with overtures of mentoring. Constand was one of at least 60 accusers who alleged that the actor and comedian acted inappropriately towards them during his career from 1980 to 2004.

Since the Weinstein scandal, a partial list of other celebrities caught up with allegations of misconduct includes the following individuals with the number of accusers in parentheses: James Franco (filmmaker, unclear number of accusers); Paul Haggis (filmmaker, 4); Ben Vereen (actor, at least 2); Peter Martins (NYC Ballet, 5); Charles Dutoit (London's Royal Philharmonic Orchestra, 4); Tavis Smiley (PBS talk show host, multiple accusers); Mario Batali (celebrity chef, 4); James Levine (NY Metropolitan Opera, multiple accusers); Garrison Keillor (radio host, 1); Matt Lauer (NBC News journalist, multiple accusers); Charlie Rose (PBS and CBS News journalist, at least 9); Glenn Thrush (New York Times political journalist, 4); Russell Simmons (hip-hop mogul, multiple accusers); Jeffrey Tambor (actor, 2); Al Franken (Senator, multiple accusers); Andrew Kreisberg (Executive Producer, 19); Roy Moore (Alabama politician, at least 9); Louis C.K. (comedian, 5); Steven Seagal (actor, 3); Ed Westwick (actor, 2); Brett Ratner (director, 7); Dustin Hoffman (actor, 6); Jeremy Piven (actor, multiple accusers); Michael Oreskes (NPR news chief, 8); Kevin Spacey (actor, multiple accusers); Mark Halperin (political analyst, 12); George H.W. Bush (former US president, 7); Terry Richardson (celebrity photographer, multiple); Leon Wieseltier (literary critic, multiple); James Toback (writer and director, 238); John Besh (celebrity chef, multiple); Bob Weinstein (movie executive, 1); Oliver Stone (director, 1); Roy Price (Amazon Studios Chief, 1); Ben Affleck (actor and director, 2); Harvey Weinstein (movie executive, more than 80); and Donald Trump (president of the USA, multiple accusers; Corey, 2017). All of these high-profile misconduct cases have the common characteristics of a powerful senior person, males in all of these cases, using their status and authority to repeatedly manipulate and harass vulnerable newcomers within the same field or profession. Donald Trump most famously, and candidly, explained the workplace harassment and bullying power dynamic to Billy Bush on the Access Hollywood tape in 2016, stating:

Trump, speaking of a past flirtation: *I moved on her like a bitch. But I couldn't get there. And she was married. Then all of a sudden I see her, she's now got the big phony tits and everything. She's totally changed her look ... [Changing topic to refer to an actress they were meeting] Yeah, that's her. With the gold. I better use some Tic Tacs just in case I start kissing her. You know, I'm automatically attracted to beautiful—I just start kissing them. It's like a magnet. Just kiss. I don't even wait. And when you're a star, they let you do it. You can do anything. Grab 'em by the pussy. You can do anything.*

While dismissed by some as "locker room talk," Trump's comments accurately reflect the power and privilege that some people use to abuse vulnerable peers and coworkers. Unfortunately, workplace harassment and bullying is not isolated to these exceptionally powerful celebrities. Indeed, bullying is recognized as a negative part of modern workplaces with long-term harmful effects for both the bullied individuals as well as their workplace (Akella, 2016; Hutchinson, Vickers, Jackson, & Wilkes, 2006). All workplaces have successful authority figures ("stars" in Trump's words) who can feel invulnerable in their status, popularity, power, prestige, and privilege. These "bully bosses" may manipulate others to further their own goals and they marshal support from coworkers against victims when they feel threatened. These playground politics function in Fortune 500 companies, in fast food franchises, or at the corner grocery store in the same fashion as they play out on the elementary school playground and middle school lunch room.

The highly publicized examples given above all focus on sexual harassment; however, that is only one form of workplace bullying. Along with unwanted physical contact, workplace bullying can be any acts or comments that intend to intimidate, offend, degrade, or humiliate the targeted victim. Katie was the manager of a busy fast food store, one location in a larger franchise. Once a month, the regional manager would randomly drop by without prior notice for site inspection. He would yell and curse at any sign of inefficiency, raising the sales targets to unreasonable goals. Armando was the only Mexican-American junior associate at his law firm. He was hired by a partner who left; the other partners never invite him to important client meetings, ask him to lunch like the other associates, or refer work his way. He was only given low-level immigration cases and his request for specialized training in corporate litigation was denied. Robin hated working in her cubicle. Her office mates in the next cubicles were constantly talking about conservative politics, making offensive jokes about Democrats, and criticizing other opinions. They would pop their heads above the cubicle walls and look at what she was doing on her computer. All of these examples show nuances of workplace bullying by using power through different types of aggression.

In this chapter, we examine bullying perpetration and victimization in the workplace. First, we set forth a definition of workplace bullying, then we discuss prevalence, costs, and the impact on victims. We relate workplace bullying to other forms of perpetration and victimization and discuss salient issues in policy and practice strategies.

9.2 Overview of Workplace Bullying

9.2.1 *Definition*

The three hallmarks of the bullying dynamic established in earlier chapters—repetition, power imbalance, and intent to harm—easily match workplace bullying, abuse, and harassment. Indeed, the playground politics and power dynamics of group formation in childhood discussed earlier strongly parallel the hierarchy, sociometry (i.e., acceptance and rejection patterns), and social interactions in many corporations and agencies. Workplace bullying is thus defined as repeated, health-harming mistreatment of one or more employees (the victims) by one or more perpetrators who are also employees and have some type of power over the victims (Dudek, 2017). "Bullying involves a desire to hurt + hurtful action + power imbalance + (typically) repetitive aggressor and a sense of being oppressed by the victim" (Rigsby, 2002, p. 51). Akella (2016) defined workplace bullying as repeated hurtful negative act or acts (physical, verbal, or psychological intimidation) that use humiliation to cause fear, distress, or harm to the individual (i.e., victim). The power imbalance can be direct, such as when the bully is a supervisor (i.e., the bully boss) or indirect, such as when a clique of coworkers excludes the victim from communications, opportunities, projects, or workplace relationships. Workplace bullying behaviors often include shifting opinions, overruling the victim's decisions, professionally attacking the victim in private or in public, flaunting one's status and power, exerting excessive monitoring, unfair criticism, judging work unfairly, blocking someone's promotion, ignoring the victim, or not returning phone calls, memos, and e-mails in order to sabotage the victim's work projects (Akella, 2016; Randle, Stsevenson, & Grayling, 2007; Yildirim, 2009).

Similar to other forms of bullying, the abusive behavior is threatening, humiliating, or intimidating to the victim and has profound consequences on self-esteem and mental health. Unlike youth school-based bullying (Chap. 3), child maltreatment (Chap. 6), college hazing (Chap. 7), and domestic violence (Chap. 6) that all have potential physical abuse, workplace bullying is predominantly characterized by verbal abuse, work interference or sabotage, harassment, and discrimination. Physical abuse in the workplace is much less common and would manifest mostly as sexual harassment, as illustrated in the examples of Harvey Weinstein, Charlie Rose, Matt Lauer, and others mentioned above. The most important thematic connection is abuse of power through aggression.

We specifically include discrimination and harassment within our definition and discussion of workplace bullying. Harassment (defined as systematic and sustained actions that include making threats and demands; creating a hostile work situation, and/or advancing unwelcome verbal or physical conduct) and discrimination are special categories within workplace bullying because state and federal civil rights laws protect specific vulnerable minority groups from maltreatment. Civil rights laws protect members of a protected status group (i.e., females, minority groups based on race, age, disability, national origin, religion) if the perpetrator was not also a member of the protected group. In these cases, the Human Relations department of an agency or organization must investigate if a harassment complaint is filed and antidiscrimination procedures codified by state and federal laws must be followed. However, according to the Workplace Bullying Institute (2018) illegal discriminatory harassment occurs in only 20% of bullying cases while 80% of workplace bullying is legal, that is the maltreatment is not a violation of any current law. Despite special circumstances for harassment and discrimination, we will include these categories within our definition and discussion of workplace bullying.

9.2.2 *Prevalence*

Unfortunately, workplace bullying is a common occurrence in the US. Using a stratified random sample of 1008 adult Americans in 2017, the Workplace Bullying Institute (WBI; Namie, 2017) asked survey respondents "At work, what has been your personal experience with the following types of repeated mistreatment: abusive conduct that is threatening, intimidating, humiliating, work sabotage or verbal abuse?" Findings indicated that one-fifth of adult Americans (19%) said they directly experienced abusive conduct at work—currently (9%) or earlier in their work life but not in the last year (10%). An additional 15% of respondents saw workplace bullying happen to others or knew about it happening to others (4%). Generalizing this random sample to the US labor force of 161,616,000 individuals gives an estimated prevalence of approximately 30 million American workers having been, or are now being, bullied at work. Another 30 million have witnessed it. Sixty million American workers who have experienced or witnessed workplace bullying is roughly equivalent to the combined total populations of California, Oregon, Washington state, Arizona, Nevada, and Utah (Namie, 2017; WBI, 2018). It is important to note that this WBI definition did not include sexual harassment or discrimination, making the 40% prevalence rate a likely underestimate of the prevalence of our definition of workplace bullying.

The U.S. Equal Employment Opportunity Commission (EEOC) created a comprehensive report on workplace harassment in the US (Feldblum & Lipnic, 2016). This government agency is responsible for processing harassment complaints that are reported. The co-chairs on the Select Task Force on the Study of Harassment in the Workplace said nearly one-third of the 90,000 complaints received in 2015 included a harassment allegation—but the agency notes that that number is far too low to reflect reality (see Table 9.1; Feldblum & Lipnic, 2016). They also estimated that 75% of all workplace harassment incidents go unreported altogether. "Anywhere from 25% to 85% of women report having experienced sexual harassment in the workplace… Roughly three out of four individuals who experienced harassment never even talked to a supervisor, manager, or union representative about the harassing conduct. Employees who experience harassment fail to report the harassing behavior or to file a complaint because they fear disbelief of their claim, inaction on their claim, blame, or social or professional retaliation" (Feldblum & Lipnic, 2016, p. V).

Table 9.1 EEOC 2015 complaints by type of harassment ($N = 90{,}000$; Feldblum & Lipnic, 2016)

Type of alleged harassment based on	Percent of complaints Private employers and state/local government	Percent of complaints Federal government employees
Sex	45	44
Race	34	36
Disability	19	34
Age	15	26
National Origin	13	12
Religion	5	5

Feldblum and Lipnic (2016) also reviewed the prevalence rates for different types of harassment in their EEOC Study of Harassment in the Workplace. Existing data shows that sexual harassment by far gets the most attention while there is very little information to draw on for harassment based on race/ethnicity, disability, age, and religion. In surveys using the most rigorous scientific methods (i.e., random probability samples), gender harassment (i.e., sexist or crude/offensive behavior to insult women) was the most common form with 80% of respondents reporting experiences in this area. Forty percent endorse experiencing unwanted sexual attention or sexual coercion, and in surveys asking about more general sex-based harassment without giving a formal definition, 25% of respondents endorsed having these experiences at work. Surveys using convenience samples (i.e., respondents come from one agency, website, or university, non-randomly selected workers) generally show higher prevalence rates; 75% for unwanted sexual attention or sexual coercion and 50% for sex-based harassment without a specific definition. There is a serious lack of information on other forms of harassment at work. Thirty-five percent of lesbian–gay–bisexual individuals who were open at work identified reported harassment in one survey and 58% of LGBT respondents reported experiencing derogatory comments. There are currently no strong estimates of harassment based on race/ethnicity, age, disability, or religion. This is troubling because racial/ethnic minorities and individuals with a disability make up large portions of the US population and are highly vulnerable to harassment. Nearly half of EEOC complaints in 2015 were based on race and national origin (see Table 9.2), but we have very limited understanding of how often these types of harassment and bullying experiences occur in the workplace.

In considering these prevalence rates, we also have to consider that studies have found only 6–13% of individuals who experienced harassment filed a formal complaint (Feldblum & Lipnic, 2016). Just like on middle school playgrounds, most victims cope with harassment by avoiding the bully, denying the situation, or trying to ignore, forget, or endure the behavior. Only 30% of victims talk to a supervisor, which is understandable because bullies are often bosses. Considering that there were 90,000 EEOC complaints in 2015 and this potentially only reflects 6–13% of actual harassment incidents, it is reasonable to estimate that there were probably between 692,307 and 1,499,999 incidents of harassment in US workplaces, but only 90,000 were reported. Assuming that the US labor force totals 161,616,000, it is a

Table 9.2 Estimates of prevalence for different harassment types from surveys

Type of harassment	Prevalence rate: survey type—random probability sample	Prevalence rate survey type—convenience sample	Notes
Sex based harassment	25%; asked about sexual harassment without giving a definition.	50%; with no definition.	Many individuals do not label certain forms of unwelcome sexually based behaviors—even if they view them as problematic or offensive—as "sexual harassment." Women report more sex and gender harassment than men.
Specific sexual behaviors, such as unwanted sexual attention or sexual coercion	40%	75%	
Gender harassment; Sexist or crude/offensive behavior to insult women	60%	No data available.	Harassment subtypes (unwanted sexual attention, sexual coercion, and gender harassment): gender harassment is the most common form of harassment for women.
Harassment on gender identity and sexual orientation	35% LGB identified respondents who were out at work reported harassment. 58% of LGBT respondents reported derogatory comments.	7% and 41% of LGBT respondents were verbally and/or physically abused at work or had their work spaces vandalized. 50% of transgender respondents reported being harassed at work. 7% physically assaulted; 6% sexually assaulted; 41% asked unwelcome questions about status; 45% repeatedly called by wrong pronouns.	Transgender individuals generally experienced higher rates of harassment than individuals who identify as LGB.
Racial and ethnic harassment	No surveys available.	40–60% of respondents reported threatening verbal comments, conduct, slurs, and jokes. Exclusionary behavior, pressured to give up race/ethnicity to fit in. 70% verbal harassment; 45% exclusionary behaviors. 69% witnessed racial/ethnic harassment in last 2 years; 39% had knowledge of harassment of coworkers.	In 2011, 35% of responding restaurant workers in Los Angeles reported verbal abuse based on race. Verbal abuse centered on language and national origin. Minorities report more racial/ethnic harassment than Whites.

(continued)

Table 9.2 (continued)

Type of harassment	Prevalence rate: survey type—random probability sample	Prevalence rate survey type—convenience sample	Notes
Disability based harassment	No data available.	20% of faculty and staff at one university experienced disability harassment; 6% observed it. At a second university, 14% experienced and 5% witnessed disability harassment.	Data is exceptionally difficult to find. Psychiatric disability 1.5 times the odds of filing EEOC complaint. People with speech impairments, learning disabilities, disfigurements, intellectual disabilities, dwarfism, traumatic brain injuries, and hearing impairments also filed more disability harassment charges than people with other disabilities.
Age harassment	No data available.	AARP: workers over 50, 8% reported unwelcome comments. In New York City, 25% of respondents or family member had unwelcome comments on age.	
Religious harassment	No data available.	No data available.	

reasonable estimate to say that harassment occurs to 1 in every 107 US workers (i.e., 161,616,000/1,499,999). Adding in the Workplace Bullying Institute's estimate that 60,000,000 American workers have experienced or witnessed workplace bullying without including harassment, we can conclude that 1 in 2.63 American workers (i.e., 161,616,000/61,499,999) experienced or witnessed workplace bullying and/or some type of harassment

9.2.3 *Cost of Workplace Bullying*

In 2015, EEOC recovered $164.5 million for workers alleging harassment and since 2010 employers have paid out $698.7 million to employees alleging harassment (Feldblum & Lipnic, 2016). According to the National Boss Day Report, in 2012, employers paid over $356 million for workplace harassment and discrimination complaints (http://blog.ebosswatch.com/2012/10/national-boss-day-reportemployers-paid-over-356-million-for-workplace-harassment-and-discrimination-complaints/). The largest sexual harassment jury award in 2012 totaled $168 million. Michigan State University had to pay out $500 million in settlement to victims of

Larry Nassar (i.e., sexual abuse of young athletes under his care). Employers have to invest time, energy, and resources from business activities to legal representation, settlements, litigation, court awards, and often pay legal fees and damages. Meanwhile, victims suffer mental, physical, and economic harm that is often not covered by settlements (Hutchinson et al., 2006). Bullying victims often lose their jobs, accrue serious economic consequences, and suffer from damaged career trajectories. Workplace bullying also affects all workers, and its true cost includes decreased productivity, increased turnover, lowered morale, reduced productivity, loyalty, and reputational harm (Quine, 1999; Raynor & Cooper, 1997). This undermines work performance and decreases profits. Indeed, workplace bullying could be a "more crippling and devastating problem for employees than all other work-related stress put together" (Einarsen, 1999, p. 16).

9.2.4 Workplace Bullying Dynamics

Workplace bullying has dynamics that are markedly similar to school-based bullying with some important nuances that are unique to adults within employment environments. Similar to school-based bullying, workplace bullying (1) is driven by perpetrators' need for power and to control the targeted individual(s); (2) is initiated by bullies who select their targets, timing, location, and methods; (3) is characterized by acts of commission (doing mean acts to others) or omission (withholding resources from others); (4) damages the victims, particularly because of humiliation, exclusion, and repetition of toxic behavior over time; and (5) commonly escalates to involve others who side with the bully, either voluntarily or through coercion (i.e., negative bystanders; WBI, 2018). Workplace bullying undermines legitimate business interests and sabotages work projects or productivity when bullies' personal agendas take precedence over work itself, just as childhood bullying undermines academic achievement.

According to WBI research by Namie (2017)

- 61% of Americans are aware of abusive conduct in the workplace
- 70% of perpetrators are men; 60% of targets are women
- Hispanics are the most frequently bullied race
- 61% of bullies are bosses, the majority (63%) operate alone
- 40% of bullied targets are believed to suffer adverse health effects
- 29% of targets remain silent about their experiences
- 71% of employer reactions are harmful to targets
- 60% of coworker reactions are harmful to targets
- To stop work place bullying, 65% of targets lose their original jobs
- 46% report worsening of work relationships, post-Trump election

Although research is limited, it is quite possible and logically coherent that middle school bullies, who find satisfaction in their dominance and power over victims, along with little effective disciplinary response from teachers or school administrators, are likely to grow up into controlling adults who adeptly use power imbalance and group dynamics to further their agendas to the detriment of others. An unknown percentage of workplace bullies have a lifelong record of disrespecting the needs of others (WBI, 2018). Indeed, a hypercompetitive work environment may feed right into the preferred style that bullies have for acting in the world. It is, once again, a scramble for resources, prestige, and power where aggressive behavior is often rewarded with promotions and raises in pay.

Bullies are strategic, adept at seeing opportunities to advance their own agendas and sabotage the efforts of their victims. This behavior could be considered to stem from a lack of empathy. Researchers divide empathy into two main components: cognitive empathy and affective empathy. Cognitive empathy refers specifically to the ability to identify and understand the emotional state of others while affective empathy relates to the ability to give the correct emotional response to others' emotions (Pöyhönen, Juvonen, & Salmivalli, 2010). Bullies often have well developed cognitive empathy, but little affective empathy. Perspective-taking refers to the ability to adopt the psychological viewpoint of others and is a main component of cognitive empathy. Workplace bullies use their cognitive empathy and perspective-taking to understand the situations of others; however, they use this information to advance their own plans rather than to respond with affective empathy. Callous-unemotional behaviors have been shown to lead to aggression, antisocial behavior, and deficits in empathic behaviors (Waller & Hyde, 2017). It is important to consider the possibility that one can use perspective-taking to understand what others are feeling and anticipate behavior but still have the desire to harm (Lamm & Majdandžić, 2014). Affective empathy generates the desire for prosocial behavior, suffering a deficit of it while having regular levels of cognitive empathy creates the possibility for perspective taking to be used negatively (e.g., rather than using perspective-taking in determining prosocial behavior, using it to determine what actions would cause harm). Both cognitive and affective aspects of empathy are critical for prosocial development and these two complementary processes must develop equally.

Strategic cognition without affect is Machiavellian or narcissistic but works well in competitive professions and in many organizational settings. Not only is harming others during the process of advancement not discouraged, but it may be rewarded. Again, consider Harvey Weinstein, Charlie Rose, or Bill Cosby whose predatory behavior was ignored for decades as they garnered increasing power from their positions. Supervisors may dismiss bullying reports because they value the assertiveness and personal relationship they have with the perpetrator; these power relationships shield bully bosses from receiving negative consequences from their behavior. Further, if bullies experience no disciplinary action, they can be emboldened to engage in more frequent and higher intensity bullying.

For victims, the detrimental social and psychological consequences of being bullied are similar to those discussed in previous chapters on childhood victimization, maltreatment, and hazing. Humiliation and social exclusion at work similarly trigger depression, anxiety, low self-esteem, PTSD symptoms, and biological chronic stress responses. According to a 2007 WBI survey, 45% of individuals targeted at work suffer from stress-related health problems. As discussed in previous chapters, chronic or extreme distress from victimization releases glucocorticoids, such as cortisol, and other hormones, such as adrenaline, that flood the brain and body. Prolonged exposure to stress response hormones can impair brain processes responsible for memory, emotional regulation, and the ability to sustain positive social relationships, as well as increase the risk for: heart disease, hypertension, strokes, immune system impairment, fibromyalgia, chronic fatigue syndrome, irritable bowel syndrome, colitis, diabetes, and skin disorders.

While child maltreatment places all developmental functioning at risk and is associated with detrimental effects on academic achievement, adult victimization at work places the victim's career trajectory in jeopardy. To stop the bullying, 65% of victims lose their original jobs, either by resigning or being forced out for one reason or another. This employment instability ruins careers that were meticulously built over time. Victims endure lost income, are blocked from advancement opportunities, and may experience extreme stress if they are providing crucial income for their families.

In many ways, the experience of workplace bullying parallels both child maltreatment and domestic violence. The bully boss or coworker inflicts pain and suffering, especially emotional abuse, on an intermittent schedule when and where she or he chooses. This keeps the victim under chronic stress, hypervigilant, and off balance because it is unclear when the next bullying attack will happen. There are periods of peace where the relationship to the bully boss or coworker may be positive, kindling the hope that the relationship can change. Just like the bond with an abusive spouse or dominating parent, the relationship between the perpetrator and the victim—parent-over-child, spouse-to-spouse, or supervisor–subordinate—feeds into the power imbalance, gives the bully reason to want the relationship manipulation to continue, discourages the victim from leaving, and keeps the toxic dynamic happening in a repeating cycle over time. Also, parallel to these other forms of intimate partner violence, in workplace bullying, the personalized, focused nature of the assault destabilizes and disassembles the victim's identity, self-esteem, ego strength, and ability to rebound from the assaults. Work plays a central part in adult identity, leaving people victimized at work to feel that their world is seriously threatened.

9.3 Workplace Culture

Numerous studies have shown that organizational conditions are the most influential predictors of whether workplace harassment and bullying will occur (Feldblum & Lipnic, 2016; Willness et al., 2007). All organizations have climate or work cultures within which employees navigate. Some work cultures are steeped in history, functioning in specific ways because it is tradition. Analogous to family traditions that are passed from generation to generation, employees inherit norms that past leaders have set for organizational functions. Employers define organizational culture and work conditions by making policies and daily practices. Norms are then reinforced by hiring new employees with commensurate values, making assignments to work groups, promoting managers to supervise work completion and behavior. Consequently, the conditions for workplace bullying to take root and grow can only be set or eliminated by employers. This is similar to school environments being central to bullying in childhood. In workplaces for example, there may be a highly competitive atmosphere (e.g., survival of the most aggressive) where promotions go to employees who are the most visible, vocal, and assertive. Dominating others through taking their ideas, keeping them subordinate, and showboating rather than collaborating may be the path forward for one's career advancement. In agencies with tight budgets, scarcity generates competition for what resources are available, making positive relationships secondary to power relationships. Work teams may become adversarial, creating a few winners and many losers, and the informal process of sociometry (i.e., relationships within a group, roles as "popular," "average," "neglected/rejected," and "controversial"), gossip, and exclusion may be just as strong in workplaces as these social processes were in middle school.

Harassment and bullying are more likely to occur in workplaces that are homogenous and lacking diversity. The risk for sexual harassment increases in male dominated workplaces and racial/ethnic discrimination may be more likely when there are few, lower status minority employees or when management has one race overrepresented. In these workplaces, the dominant social group (i.e., males, Caucasians) that has power may feel threatened by female or minority newcomers and bands together against these "others." Further, these new interlopers may not conform to workplace norms or organizational culture. A female firefighter may have to prove that she is "tough enough" to be accepted. The annual BBQ has to be changed because some new employees are vegetarian. A parochial not for profit agency that accepts federal funding has to hire gay or lesbian applicants, but it does not have to make them feel welcome. These newcomers who are different threaten historical organizational norms and climate, making current employees uncomfortable and frightened about change.

Age is also a risk factor for discrimination at both ends of the spectrum. Young workers may not understand appropriate workplace behavior and can unknowingly violate norms and policies. Youth in beginning entry-level positions are vulnerable to be targets for abuse and harassment, having little power or recourse against such behavior from supervisors or more senior coworkers. At the other end of the spectrum, older workers are also vulnerable because they fear the loss of their jobs to younger applicants with newer skills. These older workers may be willing to endure offensive comments and disrespect based on their age in order to keep their jobs. In some cases, older workers may be bullied until they leave as a way to force them into retiring.

Workplaces with "high-value" employees may also breed abuse (Feldblum & Lipnic, 2016). A senior partner who brings in many clients, a salesman who leads all the others in productivity each month, a football coach who wins championships, a doctor with tens of millions of dollars in grants; all of these high-value employees may grow to feel invulnerable, like the rules do not apply to them, and management will not challenge them for fear of losing the goose that lays the golden egg. In many high-profile cases, shielding the high-status employee may seem advantageous in the short term but is disastrous for the organization in the long term. For example, celebrity doctor Larry Nassar's abuse of elite Olympic gymnasts cost Michigan State University $500 million in settlements with victims. And Jerry Sandusky, a defensive coordinator for Penn State's football team was found guilty of sexually abusing ten boys over the course of 15 years. Although officials knew of the behavior, they failed to notify law enforcement. Penn State President Spanier and two other administrators were sentenced to short prison terms and monetary settlements totaled $109 million. Endemic issues of child sexual abuse perpetrated by Catholic priests, who were shielded for decades by church leaders, were revealed in the US (more than 3000 civil lawsuits), Ireland, Australia, Austria, Poland, Chile, Guam, Norway, India, Canada, Belgium, and the Dominican Republic. By 2009, US dioceses have paid more than $2.6 billion in abuse-related costs since 1950. It is clear that changing the workplace culture, though difficult, is ultimately better for the bottom line.

Workplace bullying is often covertly accepted by management and directed toward a victim who is unable to defend himself or herself because of his or her lower position in the organization (Akella, 2016). According to the 2017 WBI US Workplace Bullying Survey results, in response to complaints of bullying, 25% of employers did nothing, 46% did a "sham" investigation, 23% helped the target, and only 6% punished the perpetrator. This lethargic response is understandable considering that 61% of bullies were bosses protected by power and status while 33% of bullies were coworkers. Considering these fixed roles and power imbalance, bully bosses can use their authority to allocate work, assess work, and provide feedback (even unwarranted, critical, and demeaning feedback) to the victim with little risk of disciplinary action. Indeed, managers can interpret complaints of anxiety, depression, or stress from the victim as signs of incompetence, neuroticism, hypersensitivity, inability to cope, and lack of efficiency (Baillien, Neyens, De Witte, & De Cuyper, 2009). Meanwhile bully bosses may be seen as driven, Type A personalities, relentless in pursuit of high quality work, domineering (but positive) characteristics which can be a little abrasive and aggressive at times (Baillien et al., 2009; Cortina, 2008; Hutchinson & Jackson, 2014). Yet this abrasive style is worth it if the organization profits. In order to ensure customer satisfaction, management may, consciously or subconsciously, tolerate harassment and bullying rather than intervene on the workers' behalf (Feldblum & Lipnic, 2016). Workers who must focus on customer satisfaction (such as restaurant servers, salespeople, airline stewards, taxi and Uber drivers, nurses) for tips or positive reviews may tolerate more harassment to maintain their job security and income. Management often errs on the side of making the sale.

Bullying and harassment are also higher in isolated workplaces where there is little supervision or risk of getting caught. Housekeepers alone in hotel rooms, agricultural workers in distant fields, night shift workers or factory workers with management in a different building may be easy targets for bullies who have access and few witnesses around. Workers who are bored or have extra time on their hands are more likely to harass others. Some workplaces have limited communication between levels of the organization, leaving limited supervision of front line workers. Senior management may be far removed in corporate offices with little knowledge of what happens between lower level supervisors and their employees. In these workplaces, communications to upper management may be directed through mid-level supervisors who have wide latitude to bully others and not report it. Front line staff, especially if they are young, inexperienced, or fear retaliation, may not understand or have skills to navigate complex organizational processes to file complaints.

Finally, alcohol may exacerbate the risk and intensity for all of these bullying dynamics. Workplaces that tolerate alcohol use during or around work hours or activities often contend with more harassment and bullying when inhibitions are low. Drinking may be expected as a part of entertaining clients; it also may be the norm for bonding with other coworkers or supervisors. Under the influence of alcohol, both bully bosses and victims make poor choices.

Akella (2016) views workplace bullying and the lack of response from organizations through the lens of labor process theory, arguing that management exploits and controls labor to generate more profits. Drawing on Marxist theory of class divisions into labor and capital, capitalists (epitomized by executives, supervisors, managers) control conception and coordination while laborers provide labor power to transform raw materials into finished products that can be sold to earn a surplus (Braverman, 1974). In a capitalist economy, the capitalist exploits the labor power to its maximum potential to generate the most profit. Milkman (1997) wrote "You [the employee] are a machine, an object, a piece of equipment. If it breaks, they will replace it. They don't care about the individual" (p. 46). The job of the capitalist class is to conceive, control, and coordinate. Conflict between labor and management cannot be avoided. In order to overcome employee resistance and to sustain profits, management lays emphasis on designing techniques and systems to control labor. Consequently, managers are most concerned with creating structures of relationships and power to implement strategies that ensure the effective subordination of labor to the demands of capital (Zeitlin, 1974). Over time, control techniques became more indirect, hegemonic, and insidious to allow and encourage learning and innovation among the employees (Akella, 2003, 2016). In workplaces where organizational climate is infused with strong needs for control, coercion undermines norms of justice and civility, and employee abuse, humiliation, and dehumanization are permitted by the management, but control strategies are cleverly masked to secure employee compliance and cooperation (Akella, 2003). The application to workplace bullying is straightforward; capitalist bully bosses use control techniques, such as harsh repetitive discipline humiliation, and close monitoring and supervision, to create quiet, docile, obedient, polite, and eager to please employees who serve supervisors without questioning their authority or decisions. In the short term, victims respond to coercive control by working harder and longer to preserve their self-worth and protect their livelihood. From a management perspective, the bullying may be effective and efficient, and when the human suffering takes its toll the laborer can always be replaced. In the long term, allowing workplace bullying moves from being an effective and efficient control mechanism to undermining organizational morale, and increasing turnover, lost productivity, worker complaints, and litigation.

Labor process theory is helpful in explaining the ubiquity of workplace bullying and in reframing the bully–victim relationship as enduring social roles (i.e., boss-employee) rather than a function of personality characteristics or psychopathology. Just as in the Zimbardo prison experiments previously discussed where normal undergraduate students rapidly became abusive when playing guards and submissive when assigned to inmate roles, the power inherent in being a supervisor may lend itself to autocratic behavior while subordinates are primed for disempowered acquiescence. It is clear that better organizational rules, regulations, and policies to protect employees from bullying and safeguard their interests are needed.

9.4 Implications for Policy and Practice

Most forms of workplace bullying are legal, with little or no recourse for victims. We explicitly include harassment and discrimination in our definition of workplace bullying. As noted above, harassment and discrimination are special categories within workplace bullying because state and federal civil rights laws protect specific vulnerable minority groups from maltreatment. Civil rights laws protect members of a protected status group (i.e., females, minority groups based on race, age, disability, national origin, religion) if the perpetrator was not also a member of the protected group. In these cases, the Human Relations department of an agency or organization must investigate if a harassment complaint is filed and antidiscrimination procedures codified by state and federal laws must be followed. Victims can, but usually do not, file a complaint or pursue litigation for systematic and sustained actions that include creating a hostile work situation and/or advancing unwelcome verbal or physical conduct. However, illegal discriminatory harassment is dramatically under-reported (6–13% of individuals who experience harassment file a formal complaint; Feldblum & Lipnic, 2016, p. 16) and occurs in only 20% of bullying cases while 80% of workplace bullying is not a violation of any current law. Federal laws are focused on remedying past forms of discrimination for specific minority groups (i.e., equal employment opportunities, disability acts, and equal pay acts). There is no US law that protects human dignity at work (Akella, 2016). In contrast, European countries have laws to protect workers' dignity, personal and human rights (Lueders, 2008).

There is currently no federal law in place to address workplace bullying, thus a movement started in 2001 and continues today to pass the Healthy Workplace Bill (Yamada, 2004), which protects the victim's right to work in a safe and collegial office environment (Carbo, 2009; Maurer, 2013). The proposed Healthy Workplace Bill has been introduced in 29 states and 2 territories with partial victories in Utah, California, and Tennessee (healthyworkplacebill.org). The full version of the HWB holds employers accountable for fostering an abusive work environment, but some critics argue that the HWB falls short of providing adequate remedial relief to the targets of bullying (Akella, 2016; Carbo, 2009). In 2010, there were discussions with members of the U.S. House of Representatives and the U.S. Senate about proposing a federal law to cover workplace bullying. Advocates are still pushing for the bill, but policy makers often loathe to place more regulations on businesses.

In the absence of guiding legislation, it is incumbent on organizations and agencies to safeguard their workplace cultures against harassment and bullying. After collecting extensive data, reviewing academic research, and hearing testimony, the EEOC's Select Task Force on the Study of Harassment in the Workplace (Feldblum & Lipnic, 2016) concluded that workplace bullying must be addressed by organizational leadership who set the tone for the entire work culture and there must be accountability for perpetrators, commonly bully bosses, that is guided by well-articulated and consistently applied policies with objective and transparent investigations of complaints. Senior leaders at the top of the organization must set the tone that harassment and bullying will not be tolerated, that their workplaces will be characterized by civility and respect for diversity in all of its forms, and that abuse of power will be punished. Employers should assess their workplaces for risk factors associated with harassment and bullying (i.e., homogenous workforces, workplace norm violations, cultural and language differences, treatment of young and older workers, status of "high value" employees, power disparities, isolated workplaces, worker boredom, decentralized workplaces, the importance of client satisfaction, and use of alcohol) and plans should be crafted for mitigating these risk factors. Climate surveys can be useful to assess the extent of current bullying and worker morale. Resources should be devoted to harassment and bullying prevention, along with evaluation of effectiveness, and when bullying and harassment has occurred, employers should enforce consistent appropriate discipline that is prompt and proportionate to the severity of the infraction and does not show favoritism to any employee. Bullying and harassment prevention should be included with diversity and inclusion strategies and mid-level managers and front-line supervisors should be held accountable for implementation of these strategies. Policies should include clear explanations of prohibited conduct and should describe complaint processes. Employees who make complaints or participate in investigations of bullying should be protected from retaliation. To the extent possible, confidentiality should be protected and investigations should be prompt, thorough, and impartial. Most importantly, violations should trigger consequences, not promotions, for bullies. According to WBI, stopping bullying requires employers to change the routine ways of doing business that have propped up bullies for years. Bullies are often very expensive to keep, but convincing executives, who might be the bully's best friends and supporters, to fire the bully is quite difficult. Currently, we have an honor system in which employers in the US marshal themselves. High-profile scandals and the #MeToo movement have shown that this system is not working. We need to move towards making our workplaces more civil, respectful, and equitable to ensure the health and well-being of our workforce and the nation.

References

Akella, D. (2003). *Unlearning the fifth discipline: Power, politics and control in organizations*. New Delhi, India: SAGE.

Akella, D. (2016). Workplace bullying: Not a manager's right? *Journal of Workplace Rights, 14*, 97–120.

Baillien, E., Neyens, I., De Witte, H., & De Cuyper, N. (2009). A qualitative study on the development of workplace bullying: Towards a three way model. *Journal of Community & Applied Social Psychology, 19*, 1–16.

Braverman, H. (1974). *Labor and monopoly capital*. London, England: Monthly Review Press.

Carbo, J. (2009). Strengthening the health workplace act: Lessons from title VII and HED litigation and stories of targets' experiences. *Journal of Workplace Rights, 14*, 97–120.

Corey, D. (2017). *Since Weinstein, here's a growing list of men accused of sexual misconduct*. Retrieved from https://www.nbcnews.com/storyline/sexual-misconduct/weinstein-here-s-growing-list-men-accused-sexual-misconduct-n816546

Cortina, L. M. (2008). Unseen injustice: Incivility as modern discrimination in organizations. *Academy of Management Review, 33*, 55–75.

Dudek, A. (2017, February 3). Workplace bullying, a form of violence pursued under Title VII. *Huffpost*. Retrieved from https://www.huffingtonpost.com/alev-dudek/workplace-bullying-a-form_b_14584766.html

Einarsen, S. (1999). The nature and causes of bullying at work. *International Journal of Manpower, 20*, 16–27.

Feldblum, C. R., & Lipnic, V. A. (2016). *Select task force of harassment in the work place*. U.S. Equal Employment Opportunity Commission. Retrieved from https://www.eeoc.gov/eeoc/task_force/harassment/report.cfm

Hutchinson, M., & Jackson, D. (2014). The construction and legitimation of workplace bullying in the public sector: Insight into power dynamics and organizational failures in health and social care. *Nursing Inquiry, 22*, 13–26.

Hutchinson, M., Vickers, M., Jackson, M., & Wilkes, L. (2006). Workplace bullying in nursing: Towards a more critical organizational perspective. *Nursing Inquiry, 13*(2), 117–126.

Lamm, C., & Majdandžić, J. (2014). The role of shared neural activations, mirror neurons, and morality in empathy—A critical comment. *Neuroscience Research*. https://doi.org/10.1016/j.neures.2014.10.008

Lueders, A. (2008). You will need more than a voltage converter: Plugging European workplace bullying laws into the American jurisprudential outlet. *Arizona Journal of International and Comparative Law, 15*, 197–262.

Maurer, R. (2013). *Workplace bullying: Laws on the horizon?* Retrieved from www.shrm.org

Milkman, R. (1997). *Farewell to the factory: Auto workers in the late twentieth century*. Berkeley, CA: University of California Press.

Namie, G. (2017). *2017 WBI U.S. Workplace Bullying Survey*. Retrieved from http://www.workplacebullying.org/wbiresearch/wbi-2017-survey/

Pöyhönen, V., Juvonen, J., & Salmivalli, C. (2010). What does it take to stand up for the victim of bullying?: The interplay between personal and social factors. *Merrill-Palmer Quarterly, 56*(2), 143–163. Project MUSE.

Quine, L. (1999). Workplace bullying in NHS community trust: Staff questionnaire survey. *British Medical Journal, 23*, 228–232.

Randle, J., Stsevenson, K., & Grayling, I. (2007). Reducing workplace bullying in healthcare organizations. *Nursing Standard, 21*(22), 49–56.

Raynor, C., & Cooper, C. (1997). Workplace bullying. Myth or reality—Can we afford to ignore it? *Leadership and Organization Development Journal, 18*, 211–214.

Rigsby, K. (2002). *New perspectives on bullying*. London, England: Jessica Kingsley Publishers Ltd.

Waller, R., & Hyde, L. W. (2017). Callous–unemotional behaviors in early childhood: Measurement, meaning, and the influence of parenting. *Child Development Perspectives, 11*(2), 120–126. https://doi.org/10.1111/cdep.12222

Willness, C. R., et al. (2007). A meta-analysis of the antecedents and consequences of workplace sexual harassment. *Personnel Psychology, 60*(1), 127.

Workplace Bullying Institute. (2018). *Workplace bullying*. Retrieved from http://www.workplacebullying.org

Yamada, D. (2004). Crafting a legislative response to workplace bullying. *Employee Rights and Employment Policy Journal, 8*, 475–521.

Yildirim, D. (2009). Bullying among nurses and its effects. *International Nursing Review, 56*(4), 504–511.

Zeitlin, M. (1974). Corporate ownership and control: The large corporation and the capitalist class. *American Journal of Sociology, 79*, 1073–1119.

Chapter 10
Playground Politics Among Older Adults: How Elder Abuse Can Ruin the Golden Years

10.1 Introduction

In her mid-80s, Alena's health care was increasingly complicated by macular degeneration and diabetes. She could no longer drive and stayed at home all the time. She gave her son, Rob, Power of Attorney after her husband of 40 years died of cancer. Alena remembers that she had much more in her savings account, but Rob says that she is having more frequent memory lapses.

Sam and Catherine were married for 53 years. At 85 years old, Sam's Alzheimer's Disease had gotten bad, but Catherine was determined to take care of him at home (where they raised their children) for as long as she could. Evenings were the hardest when his personality seemed to change and Sam became argumentative. He called Catherine names and shouted at her to take him back to his mother. When Catherine told him that his mother died 20 years ago, he became more aggressive. She counted the minutes until he would go to bed.

Sonia dreaded going to the nursing home's dining hall for dinner. She would sit in her assigned seat and the other women would insult her clothes. She told them that she could not afford new blouses like theirs, but then they would spend the rest of the dinner lecturing her on making better investment choices "so that her money worked for her." Sonia decided to make a slice of toast and eat in bed again.

Cassandra was despondent because her grandson called and was in trouble while studying abroad in Mexico. She wired $10,000 from her bank account to help him get his passport back. He said not to tell because he was embarrassed. Cassandra's real grandson never left the US.

Robin was helping her mother organize financial records. She became concerned when she saw checks her mother paid for three colonoscopies in the past year and two pairs of hearing aids at $15,000 each for her father. He was 88 years old and had dementia. Robin told her mother to be careful with their money, but her mother was adamant about listening to all of their doctors because "they know best."

© Springer Nature Switzerland AG 2019

P. R. Smokowski, C. B. R. Evans, *Bullying and Victimization Across the Lifespan*, https://doi.org/10.1007/978-3-030-20293-4_10

Each of these examples illustrates elder abuse, bullying, and/or maltreatment (these terms can be used interchangeably), a serious situation that has a host of negative consequences for elderly victims. Elder abuse has received almost negligible attention compared with other forms of abuse, such as child abuse and spousal abuse (Giles & Helmle, 2011; Lin & Giles, 2013). In this chapter, we will first provide an overview of elder maltreatment by offering a definition of elder abuse and discussing prevalence rates as well as negative consequences. We will then discuss elder abuse in the context of community settings when elders live with their families or on their own and are at risk of being abused by family and/or friends physically, emotionally, and financially. Elder maltreatment in institutional settings (i.e., nursing homes) will be discussed as both staff and other residents can be perpetrators. Finally, we will apply the bullying definitional framework (i.e., repetition, power imbalance, intent to harm) to elder abuse.

10.2 Elder Abuse Overview: Definition, Prevalence Rates, Negative Consequences

Academic discussions of elder maltreatment began in the 1970s with references to "granny battering" or "battered older person syndrome" (Burston, 1975; Butler, 1975; Choi & Mayer, 2000). Elder abuse is the exploitation of adults over age 60, including physical, sexual, and emotional abuse, neglect and abandonment, and financial exploitation (National Institute on Aging [NIA], 2018). Parallel to other types of abuse and maltreatment in different life stages: elder physical abuse includes hitting, slapping, pushing; emotional abuse is psychological (e.g., yelling, threatening, belittling, ignoring, restricting access to relatives or friends); sexual abuse is being forced to watch or engage in sexual acts; neglect and abandonment include not responding to the older person's needs or leaving them alone without planning to meet needs. According to the NIA (2018), elder financial abuse is happening with increasing frequency and includes stealing money or belongings, forging checks, taking retirement and Social Security benefits, using the older person's credit cards or bank accounts without authorization. In addition to these types of abuse and neglect, health care fraud occurs when doctors, hospital staff, and other healthcare workers overcharge, bill repeatedly for the same service, falsify claims to Medicaid or Medicare, or charge when care was not actually provided.

Each year approximately one in ten older adults in the US are abused, neglected, or financially exploited, resulting in hundreds of thousands of cases. The World Health Organization cites even higher rates with one in six people 60 years and older experiencing some form of abuse in community settings during the past year (World Health Organization, 2018). Considering that many countries, including the US, are experiencing rapidly aging populations, problems concerning elder maltreatment are likely to increase. The global population of people aged 60 years and older will more than double, from 900 million in 2015 to about 2 billion in 2050. With an overall elder maltreatment prevalence rate of 15.7%, it is reasonable to extrapolate the number of victims to reach 320 million worldwide by 2050 (Yon, Mikton, Gassoumis, & Wilber, 2017). This rapid growth precipitates a worldwide crisis of conscience in which we all have to plan how to treat our most senior members of society.

There are a variety of negative consequences from experiencing elder abuse that often serve as signs that elder abuse is occurring: the older adult (1) has trouble sleeping; (2) seems depressed or confused; (3) loses weight for no reason; (4) displays signs of trauma, like rocking back and forth; (5) acts agitated or violent; (6) becomes withdrawn; (7) stops taking part in activities he or she enjoys; (8) has unexplained bruises, burns, or scars; (9) looks messy, with unwashed hair or dirty clothes; or (10) develops bed sores or other preventable conditions (NIA, 2018). Victims of elder abuse have twice or three times the chances of dying prematurely than people who are not victims of elder abuse (Choi & Mayer, 2000; Doug et al., 2009; Lachs, Williams, O'Brien, Pillemer, & Charlson, 1998). Minor injuries like scratches, bruises, or broken bones can take significantly longer to heal in older adults and neglect can have profound consequences physically (e.g., bed sores that become infected, untreated flu or pneumonia) or mentally (e.g., depression, anxiety, severe loneliness). It is likely that victims of elder maltreatment and abuse experience psychological consequences such as learned helplessness, alienation, guilt, shame, fear, and posttraumatic stress; however, few studies have investigated these impacts (Choi & Mayer, 2000; Wolf, 1997). As evidenced in many areas of risk and protective factor research, the odds of elder abuse grow considerably with the number of risk factors in the elder's life. Dong, Chen, & Simon (2014) reported that the odds of elder abuse doubled for each additional risk factor in an elder's life (i.e., risk factors included age, African American race, female gender, medical conditions, low income, social isolation). Having more risk factors increased the odds of suffering from elder abuse. For example, endorsing three to four risk factors nearly quadrupled the odds of confirmed elder abuse while having five or more risk factors made elder abuse 18 times more likely.

Choi and Mayer (2000, p. 6) underscore that elder maltreatment and abuse is a particularly difficult problem to discuss, prevent, and intervene in because:

> "(1) Elder maltreatment is largely a hidden problem, committed in the privacy of the elder's home, mostly by his/her family members (Administration on Aging [AoA], 1998).
>
> (2) Both abused elders and perpetrators often feel ashamed of abusive behaviors and thus hide the incidents from investigators (Quinn & Tomita, 1997). Victims fear losing their only social support, especially if the perpetrator is a relative, being forced into an institution, or future retaliation by the perpetrator(s) (Kosberg & Garcia, 1995).
>
> (3) The victim's mental and cognitive impairments and ill health and the resulting lack of cooperation may interfere with the identification and substantiation of abuse and neglect.
>
> (4) Because of mental and cognitive impairments, ill health, and/or depression, abused and neglected elders may engage in self-neglecting behaviors, making it difficult to separate abuse and neglect by others from self-neglect.
>
> (5) Even mentally lucid victims are often unaware of available resources.
>
> (6) Elder abuse and neglect encompasses a wide variety of maltreatment—physical, sexual, and emotional or psychological abuse, financial/material exploitation, passive or active neglect by caregivers, and self-neglect by the elder him/herself."

Indeed, after studying elders receiving visiting nursing care in their homes, Friedman, Santos, Liebel, Russ, and Conwell (2015) reported that it took nurses an average of 10.5 monthly visits, nearly a year, to discern elder maltreatment. Substantial damage can occur while the abuse goes undetected. Considering the hidden and covert nature of elder maltreatment and abuse, it is critical to raise awareness about this problem so that many older adults do not suffer in silence.

10.3 Elder Abuse as a Form of Bullying

The application of our bullying dynamic to elders is straightforward. The three components inherent in bullying are repetition in aggressive behavior, power imbalance, and intent to harm. There is little controversy that each of these elements plays an important role in manifestations of elder maltreatment.

Some researchers include self neglect in their definitions of elder abuse and maltreatment (Choi & Mayer, 2000). Although we acknowledge that self-neglect is a significant offshoot and may be intricately connected to interpersonal abuse (i.e., "My daughter says I should eat one meal a day because of my cholesterol"), self-neglect is tangential to our discussion of elder abuse and maltreatment as a form of bullying. Bullying is inherently relational with victim and perpetrator roles interacting. In our view, self-neglect may be an important consequence of internalized messages from abusive interpersonal relationships (i.e., "My son makes all my financial decisions because he says I am no good at it").

10.3.1 Repetition

Repetition is usually present because elders tend to become more vulnerable over time, making it easier to perpetuate the abuse with impunity. A teenager stealing money from her grandmother is reinforced by the ease of getting away with it, increasing the probability of trying again with more intensity and brazenness. The repetition criterion may also surface due to the elder's dependence and decreased capacity for decision-making. More medical tests may be justified because the risk of health problems always increases with age. Yet when does performing multiple colonoscopies on an 88-year-old patient move from following prudent practice to unnecessary abundance of concern to abuse? In this example of medical overbilling through overuse of expensive procedures, the intent to harm may not be focused on the patient as much as manipulating the elder's acquiescence to take advantage of the health care system. The elder is still victimized.

10.3.2 *Power Imbalance*

Older adults can be particularly vulnerable to abuse and serve as easy targets for bullies because they may lack support from family or friends nearby, may have cognitive problems such as memory loss or dementia, and may have disabilities that increase their dependence on caregivers for assisting with activities of daily living. With increasing frailty, some older adults may have to trust family members, financial planners, home health aides, or neighbors with important decisions. The power dynamic that we have emphasized in all of the reflections of the bullying dynamic clearly comes into play as older adults designate executors of their estate, health care proxies, beneficiaries, heirs in wills, and doctors who lead them through complicated health care situations. Loss of a spouse who was in charge of financial planning or home repairs, for example, may compound the older adult's vulnerability and reliance on others. Illness, disability, frailty, and, in many situations, isolation may lead to a disempowered state for elders; reliance on others feeds into a profound power imbalance that can be manipulated by bullies.

Researchers have used a number of social science theories to interpret elder abuse dynamics, in general, and the power imbalance, in particular (Mosqueda et al., 2016). Caregiver stress theory suggests maltreatment results from unmanageable burden on caregivers. Social exchange theory posits that negotiated exchanges between people potentiate stress (e.g., "I am taking care of Mom so I should have access to spending her money"). Dyadic discord theory sees dysfunctional relationships (e.g., history of family violence, lack of satisfaction, low bonding) at the core of maltreatment. Social learning theory views violence as a learned behavior; bullies not stopped on the playground bring their coercive behavior to their marriages, workplaces, and caretaking roles. Sociocultural power and control theory suggests that abusers seek power and domination over others, enjoying the resulting status, prestige, and control of resources. In all of these theories, the power imbalance is a key to bullying dynamics, but there are different explanations for what drives the imbalance and search for power.

Having established the relevance of intent to harm, repetition, and power imbalance to elder maltreatment, we will now concentrate our discussion on two primary contexts where bullying happens for older adults—in community settings while elders are trying to maintain their independence and in institutional settings where elders are in the role of patients.

10.3.3 *Intent to Harm*

For elders, intent to harm is clear in physical, social, psychological, or emotional altercations with caregivers who become aggressive. Intent to harm can also be covert and subversive, as in situations of secret financial abuse or failure to attend to unmet needs for the elder person. One nuance with the intent to harm criterion when applied to elders is that it may be rationalized or minimized by perpetrators more readily than other forms of abuse. Maltreatment of a child or intimate partner often generates remorse and is difficult to justify when confronted with the impact (e.g., bruises on a child or spouse after a fight raise immediate questions about inappropriate aggression). Yet with frail elders, broken bones could be from osteoporosis, bruises and burns from absentmindedness, and financial loss may be due to mistaken memory that the victim is not recollecting correctly how much money he really had. Another subtlety may come in the form of neglect. Parents leaving small children on their own for any length of time will often raise concerns. Yet many adult children living a distance from a frail parent may check in every so often or infrequently due to busy schedules. Meanwhile the elder is missing medical treatment, experiencing increasing anxiety, depression, loneliness, or accidents while not wanting to bother her or his busy children. This intent to harm may be passive, yet it often leads to the same deleterious results for the neglected elder. Consequently, the intent to harm has significant ambiguity for perpetrators to explain their way out of scrutiny for long periods of time.

10.4 Elder Abuse in Community Settings

Elders in community settings typically are living independently or with relatives. Depending upon functional capacities and challenges to activities of daily living, they may receive services such as Meals on Wheels, home health care, or visits from members of their church congregations. Community living situations may often be optimal until poor physical and/or mental health of the elder places her or him at risk for victimization and maltreatment. Life transitions, such as death of a spouse or having an adult child move away for a new job, also heighten the vulnerability for elders. In cultures where women have inferior social status, becoming widowed may lead to seizure of property, financial abuse, and neglect. Increasing use of technology (e.g., cell phones, e-mail, Internet-connected televisions, online banking) and complex bureaucracies (e.g., managed care conglomerates, the Social Security Administration) can also generate daily stress and hassles for many elderly individuals who are "digital immigrants."

Analyzing the National Elder Mistreatment Study, Acierno et al. (2010) reported that 11.4% of adults age 60 years and older living in the community in 2008 reported emotional, physical, or sexual mistreatment in the past year. In the past year, many community-based elders have suffered from abuse in the US; between 1.1% and 9.0% suffered from emotional abuse, 0.2–1.8% from physical abuse, and 0.4–5.4% from neglect. Studies of home visiting nurses identified 7.4% of elders (54 of 724) in community settings experienced maltreatment in the last 19 months (Friedman et al., 2015). Rates may be profoundly underestimated because elders have to be both cognitively aware and willing to disclose highly sensitive information about victimization, often committed by loved ones. Burnes et al. (2015) conducted telephone surveys with 4156 community-dwelling elders and in the past year 1.9% endorsed emotional abuse, 1.8% endorsed physical abuse and neglect, with an aggregate prevalence of 4.6%. In another US study of 5777 elders, the 1-year prevalence for financial abuse by a family member was 5.2% (Acierno et al., 2010).

International studies have also found elder maltreatment to be a common problem. In the UK, Biggs, Manthorpe, Tinker, Doyle, and Erens (2009) found that 2.6% of 2111 elders reported mistreatment by family members, close friends, or care workers during a face-to-face survey. Financial abuse was the second most common form of abuse (0.6%) after neglect (1.1%). In Israel, the most common form of abuse was verbal abuse (11.5%), followed by financial exploitation (9.3%; Lowenstein, Eisikovits, Band-Winterstein, & Enosh, 2009). In Ireland, the overall prevalence of elder abuse and neglect was 2.2%, with financial abuse the most frequent type of mistreatment at 1.3% (Naughton et al., 2012). Although these rates are lower than prevalence for other types of bullying, these studies show that elder abuse is a significant societal problem worldwide. Similar to other forms of abuse, it is highly likely that many cases are not reported in telephone or face-to-face interviews due to the sensitivity and privacy of these issues. Many victims are reluctant to report the abuse, creating much lower prevalence estimates than actual occurrences.

Independent community living may sustain the elder through routine interactions with family, neighbors, friends, service workers, and others. At the same time, social isolation of caregivers and older persons, and the ensuing lack of social support, is a significant risk factor for elder abuse by caregivers (World Health Organization, 2018). Many elderly people are isolated because of loss of physical or mental capacity, or through the loss of friends and family members. These mounting losses can take a toll on the grieving elder psychologically, heighten feelings of loneliness, and create new demands to manage money, home repairs, health care decisions, or other areas that the person is not comfortable navigating. Mounting losses of peers and spouses, along with growing demands from physical and mental concerns, may undermine the elder's sense of competence, heightening vulnerability to power imbalances. Older adults are increasingly given directions by health care providers, adult children, financial planners, and others who may or may not have their best interests in mind (e.g., intent to harm may be covert and increasingly overt as physical and mental health concerns become more challenging).

10.4.1 Elder Abuse and Family Relationships

A shared living situation is a risk factor for elder abuse and bullying by family members. It is not yet clear whether spouses or adult children of older people are more likely to perpetrate abuse. In spousal relationships, one elder may be overwhelmed taking care of the other and revert to bullying out of frustration and impatience. This is often the case when dementia or Alzheimer's disease becomes unmanageable and the caretaker does not have adequate support or respite. It is important to assess the subtleties of the situation. It is well known that Alzheimer's patients can become particularly difficult and aggressive at certain times of day (i.e., "sundowning") as a symptom of the disease. The elder with Alzheimer's could be the bully or the victim or a bully-victim. The caretaking spouse may be physically, verbally, and emotionally abused by the spouse with dementia or the caretaker may bully the disempowered dementia patient; sometimes both dynamics are present in situations where the chronic stress of caretaking take a particularly high toll on family relationships.

Financial abuse includes changing names on a will, bank account, life insurance policy, or title to a house without permission from the older person (Payne & Strasser, 2012). This type of abuse is becoming a widespread and hard-to-detect issue. Even someone the elder never met can steal financial information using the telephone or e-mail. Financial abuse by a family member is a common form of abuse experienced by older adults. Although service providers are well placed to recognize financial abuse, it was often difficult to detect abuse and intervene successfully (Adams, Bagshaw, Wendt, & Zannettino, 2014). The elder's adult children are most likely to commit financial abuse (Boldy, Webb, Horner, Davey, & Kingley, 2002; Brill, 1999; Cripps, 2001; Faye & Sellick, 2003; Livermore, Bunt, & Biscan, 2001), and older females are more vulnerable to financial abuse than older males (Adams et al., 2014; Rabiner, O'Keeffe, & Brown, 2004). Because the abuser is often a close family member or friend (Boldy, Horner, Crouchley, Davey, & Boylen, 2005; Faye & Sellick, 2003; Wilson, Tilse, Setterlund, & Rosenman, 2009), the elder victim is unlikely to report this abuse. Mukherjee (2013) surveyed caregiver attitudes about financial exploitation of older adults in rural settings and reported that caregivers overestimate their parents' ability to manage finances, prefer to manage their parents' finances informally without legal options (i.e., power of attorney status), and views their parents' finances as "almost theirs," meaning that anticipation of inheritance blurs the boundaries of ownership and use of assets.

Financial abuse commonly goes undetected to outsiders or even to the elder victim for significant periods of time. The victim's mental or cognitive impairment and physical illness allows the financial abuse to be easily hidden. The abuser's financial dependency on the victim, greed, and substance abuse are significant factors that raise the risk for financial abuse (Berman, 1994; Giordano, Yegidis, & Giordano, 1992; Hwalek, Neale, Goodrich, & Quinn, 1996). Choi and Mayer (2000) also show that financial exploitation commonly comes in combination with other forms of abuse and/or neglect. Friedman et al. (2015) reported that more than half (52%) of maltreated elders experienced multiple forms of abuse, with emotional maltreatment often combining with neglect and/or financial maltreatment.

Providers need consent before they can take action and perpetrating family members (and sometimes the victim) will not necessarily agree. Abusive family members can withdraw the client from service when scrutiny becomes intense, which places the victim in worse circumstances. An abuser's dependency on the older person (often financial) also increases the risk of abuse. The family perpetrator may be the only link for the elder adult to receive needed treatment (e.g., driving to doctor's appointments, to the Adult Day Care Center). Unfortunately, as impairments with activities of daily living and cognitive deficits increase with the elder's age, the chances for maltreatment and abuse also increase as a function of these higher dependency needs and social isolation (Godkin, Wolf, & Pillemer, 1989; Lachs, Williams, O'Brien, Hurst, & Horwitz, 1997; Pillemer & Finkelhor, 1989; Sharon, 1991).

In some cases, a long history of poor family relationships and/or communication deficits may worsen as a result of stress when the older person becomes more care dependent. Grievances between the elder and adult children may worsen and lead to neglect of important needs (e.g., "Mom is alone because she drove everyone away") or rationalization of active abuse (e.g., "I deserve this money because it is my inheritance anyway"). As more women enter the workforce and have less spare time, caring for older relatives becomes a greater burden, increasing the risk of abuse. Family members may be thrust into caretaking roles when they have little capacity, patience, or skills to play the caretaker role; however, the high cost of institutional care precludes other arrangements. Consequently, caregiver stress is a significant risk factor for elder abuse (Coyne, Reichman, & Berbig, 1993; Paveza et al., 1992). Caregiver life stress, including mental illness and substance abuse, along with the abuser's dependence on the victim (e.g., an adult child living in the elder victim's home) are key predictors of physical and psychological abuse (Choi & Mayer, 2000; Godkin et al., 1989; Pillemer & Finkelhor, 1989; Wolf & Pillemer, 1994). Neglect has been linked to the victim's overwhelming dependency needs (i.e., "I can't handle mom's needing me all the time; I am out of here"; Wolf, 1997) while abuse is a stronger function of the problems of the perpetrator (Choi & Mayer, 2000).

Lin and Giles (2013) constructed a dyadic communications model of elder abuse to explain how dysfunctional intergenerational communication between caregivers and care receivers may increase the chances of elder abuse. Caregivers may be placed in the role of providing assistance to their aged relative with no training or support. Indeed, caregivers may have histories of mental health problems, substance use, social isolation, financial dependency, lack of knowledge of caregiving, propensity for verbal aggressiveness, and a history of other abusive behavior (e.g., child maltreatment, intimate partner violence), but none of these red flags stops them from taking the caregiver role. In many cases, it may be a role the person does not want, but the family cannot afford institutional care. With these antecedents in place for a rocky caregiver-care receiver relationship, caregiver stress results in mood disturbance (Bendik, 1992) or anger (Garcia & Kosberg, 1992), increasing the chances for the situation to turn violent. Interestingly, this communications model suggests that deficits in communication skills and abusive behaviors are bidirectional. Negative interactions block positive communication and create feelings of fear, unworthiness, guilt, and shame for both caregivers and care receivers that provoke further destructive interactions.

In a subtle twist from our previous discussions of the power differential in abusive relationships, Lin and Giles (2013) put forth a "power deficit hypothesis" that suggests the caregiver who feels powerless in the relationship (e.g., due to stress, constant demands from the care receiver, aggravation from poor communication, or the elder's noncompliance with commands) may resort to violence or coercive behaviors to regain control (see also Baucom et al., 2011). Importantly, the overburdened and poorly matched caregiver perceives a sense of powerlessness and interprets the situation with hostility, threat, danger, anxiety, and fear. The elder's noncompliance, lack of responsivity, or overly demanding behaviors become a mounting threat, activating negative emotions. This dyadic recipe may explode in abuse when the caregiver reacts against his or her perception of powerlessness by lashing out physically, verbally, emotionally or by withdrawing (i.e., neglect) to regain control. Patronizing talk, painful self-disclosures (e.g., "You never were as organized as your sister"), verbosity, redundancy (e.g., "Mom goes on and on and on"), insults, and aggravation may act as the dry kindling for a dyadic power struggle. The resulting maltreatment remains a function of a key power differential (i.e., the caregiver is younger, stronger, healthier, with sharper cognitions); however, this communications hypothesis is helpful in considering how the caregiver's intent to harm may derive from feeling flooded, overwhelmed, threatened, aggravated, and powerless. While this perspective is illuminating in understanding the abuser's psychology and relative contributions of both roles, it is still the caregiver's responsibility to recognize his or her reactions and seek help before becoming abusive.

While it is more difficult to reconcile with our definition of bullying, elder abandonment is also a significant concern. According to Rzeszut (2017), elder abandonment occurs when an elderly person is deserted by a caretaker or by a person with physical custody of an elder. While elder neglect is withholding services or assistance, abandonment is desertion by abusers who are divesting themselves of the responsibility of providing care. This dereliction of duties can bring about harm, injury, or even death as the elder is left to fend for him or herself. The majority of state laws do not recognize elder abandonment as a form of elder abuse. Caregivers who abandon their duties often do not face criminal or civil liability. Little information on elder abandonment is available because most states categorize abandonment as a form of neglect. Dropping an elder off at an emergency room with no follow-up information may attract attention; however, many less dramatic cases may involve adult children leaving town or never visiting elderly parents without setting up alternative care that is necessary. Like other forms of elder maltreatment, abandonment is very likely underreported, has few consequences for abusers, and requires policy-level initiatives to create coherent statutes across states.

To summarize, elders living in community settings experience daily and increasingly intense challenges to maintain their independence as aging takes its toll. Studies of substantiated cases from Adult Protective Service indicate that neglect was the most common form of maltreatment (48.7%), followed by emotional/psychological abuse (35.4%), financial/material exploitation (30.2%), physical abuse (25.6%), abandonment (3.6%), sexual abuse (0.3%), and other (1.4%; AoA, 1998; Choi & Mayer, 2000). In community settings, abuse is usually perpetrated by a close family member, often in a shared living situation. Family members who are ill equipped to take caregiving roles may be placed in the situation because of lack of funds to pay for care, migration of other family members, erosion of the bonds between family generations, or societal stereotypes (e.g., unmarried daughters should take care of elders). Under the escalating stress of dependency, dyadic power struggles between caregiver and care receiver can erupt into overt physical and emotional abuse or quietly fester as covert neglect, abandonment, or financial exploitation. Considering that most community-based abuse is perpetrated by close family members often in shared housing situations, elder maltreatment prevalence rates are likely to be highly underestimated with many cases taking many months to surface. This is a highly sensitive area for the dependent elder to disclose. Family relationships are the strongest attachments that many people have, making abuse from those relationships particularly shameful and psychologically traumatic. Experiencing elder abuse in community settings more than doubles the odds of the older adult being admitted to a skilled nursing facility and neglect raises this risk of institutionalization by nearly 5 times (Dong & Simon, 2013). Unfortunately, institutional living also has the potential for abuse.

10.5 Elder Abuse in Institutional Settings

Elder abuse that occurs in institutional settings has been well documented (Thobaben & Duncan, 2003). With the burgeoning population of older adults and lengthening life spans, it is increasingly likely that individuals spend a portion of their later lives in nursing homes or assisted living facilities. In 2014, there were 15,640 nursing homes in the US; 10,913 were for profit, 3756 were not for profit, and 971 were run by the government (Statista, n.d.). Forty four percent of these nursing homes had 100–199 beds, 37% had 50–99 beds, 6% had more than 199 beds, leaving only 13% of nursing homes with fewer than 50 beds. In 2015, the average length of stay in a nursing home was 180 days. It is estimated that 70% of Americans over age 65 will need long term care at some point in their lives.

Caring for the elderly is big, profitable business. Annual median costs for a private room in a nursing home in 2018 were highest in Alaska ($330,873), Connecticut ($164,798), Hawaii ($163,885), Massachusetts ($153,300), New York ($146,274), New Jersey ($142,350), North Dakota ($140,277), New Hampshire ($133,225), Delaware ($131,400), and Minnesota ($122,260). Revenues from nursing and residential care facilities are projected to reach $248 billion in 2018 (BEA.gov); 73% of this revenue is paid for by public programs, primarily Medicare and Medicaid.

Nursing home profits are maximized by hiring low-wage, part-time and hourly workers. In 2015, these facilities employed 3.32 million people (47% full-time workers). There were 612,120 nursing assistants employed in 2015 (37% of nursing home employees) making a median hourly wage of $11.87 per hour ($19,000 per year) caring for 1.4 million residents. Indeed, 17% of nursing assistants were living below the federal poverty level, 38% received public assistance, and 20% had no health insurance of their own. Nursing Assistants tend to be female (91%), young (21% 16–24 years old, 26% 25–34), and minority (53% African American, Latino, or Other Race), and have low educational attainment (94% less than a bachelor's degree; 51% high school degree or less; PHI, n.d.). Due to the poor quality work environment and high number of hands-on hours (2.4 h per resident per day), nursing assistants are 3.5 times more likely to be injured on the job than the typical US worker (372 injuries per 10,000 nursing assistants vs. 107 per 10,000 other occupations), including sprains, strains, and tears (205 per 10,000 nursing assistants vs. 39 per 10,000 other occupations), musculoskeletal disorders (200 per 10,000 nursing assistants vs. 34 other occupations), and back injuries (124 per 10,000 nursing assistants vs. 18 other occupations). Along with low pay and high stress, nursing home and assisted living staff must handle residents' high dependency needs. Out of the 1.4 million US nursing home residents in 2015, 63% had bladder incontinence, 52% had documented depression, 51% had Alzheimer's dementia, 50% had bowel incontinence, 30% had psychiatric diagnoses, 26% had behavioral symptoms, 7% had weight loss, 6.5% had pressure sores, and 4% had skin rashes. These statistics describe a situation where young, low-paid, highly stressed, untrained nursing assistants are asked to spend a very high number of contact hours caring for incontinent residents with dementia with little supervision from licensed nurses and high risk of personal injury.

10.5.1 Staff-to-Resident Bullying

It is no surprise that this environment is fertile ground for maltreatment. Staff burnout and low job satisfaction further exacerbate this risk for stress-induced abuse by caregivers particularly when nursing home residents display behavior problems, lack of compliance, and low physical capacities (Baker & Heitkemper, 2005; Shinan-Altman & Cohen, 2009). Further, residents may abuse nursing staff (Lachs et al., 2012; Zeller et al., 2009), which heightens stress and may trigger retaliation (Castle, Ferguson-Rome, & Teresi, 2015). These negative feedback loops of stress and abuse between caregivers and care receivers once again place both actors within our definition of bully-victims (i.e., those who both bully and are bullied).

Few studies have been able to estimate the prevalence of elder abuse in institutional settings. In a telephone survey of relatives of long-term care residents in Michigan (718 respondents), Page, Conner, Prokhorov, Fang, and Post (2009) reported that neglect (9.8%) and caretaking abuse (17.4%) were the most common forms of abuse in nursing homes while emotional abuse (10.0%) and neglect (9.8%) were the most common in assisted living facilities (see also Castle et al., 2015 for a review). Some research indicates that physical abuse is more likely in larger facilities, while psychological abuse and neglect were more likely in smaller facilities (Phillips & Guo, 2011). Castle et al. (2015) also report that 20% of nursing homes per year receive deficiency citations for abuse that had caused actual harm to at least one resident. These deficiency citations only capture physical abuse that is severe enough to cause "actual harm."

Surveys of nurse aides indicate that 36% of nurse aides observed staff abuse of residents in the forms of argumentative behavior with residents and 28% intimidation (i.e., verbal and psychological abuse; 4451 respondents; Castle, 2012a). In a second survey of reports from nurse aides (N = 855) working in assisted living facilities, 59% of nurse aides observed or had evidence of staff verbal abuse of residents (i.e., cursing at residents) and 52% of nurse aides suspected other staff of physical abuse (i.e., pulling the hair of residents; Castle, 2012a). Natan, Lowenstein, and Eisikovits (2010) analyzed a questionnaire filled out by 510 nursing home staff and 22 directors in 22 nursing facilities. The 532 respondents reported 513 accounts of maltreatment, about two thirds were neglect, and 70% of participants reported witnessing psychological abuse and neglect.

Charpentier and Soulières (2013) provide the resident's perspective after interviewing 20 Canadian elders in institutional care. Media coverage of tragic and intense elder abuse cases served to desensitize residents to lower level maltreatment in their nursing homes. In comparison to instances of being scalded while bathing or left to bleed in bed, residents assess their personal vulnerability and often decide to stay quiet. Day to day transgressions are discounted when compared to media tragedies; disrespect, impolite, and rough treatment may be written off as the overworked, overtired staff having a bad day. Standing up for oneself, rather than taking the abuse silently, may make living situations worse from retaliation. Coping strategies emphasized avoidance of direct confrontations with staff or other residents, leaving well enough alone by not voicing dissent, staying in their rooms (i.e., self-isolation), using humor, making friends with the staff, taking care of their own housekeeping tasks, and/or making special arrangements with certain employees. These are strikingly similar to the strategies an inmate might use to get along in a prison.

Few of these data sources have estimated the prevalence of neglect and underreporting is highly likely. With one in five nursing homes cited for physical abuse annually and more than 50% of nurse aides reporting evidence of verbal and physical abuse that is not likely to rise to the severity of a deficiency citation, it is clear that resident maltreatment in institutional settings is a common problem. This is a cause for concern, especially when considering that resident abuse in institutional settings has been linked to elder dehydration, undernourishment, pressure sores, inadequate management of chronic diseases and functional disability, gynecological and gastrointestinal ailments, headaches, depression, anxiety, increased dementia, and increased mortality (Castle et al., 2015; Rodriguez, Wallace, Woolf, & Mangione, 2006; Schofield & Mishra, 2004).

10.5.2 Resident-to-Resident Bullying

There is a small but emerging line of research on resident-to-resident abuse that is of particular interest to our discussion of bullying dynamics. Resident-to-resident abuse occurs when one resident in an institutional facility is abused by another resident (Lachs et al., 2005). If elder abuse by a family member is similar to domestic violence and staff-to-resident abuse is similar to workplace abuse by a supervisor, resident-to-resident bullying of elders is most similar to the playground politics we described for middle school youth. With estimates of 4.8% of residents experiencing physical abuse resulting in police investigations (Lachs, Bachman, Williams, & O'Leary, 2007) and 5.2% of retrospective case reports of maltreatment (Allen, Kallett, & Gruman, 2003), resident-to-resident abuse is possibly the most common form of abuse in institutional facilities.

While most of this research has used qualitative interviews, focus groups, or case records rather than quantitative methods, it is informative to consider the bullying social processes found among residents. Rosen, Pillemer, and Lachs' (2008) focus groups uncovered 35 different types of abuse (e.g., physical, verbal, and sexual), with verbal aggression the most frequent. Qualitative work by Pillemer and associates (2012) discovered five themes: (1) invasion of privacy or personal integrity; (2) roommate problems; (3) hostile interpersonal interactions such as teasing; (4) unprovoked actions; and (5) inappropriate sexual behavior. In a study of 4451 nursing aides, Castle (2012a) reported that 97% observed residents yelling at each other and 94% observed residents pushing, grabbing, or pinching each other in the prior 3 months. Resident bullies were described by nurse aides as being more cognitively aware, with strong personalities, short fuses, and rougher life histories (Sifford-Snellgrove, Beck, Green, & McSweeney, 2012). Victims were vulnerable to abuse due to limited mobility, difficulty communicating, and impaired cognition (i.e., dementia or difficulties remembering). Rosen et al. (2008) found resident-to-resident abuse most commonly happened in the dining room or in residents' rooms, often in the afternoon.

In another study of 832 nurse aides in Pennsylvania (Castle, 2012b), 16% reported observing residents throwing objects at other residents (physical abuse) and 35% reported witnessing residents trading insulting remarks (verbal abuse) in the past 3 months. Studies including police records showed that most reports were for simple assault and violent episodes were more likely in nursing homes than in community settings (Lachs et al., 2005, 2007). In an examination of 294 serious injuries resulting in official complaints in Massachusetts, Shinoda-Tagawa, Leonard, and Pontikas (2004) reported that victims were often cognitively impaired, wanderers, exhibited socially inappropriate behaviors, and verbally abusive. Alzheimer's patients were three times more likely to suffer an injury. Conner et al. (2011) also found age, physical impairment, and behavior problems significant predictors of susceptibility to abuse.

Resident-to-resident abuse negatively impacted the quality of life and safety of many residents (Castle, 2012a; Castle et al., 2015). Indeed, these bullying dynamics dominated by obnoxious, disruptive, and toxic verbal and physical behavior make nursing homes and assisted living facilities sound strikingly similar to poorly managed middle schools. Overall, within institutions, abuse is more likely to occur: if standards, supervision, and oversight are low; staff are poorly trained, paid little, and overworked; the physical environment is deficient; and policies operate in the interests of the institution rather than the residents.

10.6 Conclusions

Research on elder abuse is developing slowly and will become increasingly critical as the population over 65 continues to mushroom. Too little is known about elder abuse and how to prevent it. States are autonomous in creating their own statutes, policies, procedures, and programs for addressing elder abuse cases, leaving the country with an incoherent patchwork of policies and practices (Jirik & Sanders, 2014; Teaster et al., 2006). Effectiveness of most prevention initiatives is limited or untested and some strategies are contraindicated due to deleterious effects (i.e., adult protective services and home visitation by police and social workers for victims; World Health Organization, 2018). Interdisciplinary collaboration is warranted for reducing elder abuse, including social workers (i.e., legal, financial, and housing support), educators (i.e., public awareness campaigns), and health care providers (detection and treatment of victims).

Extant data clearly shows that abused and/or neglected frail elders are at risk for increased morbidity, functional disabilities, worsening cognitive impairment, and depression because they receive physical injury and/or are deprived of proper care, including having access to food and medicine (Castle et al., 2015). Financial abuse is increasingly common, drains elderly victims of lifetime savings and assets, and robs them of economic independence. The consequences of community-based victimization by family or friends, including decreased physical, functional, mental, and economic capacities, can trigger premature institutionalization where abuse and maltreatment may continue, perpetrated by either overly stressed staff or aggressive fellow residents. The end result is an unacceptable level of suffering, an overall low quality of life and sense of well-being, and an increased risk of death (Choi & Mayer, 2000).

References

Acierno, R., Hernandez, M. A., Amsadter, A. B., Resnick, H. S., Steve, K., Muzzy, W., & Kilpatrick, D. G. (2010). Prevalence and correlates of emotional, psychical, sexual, and financial abuse and potential neglect in the United States: The National Elder Mistreatment Study. *American Journal Public Health, 100*(2), 292–297.

Adams, M. V., Bagshaw, D., Wendt, S., & Zannettino, L. (2014). Financial abuse of older people by a family member: A difficult terrain for service providers in Australia. *Journal of Elder Abuse & Neglect, 26*(3), 270–290.

Administration on Aging [AoA]. (1998). *The national elder abuse incidence study: Final report.* Retrieved from https://acl.gov/sites/default/files/programs/2016-09/ABuseReport_Full.pdf

Allen, P., Kallett, K., & Gruman, C. (2003). Elder abuse in Connecticut's nursing homes. *Journal of Elder Abuse & Neglect, 15*(1), 19–42.

Baker, M. W., & Heitkemper, M. M. (2005). The roles of nurses on interprofessional teams to combat elder mistreatment. *Nursing Outlook, 53*, 253–259.

Baucom, B. R., Atkins, D. C., Eldridge, K., McFarland, P., Sevier, M., & Christensen, A. (2011). The language of demand/withdraw: Verbal and vocal expression in dyadic interactions. *Journal of Family Psychology, 25*, 570–580.

Bendik, M. F. (1992). Reaching the breaking point: Dangers of mistreatment in elder caregiving situations. *Journal of Elder Abuse & Neglect, 4*, 39–60.

Berman, J. (1994). *Maladaptive networks: Elder abuse victims' experience within the service delivery system.* Doctoral dissertation, Columbia University School of Social Work.

Biggs, S., Manthorpe, J., Tinker, A., Doyle, M., & Erens, B. (2009). Mistreatment of older people in the United Kingdom: Findings from the first national prevalence study. *Journal of Elder Abuse & Neglect, 21*(1), 1–14.

Boldy, D., Horner, B., Crouchley, K., Davey, M., & Boylen, S. (2005). Addressing elder abuse: Western Australian case study. *Australasian Journal on Ageing, 24*(1), 3–8.

Boldy, D., Webb, M., Horner, B., Davey, M., & Kingley, B. (2002). *Elder abuse in Western Australia*. Report of a survey conducted for The Department for Community Development, Seniors Interest, Freemasons Centre for Research Into Aged Care Services. Retrieved from http://apeawa.advocare.org.au/publications/Elder%20Abuse%20in%20WA.pdfBrill

Brill, D. (1999). *Safeguarding the financial interests of vulnerable seniors*. Paper presented at the 7th National Guardianship & Administration Conference, Wesley Conference Centre, Sydney, Australia.

Burnes, D., Pillemer, K., Caccamise, P. L., Mason, A., Henderson, C. R., Berman, J., … Lachs, M. S. (2015). Prevalence of the risk factors for elder abuse and neglect in the community: A population-based study. *Journal of American Geriatric Society, 63*, 1906–1912.

Burston, G. R. (1975). Granny battering. *British Medical Journal, 6*, 592.

Butler, R. N. (1975). *Why survive? Growing old in America*. New York, NY: Harper & Row.

Castle, N. G. (2012a). Nurse aides' reports of resident abuse in nursing homes. *Journal of Applied Gerontology, 31*(3), 402–422.

Castle, N. G. (2012b). Resident-to-resident abuse in nursing homes as reported by nurse aides. *Journal of Elder Abuse & Neglect, 24*, 340–356.

Castle, N. G., Ferguson-Rome, J. C., & Teresi, J. A. (2015). Elder abuse in residential long-term care: An update to the 2003 National Research Council Report. *Journal of Applied Gerontology, 34*(4), 407–443.

Charpentier, M., & Soulières, M, (2013). Elder abuse and neglect in institutional settings: The resident's perspective. *Journal of Elder Abuse & Neglect, 25*(4), 339–354.

Choi, N. G., & Mayer, J. (2000). Elder abuse, neglect, and exploitation. *Journal of Gerontological Social Work, 33*(2), 5–25.

Conner, T., Prokhorov, A., Page, C., Fang, Y., Xiao, Y., & Post, L. A. (2011). Impairment and abuse of elderly by staff in long-term care in Michigan: Evidence from structural equation modeling. *Journal Interpersonal Violence, 26*(1), 21–33.

Coyne, A., Reichman, W., & Berbig, L. (1993). The relationship between dementia and elder abuse. *American Journal of Psychiatry, 150*(4), 643–646.

Cripps, D. (2001). Rights focused advocacy and elder abuse. *Australasian Journal on Ageing, 20*(1), 17–22.

Dong, X., & Simon, M. A. (2013). Association between reported elder abuse and rates of admission to skilled nursing facilities: Findings from a longitudinal population-based cohort study. *Gerontology, 59*, 464–472.

Dong, X., Chen, R., & Simon, M. A. (2014). Elder abuse and dementia: A review of the research and health policy. *Health Affairs (Millwood), 33*(4), 642–649. https://doi.org/10.1377/hlthaff.2013.1261. PMID: 24711326.

Faye, B., & Sellick, M. (2003). *Advocare's speak out survey "S.O.S." on elder abuse*. Retrieved from http://apeawa.advocare.org.au/publications/Speak%20Out%20Survey%20Final%20Report.PDF

Friedman, B., Santos, E. J., Liebel, D. V., Russ, A. J., & Conwell, Y. (2015). Longitudinal prevalence and correlates of elder mistreatment among older adults receiving home visiting nursing. *Journal of Elder Abuse & Neglect, 27*(1), 34–64.

Garcia, J. L., & Kosberg, J. I. (1992). Understanding anger: Implications for formal and informal caregivers. *Journal of Elder Abuse & Neglect, 4*(4), 87–99.

Giles, H., & Helmle, J. (2011). Elder abuse and neglect: A communication framework. In A. Duszak & U. Okulska (Eds.), *Language, culture and the dynamics of age* (pp. 223–252). Berlin, Germany: Mouton de Gruyter.

Giordano, J. A., Yegidis, B. L., & Giordano, N. H. (1992). Victimization of the elderly: Individual and family characteristics of financial abuse. *Arete, 17*, 26–37.

Godkin, M. A., Wolf, R. S., & Pillemer, K. A. (1989). A case-comparison analysis of elder abuse and neglect. *International Journal on Aging and Human Development, 28*(3), 207–225.

Hwalek, M. A., Neale, A. V., Goodrich, C. S., & Quinn, K. (1996). The association of elder abuse and substance abuse in the Illinois elder abuse system. *The Gerontologist, 36*, 694–700.

Jirik, S., & Sanders, S. (2014). Analysis of elder abuse statutes across the United States, 2011–2012. *Journal of Gerontological Social Work, 57*(5), 478–497.

Kosberg, J. I., & Garcia, J. A. (1995). Confronting maltreatment of elders by their family. In G. C. Smith, S. S. Tobin, E. A. Robertson-Tchabo, & P. W. Power (Eds.), *Strengthening aging families* (pp. 63–79). Thousand Oaks, CA: Sage.

Lachs, M., Bachman, R., Williams, C., Kossack, A., Bove, C., & O'Leary, J. (2005). Older adults as crime victims, perpetrators, witnesses, and complainants: A population-based study of police interactions. *Journal of Elder Abuse & Neglect, 16*(4), 25–40.

Lachs, M., Bachman, R., Williams, C. S., & O'Leary, J. R. (2007). Resident-to-resident elder mistreatment and police contact in nursing homes: Findings from a population-based cohort. *Journal of American Geriatrics Society, 55*(6), 840–845.

Lachs, M. S., Rosen, T., Teresi, J. A., Eimicke, J. P., Ramirez, M., Silver, S., & Pillemer, K. (2012). Verbal and physical aggression directed at nursing home staff by residents. *Journal of General Internal Medicine, 28*(5), 660–667.

Lachs, M. S., Williams, C., O'Brien, S., Hurst, L., & Horwitz, R. (1997). Risk factors for reported elder abuse and neglect: A nine-year observational cohort study. *The Gerontologist, 37*, 469–474.

Lachs, M. S., Williams, C. S., O'Brien, S., Pillemer, K. A., & Charlson, M. E. (1998). The mortality of elder mistreatment. *JAMA, 280*(5), 428–432.

Lin, M., & Giles, H. (2013). The dark side of family communication: A communication model of elder abuse and neglect. *International Psychogeriatrics, 25*(8), 1275–1290.

Livermore, P., Bunt, R., & Biscan, K. (2001). Elder abuse among clients and carers referred to the Central Coast ACAT: A descriptive analysis. *Australasian Journal on Ageing, 20*(1), 41–47.

Lowenstein, A., Eisikovits, Z., Band-Winterstein, T., & Enosh, G. (2009). Is elder abuse and neglect a social phenomenon? Data from the first national prevalence survey in Israel. *Journal of Elder Abuse & Neglect, 21*(3), 253–277. https://doi.org/10.1080/08946560902997629

Mosqueda, L., Burnight, K., Gironda, M. W., Moore, A. A., Robinson, J., & Olsen, B. (2016). The abuse intervention model: A pragmatic approach to intervention for elder mistreatment. *Journal of the American Geriatrics Society, 64*(9), 1879–1883.

Mukherjee, D. (2013). Financial exploitation of older adults in rural settings: Family perspective. *Journal of Elder Abuse & Neglect, 25*(5), 425–437.

Natan, M. B., Lowenstein, A., & Eisikovits, Z. (2010). Psycho-social factors affecting elders' maltreatment in long-term care facilities. *International Nursing Review, 57*, 113–120.

National Institute on Aging (NIA). (2018). *Elder abuse.* Retrieved from https://www.nia.nih.gov/health/elder-abuse

Naughton, C., Drennan, J., Lyons, I., Lafferty, A., Treacy, M., Phelan, A., … Delaney, L. (2012). Elder abuse and neglect in Ireland: Results from a national prevalence survey. *Age Aging, 41*(1), 98–103.

Page, C., Conner, T., Prokhorov, A., Fang, Y., & Post, L. (2009). The effect of care setting on elder abuse: Results from a Michigan survey. *Journal of Elder Abuse & Neglect, 21*, 239–252.

Paveza, G., Cohen, D., Eisdorfer, C., Freels, S., Semla, T., Ashford, J. W., … Levy, P. (1992). Severe family violence and Alzheimer's disease: Prevalence and risk factors. *The Gerontologist, 32*(4), 493–497.

Payne, B. K., & Strasser, S. M. (2012). Financial exploitation of older persons in adult care settings: Comparisons to physical abuse and the justice system's response. *Journal of Elder Abuse & neglect, 24*(3), 231–250.

PHI. (n.d.). *U.S. nursing assistants employed in nursing homes: Key facts*. Retrieved from https://phinational.org/wp-content/uploads/legacy/phi-nursing-assistants-key-facts.pdf

Phillips, L. R., & Guo, G. (2011). Mistreatment in assisted living facilities: Complaints, substantiations, and risk factors. *The Gerontologist, 51*, 343–353.

Pillemer, K., Chen, E. K., Van Haitsma, K. S., Teresi, J., Ramirex, M., Silver, S., … Lachs, M. S. (2012). Resident-to-resident aggression in nursing homes: Results from a qualitative event reconstruction study. *The Gerontologist, 52*(1), 24–33.

Pillemer, K., & Finkelhor, D. (1989). Causes of elder abuse: Caregiver stress versus problem relatives. *American Journal of Orthopsychiatry, 59*(2), 179–187.

Quinn, J. Q., & Tomita, S. K. (1997). *Elder abuse and neglect: Causes, diagnosis, intervention strategies*. New York, NY: Springer Publishing Company.

Rabiner, D. J., O'Keeffe, J., & Brown, D. (2004). A conceptual framework of financial exploitation of older persons. *Journal of Elder Abuse and Neglect, 16*(2), 53–72.

Rodriguez, M. A., Wallace, S. P., Woolf, N. H., & Mangione, C. M. (2006). Mandatory reporting of elder abuse: Between a rock and a hard place. *Annals of Family Medicine, 4*, 403–409.

Rosen, T., Pillemer, K., & Lachs, M. (2008). Resident-to-resident aggression in long-term care facilities: An understudied problem. *Aggression and Violent Behavior, 13*, 77–87.

Rzeszut, S. M. (2017). The need for a stronger definition: Recognizing abandonment as a form of elder abuse across the United States. *Family Court Review, 55*(3), 444–457.

Schofield, M. J., & Mishra, G. D. (2004). Three year health outcomes among older women at risk of elder abuse: Women's Health Australia. *Quality of Life Research, 13*, 1043–1052.

Sharon, N. (1991). Elder abuse and neglect substantiations: What they tell us about the problem. *Journal of Elder Abuse & Neglect, 3*, 91–108.

Shinan-Altman, S., & Cohen, M. (2009). Nursing aides' attitudes to elder abuse in nursing homes: The effect of work stressors and burnout. *The Gerontologist, 49*, 674–684.

Shinoda-Tagawa, T., Leonard, R., & Pontikas, J. (2004). Resident-to-resident violent incidents in nursing homes. *Journal of the American Medical Association, 291*, 591–598.

Sifford-Snellgrove, K. S., Beck, C., Green, A., & McSweeney, J. C. (2012). Victim or initiator? Certified nursing assistants' perceptions of resident characteristics that contribute to resident-to-resident violence in nursing homes. *Research in Gerontological Nursing, 5*, 55–63.

Statista. (n.d.). *Care & support*. Retrieved from https://www.statista.com/statistics/716813/total-number-of-nursing-homes-in-us-by-ownership-type/

Teaster, P. B., Otto, J. M., Dugar, T. D., Mendiondo, M. S., Abner, E. L., & Cecil, K. A. (2006). *The 2004 survey of state Adult Protective Services: Abuse of adults 60 years of age and older. Report to the National Center on Elder Abuse*. Washington, DC: Administration on Aging.

Thobaben, M., & Duncan, R. (2003). Domestic elder abuse by health care providers. *Home Health Care Management & Practice, 15*(2), 168–169.

Wilson, J., Tilse, C., Setterlund, D., & Rosenman, L. (2009). Older people and their assets: A range of roles and issues for social workers. *Australian Social Work, 62*(2), 155–167.

Wolf, R. S. (1997). Elder abuse and neglect: Causes and consequences. *Journal of Geriatric Psychiatry, 30*, 153–174.

Wolf, R. S., & Pillemer, K. (1994). What's new in elder abuse programming? Four bright ideas. *The Gerontologist, 34*, 126–129.

World Health Organization. (2018). *Elder abuse*. Retrieved from http://www.who.int/news-room/fact-sheets/detail/elder-abuse

Yon, Y., Mikton, C. R., Gassoumis, Z. D., & Wilber, K. H. (2017). Elder abuse prevalence in community settings: A systematic review and meta-analysis. *Lancet Global Health, 5*(2), e147–e156.

Zeller, A., Hahn, S., Needham, I., Kok, G., Dassen, T., & Halfens, R. J. (2009). Aggressive behavior of nursing home residents toward caregivers: A systematic literature review. *Geriatric Nursing, 30*, 174–187.

Chapter 11
Bullying Between Societal Groups: Playground Politics on a Grand Scale

11.1 Introduction

Not only does bullying happen among individuals on the playground, in families, in organizations or nursing homes, but the bullying dynamic can be applied to larger-scale social groups. At the foundation of our definition of bullying is repeated aggressive behavior that occurs over time, a power differential between perpetrator and victim, and intent to harm. These criteria can be applied to social groups, organizations, and countries to reframe bullying as a global sociological dynamic with deep historical roots. To borrow language from ecological systems theory (Bronfenbrenner, 1989), bullying is easily detected in microsystems (i.e., the individual and immediate environment she or he interacts with—children maltreated by parents, sibling aggression), mesosystems (i.e., relationships between systems—a child and his peer group, a worker and her organization), and macrosystems (i.e., cultures, social institutions, countries). This chapter applies the bullying dynamic to macrosystem conflicts among social groups and societies. Individuals may serve as perpetrators and victims; however, these roles are played out because of group membership, with more powerful groups victimizing less powerful groups.

In group-level bullying, victims can still be individuals, but they are targeted for abuse because they are members of minority social groups that often lack power and/or access to resources. This victimization is overlooked due to the group's marginalization and may require focused social activism over extended periods of time to change the societal power structure. Further, targeted bullying is often institutionalized in the form of discriminatory policies that keep the disempowered group in its place with low social standing and provide few, if any, protections against harm. The legal capacity to own slaves that guided the sociopolitical context in the US from 1776 to 1865 (and then more covertly into the late twentieth century's Civil Rights Movement) is a poignant example of group-level bullying that caused immeasurable human suffering for African Americans. On August 18, 1920, the

© Springer Nature Switzerland AG 2019
P. R. Smokowski, C. B. R. Evans, *Bullying and Victimization Across the Lifespan*, https://doi.org/10.1007/978-3-030-20293-4_11

19th Amendment to the US Constitution granted American women the right to vote (i.e., women's suffrage) after almost a century of protest. Previously, women were expected to focus on housework and motherhood, having no legal claim to money or property. Indeed, after ratification in 1920, it took over 60 years for the remaining 12 US states to ratify the 19th Amendment; Mississippi finally acquiesced on March 22, 1984! Although this was hard-fought progress, a gender pay gap continues to the present with average woman's unadjusted annual salary estimated as 78–82% of that of the average man's. Access to the labor force and college has expanded for women over the past 70 years. Yet women continue to have a higher likelihood of working in female dominated jobs, which typically have below average wages (Boraas & Rodgers, 2003). Figure 11.1 uses data from the U.S. Bureau of Labor Statistics (2000) to illustrate that the gender wage gap varies by state and occupation. Is this a reflection of group-level bullying, males dominating females in a power imbalance repeated over time? We believe that it is.

Similarly, bullies often have power and access due to their affiliation with higher status social groups and use this to exploit others. Perpetrators often escape detection and discipline for long periods of time because of their social affiliations and privilege. As members of the dominant or ruling class, these bullies use their power to enact those policies that create or continue disparity and disadvantage for victimized groups. The resulting institutionalized discrimination is rationalized by group-level attitudes, beliefs, and fears that prompt one group to act against another in service of its survival-and-growth needs. The discriminatory policies set in place by the group protect the dominant group and furthers its goals.

According to the Southern Poverty Law Center (SPLC, n.d.-a), there are 954 hate groups currently operating in the US, enough to have to track all these activities on a national map (https://www.splcenter.org/hate-map). All hate groups have beliefs or practices that attack or malign an entire class of people, typically for their immutable characteristics (e.g., race, religion). Hate group activities can include criminal acts, marches, rallies, speeches, meetings, leafleting, or publishing (SPLC, n.d.-b).

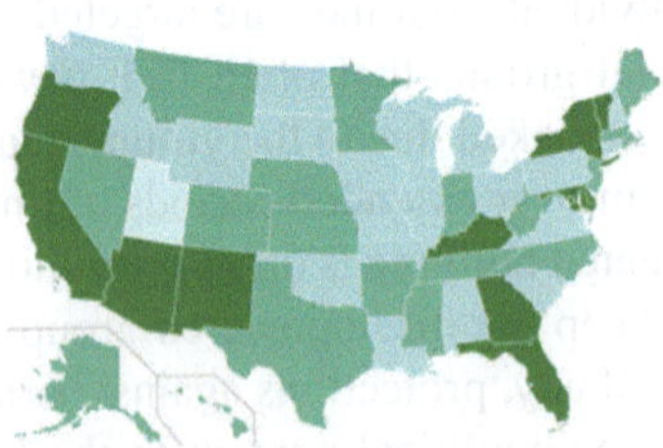

Women's earnings as a percentage of men's earnings, by state, 2016. Data from U.S. Census Bureau.

Green:	85.0–90.2%
Light Green:	80.0–85.0%
Light Blue:	70.0–80.0%
White:	<70.0%

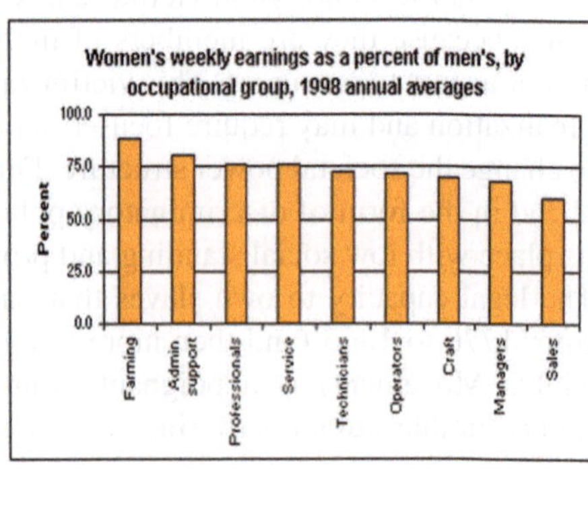

Fig. 11.1 U.S. Bureau of Labor Statistics: gender wage gap varies by occupation and geography

SPLC tracking indicates that the number of hate groups rose to 954 in 2017, from 457 in 1999 (a 52% increase over 18 years) and up from 917 in 2016. Within the white supremacist movement, neo-Nazi groups saw the most growth—increasing by 22%. Anti-Muslim groups increased for a third straight year, while Ku Klux Klan groups decreased from 130 groups to 72. Table 11.1 provides a snapshot of hate groups in the US, according to the SPLC.

It is disheartening to think of group-level bullying as a global dynamic that characterizes social behavior for humans; however, there are innumerable examples spanning historical time and place. The United Nations Genocide Convention defines genocide as "acts committed with intent to destroy, in whole or in part, a national, ethnical, racial or religious group" (Office of the UN Special Adviser on the Prevention of Genocide [OSAPG], 2017). Various other definitions can be found in scholarly literature and national law of different countries; however, the specific definition is less important than the phenomenon fitting into our bullying dynamic of intent to harm, repeated aggression, and power differential. Our bullying definition, when pushed to an extreme, would include genocide, mass murder, crimes against humanity, politicide (destruction of a victim group that shares political beliefs), policide (destruction of a city or nation), classicide (persecution of a social class), and war crimes (e.g., torture, rape during war). While we concede that all of these sociopolitical conflicts would have extensive background and contextual influences, we also believe that it is instructive to see these macrosystem conflicts as massively magnified reflections of basic dynamics of perpetration and victimization rooted in social psychology and intergroup dynamics that are applicable on middle school playgrounds and within the United Nations Security Council. Viewing these serious forms of sociopolitical violence through the lens of the bullying definition is not meant to undermine their severity. Our intent is to provide an innovative means of examining large scale aggression and violence while simultaneously highlighting that bullying behavior can be taken to the extreme with serious consequences. Engaging in bullying behavior on the elementary school playground can set the stage for more serious forms of bullying and violence down the road.

11.2 Genocide

During the Holocaust from 1937 to 1945, Adolf Hitler's German army tried to eliminate Jewish people on the European continent. Nearly six million Jewish people (58% of the Jewish population at the time) from 22 different countries were hunted down and killed. Legislative discriminatory policies targeting genocide based on ethnicity, religion, politics, and/or sexual orientation were enacted, resulting in incarceration without legal proceedings, confiscation of property, forced labor, sexual slavery, medical experimentation, torture, and death. Along with Jewish people, Soviet citizens and POWs (approximately 7.5 million), Polish people (3 million), Serbs (600,000), people with disabilities (270,000), Romani (500,000), Freemasons (200,000), Slovenes (25,000), Spanish Republicans (7000), homosexuals (15,000),

Table 11.1 Hate groups in the USA 2017 by ideology—SPLC

Type of group	Belief or ideology	Number of organizations/ branches	Examples
Alt-Right (Alternative Right)	White identity is being attacked by multicultural groups using political correctness and social justice to undermine white people and their civilization.	1; ghost headquarters, Statewide Virginia	Charlottesville rally 2017 where one woman was killed; heavy use of social media.
Anti-immigrant	Nativist and vigilante groups that target immigrants and their supporters.	22 nationwide	President Trump: Family separations of immigrant parents from children at border, calling Mexicans "rapists"; "shithole countries" in Africa.
Anti-LGBT	Opposition to LGBT rights, vilify LGBT individuals as threats to children, society, and public health.	51 nationwide	Christian Right groups, oppose gay marriage, LGBT rights, rhetoric that LGBT people are perverts and pedophiles.
Anti-Muslim	Extreme hostility towards Muslims.	113 nationwide	Anti-Muslim groups mushroomed after World Trade Center bombing. Rhetoric that Muslims are terrorists.
Black Nationalist	The solution to white racism is to create separate institutions—or even a separate nation—for black people; anti-white and anti-Semitic.	233 nationwide	Should not be confused with the many non-racist African American organizations that work for social justice and the elimination of institutional racism in America.
Christian Identity	Anti-Semitic and racist theology; Christian in name only.	20 nationwide	White racists hostile to Evangelicals and Fundamentalist Christians.
General Hate Groups	Miscellaneous hate attitudes from a variety of White Supremacist materials.	53 nationwide	Cultural Studies Press, NY, NY. General hate groups were early adopters of bitcoin because no government can intervene in the fundraising.
Hate Music	White Power music labels.	15 nationwide	Record, publish, and distribute music with racist themes.
Holocaust Denial	Deny that 6 million Jews were killed in World War II.	10 nationwide	Call themselves "historical revisionists." Try to rehabilitate the German Nazis' image to make national socialism more acceptable.

(continued)

Table 11.1 (continued)

Type of group	Belief or ideology	Number of organizations/ branches	Examples
Klu Klux Klan	Attacked Blacks, Jews, immigrants, gays and lesbians and Catholics.	72 nationwide	Oldest and most violent hate group; Lynchings, tar-and-featherings, rapes and other violent attacks on southern Blacks.
Male Supremacy	Subjugation of women.	2	A Voice For Men (Statewide, Texas). Return of Kings (Statewide, District of Columbia).
Neo-Confederate	Espouse symbols of the Confederate States of America, secession.	31, mostly in southern US	Protection of Confederate symbols and monuments.
Neo-Nazi	Hate minorities, gays and lesbians and sometimes Christians, but they view "the Jew" as their ultimate enemy.	121 nationwide	Love Adolf Hitler and Nazi Germany.
Neo-Volkisch	Worship the Norse or Germanic gods, spirituality premised on the survival of white Europeans and the preservation of dead or dying cultures they presume to embody.	28 nationwide	Spirituality such as Odinism or Wotanism, Odalism, heathenism, Ásatrú, or even paganism.
Racist Skinhead	Violent element of the white supremacist movement.	71 nationwide	Confederate Hammerskins, Crew 38, Confederate 28.
Radical Traditional Catholicism	See Jews as "the perpetual enemy of Christ," reject the ecumenical efforts of the Vatican, and even assert that recent popes have all been illegitimate.	11 sparse distribution nationwide	Culture Wars/Fidelity Press in South Bend, IN.
White Nationalist	Believe in White supremacy and inferiority of nonwhites.	100 nationwide	Other groups including the Ku Klux Klan, neo-Confederate, neo-Nazi, racist skinhead, and Christian Identity—could also be described as white nationalist.

Catholics (no estimate), and Jehovah's Witnesses (5000) were also killed. Individuals considered Aryan or members of the "master race" were empowered to kill off those victims they considered to be burdens on society. Children and adults with disabilities, and those with mental illness, were among the first to be killed beginning in 1939. Indeed, some historians suggest that when Hitler's goal of dominating Europe became unachievable, he turned his attention to exterminating weaker minority groups; he bullied those social groups that were easier to victimize and least able to retaliate. Further, the death toll might have been so high for so long because the Nazis were abusing marginalized groups who had far less power and influence to generate resistance or retaliate. Picking on the powerless is at the heart of all bullying behavior.

The Holocaust was exceptionally tragic and shameful in ways that defy human explanation. Yet the hatred, discrimination, and abuse among societal groups vying for power and control that characterized that dark time in history is not isolated or overly idiosyncratic. Up to 7.5 million Ukrainians died from artificial starvation during the Soviet famine of 1932–1933, although the exact circumstances are controversial. Cambodian genocide was carried out by the Khmer Rouge led by Pol Pot who forced the urban population of an estimated three million Cambodian Chinese, Cham, Lao, and Thai to relocate to the countryside, experiencing savage torture, mass executions, forced labor, and starvation. At least 50% of Armenians (1.5 million) in Turkey were killed from 1915 to 1922 by the Ottoman Empire. From 1949 to 1951, Mao Zedong conducted mass killings of millions of landlords (classicide) to redistribute land to peasants during the Chinese Civil War and up to possibly 14 million deaths occurred from 1947 to 1976. In 1994, 70% of (an estimated one million) Tutsis in Rwanda were killed, representing 20% of Rwanda's total population.

Genocide is not simply a historical phenomenon; there are ongoing genocides happening today in Darfur, Sudan (estimate 500,000 deaths and counting), Rohingya (43,000 deaths), and northern Iraq and Syria (4400 deaths). China invaded neighboring Tibet in 1950 based on claims of past ownership. Occupation has lasted more than 60 years (and continues) with more than one million Tibetans killed, a vast network of monasteries destroyed, thousands of monks jailed, and forced sterilization of Tibetan women to keep the population from reproducing (Free Tibet, n.d.). Expression of political and religious ideas is harshly repressed, resulting in imprisonment and torture. To enable access to natural resources and to improve control over Tibetans, China has moved more than two million Tibetan nomads from the land they have lived off for generations to barrack-like urban settlements. Facing institutionalized discrimination and lacking skills to obtain work in an urban environment, nomads face poverty, unemployment, and social exclusion (Free Tibet, n.d.).

Indeed, the Freedom House (2016) *Freedom in the World Report* documented that 40% of the world's population lives in free countries, 24% in partly free countries, and 36% in areas that are not free. Areas considered not free are characterized by authoritarian regimes, anxious dictators cracking down on dissent, and/or wavering democracies. In 2017, global freedom declined for the tenth consecutive year, with 72 countries declining in freedom while 42 made gains (Freedom House, 2016). Historical and contemporary genocide and intergroup conflicts are often fueled by hate based on race, religion, gender, disability, and sexual orientation. Physical indicators of group affiliation (such as skin color or primary sex characteristics defining males/females) may play into group separation and "us versus them" cognitive scripts.

11.3 Income Inequality and Power

Societies consistently craft norms and values that prioritize particularly prized attributes over lower-value attributes. In the US, there are clear inequalities in income, resources, and wealth that favor males, those with higher education, Caucasians, size (thin rather than heavy, with "fat" people receiving harsh social criticism), and even stature (i.e., tall rather than shorter individuals). Despite a progressive tax system meant to redistribute some wealth from top earners to lower income workers, the World Factbook (Central Intelligence Agency, n.d.) states that 70% of countries have a more equal income distribution than the US does. Figure 11.2 shows indicators of income inequality suggesting that the top 1% of earners garner nearly 20% of the nation's income. This suggests a consolidation of wealth and power that lends itself to bullying by high status individuals/groups against those with less status in order to maintain their advantages. This is not to say that all wealthy individuals are bullies, like most attributes there is considerable variation within social group or strata. Noteworthy examples of billionaires, such as Bill Gates or Warren Buffet, giving away fortunes through philanthropy certainly exist. However, examples of corruption and manipulation are also easy to find and are the focus for our group level bullying discussion.

Because political power often follows wealth, high-status groups are in the position to set policy and impact social programs through budgetary processes. Donald Trump became the first billionaire to be president of the US in 2017 and filled his cabinet with friends and donors worth $4.3 billion. The richest cabinet in modern history includes Wilbur Ross, Secretary of Commerce—$2.5 billion; Betsy Devos, Secretary of Education—$1 billion; Stephen Mnuchin, Secretary of Treasury—$385 million; Rex Tillerson, former Secretary of State—$300 million; Ben Carson, Secretary of Housing and Urban Development—$22 million; Elaine Chao, Secretary of Transportation—$22 million; David Shulkin, Secretary of Veteran's Affairs—$17 million; and a number of other wealthy appointees who brought controversial

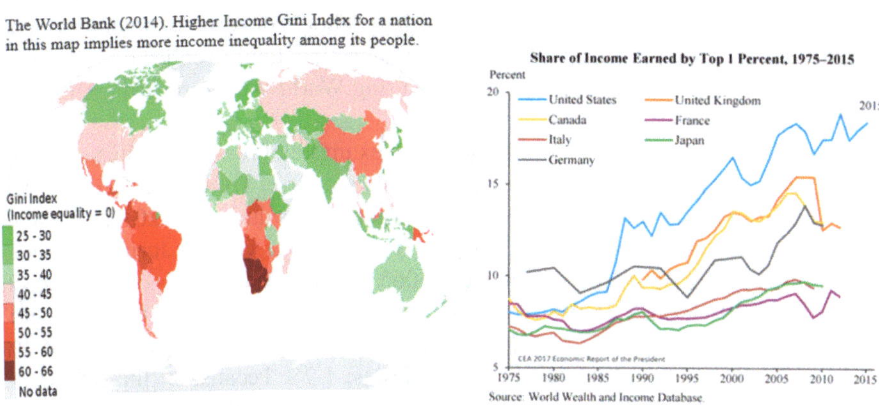

Fig. 11.2 Income inequality and share of income earned by top 1%

conflicts of interest and low levels of specific experience relevant to their posts. The major accomplishment that the Republican-controlled Congress and White House made in the first 2 years of the Trump administration was passing a major tax cut in December of 2017 that disproportionately aids the wealthy and adds $1.4 trillion to the national debt over the next 10 years that all citizens and future generations have to shoulder. Eighty percent of the tax cut benefit would go to the top 1% of households making $730,000 or more annually. These 1%-ers already control 40% of the country's wealth. It is hard not to interpret this as overt classism, favoring the rich.

11.4 Political Bullying

In 2018, the Trump administration also showed a propensity toward bullying by roughing up the most powerless segment of society, immigrants. Immigrants and refugees typically have no rights that come with citizenship, no resources, and few interpersonal connections within the new country. Those coming without legal documentation must evade the authorities and start a new life, often without speaking the language, in the shadows of society to avoid detection. In the now infamous "family separation" policy, Attorney General Jeff Sessions pursued a new "zero tolerance" policy of treating all border crossings by immigrants as federal criminal offenses that would be prosecuted. More than 2500 immigrant children were separated from their parents, sending parents to jail to await judicial hearings and children went to facilities run by the Office of Refugee Resettlement within the Department of Health and Human Services, such as a converted Walmart in Texas. Children were sent to facilities across the country with no information given to parents about their whereabouts or when they would be reunited, siblings were split up, and photos emerged of youth huddled in cages, sleeping on the floor. Protests and litigation ensued from immigrant advocacy groups; news reports described child trauma and abuse at detention facilities. This inhumane treatment of families paralleled historical use of similar strategies when Native American children were taken away from their families to be raised in boarding schools or when African American families were split up by slaveowners to undermine family cohesion. Japanese American families were interred in camps during World War II, regardless of their citizenship.

Trump's family separation policy is a good example of how low-status minority groups are at high risk of victimization with little recourse. Trump repeatedly called Mexicans, and then Latinos in general, rapists and killers during his 2016 campaign rallies to fire up his xenophobic supporters. Hate speech escalated during this time. According to the FBI, in 2016, there were 6063 single-bias incidents of hate speech involving 7509 victims: 58.9% of victims were targeted because of the offenders' race/ethnicity/ancestry bias; 21.1% because of the offenders' religious bias; 16.7% because of the offenders' sexual-orientation bias; 1.7% because of the offenders' gender identity bias; 1.0% because of the offenders' disability bias; and 0.5% because of the offenders' gender bias (Federal Bureau of Investigations, 2016).

After the 2016 election, hate crimes overall increased by 92%, anti-Black 77%, anti-White 62%, anti-Hispanic/Latino 176%, anti-Muslim/Arab 78% (Federal Bureau of Investigations, 2016). This illustrates how the leadership of a vocal bully, in this case Donald Trump, can dramatically impact intergroup conflict.

We will use these examples of bullying against immigrants to lead into a more theoretical discussion of intergroup conflict over culture. The process of acculturation in general and assimilation of immigrants into the dominant host culture in particular provides a relevant example of bullying across cultural groups.

11.5 Assimilation and Eugenics: Immigrants Bullied by the Dominant Cultural Group to Become Like Us, Leave, or Die

After immigration to a new country, the central issue for immigrant families becomes how to adjust to the new sociocultural environment. Within the new country, immigrants are a particularly disempowered group with few rights and privileges that come with citizenship and little access to societal resources. Policies may even restrict access to basic educational institutions, social services, and/or health care, leaving immigrants, individually and as a group, vulnerable to abuse and exploitation. This leads to a significant example of group-level bullying where the same issues characterizing playground politics (i.e., who has power and control, and how the dominant people in high status roles will use that power) are reflected in how dominant and vulnerable social groups treat each other. In group level bullying, the nondominant or vulnerable group is strongly influenced to take on norms, values, and behaviors espoused by the dominant group. The intensity and negativity associated with this process are largely contingent upon the receptivity of the dominant group in welcoming, respecting, or stigmatizing the nondominant group (Berry, 1998). Further, the attitudes held by the dominant group influence the adoption of policies for relating to the nondominant group. For example, dominant group attitudes towards immigrants that influence policy are reflected in the debate in the US regarding whether English should be declared the country's official language, in the question of whether school districts support English immersion or bilingual education programs, and in restrictions requiring certain forms of identification that are difficult for some immigrants to obtain in order for them to receive a driver's license. Cutting off social resources (e.g., education, health care) gives the strong assimilationist message to conform (e.g., learn English, abandon your culture of origin norms), leave (e.g., many immigrants are frequently told to go back to their own countries), or die (e.g., from lack of health care, exploitation, or in rare cases through homicide).

Antagonistic attitudes from the dominant group towards immigrants often prompt calls for assimilation or elimination. The term "assimilation," refers to unidirectional adaptations made by minority individuals to conform to the dominant group. Such change is commonly characterized by nondominant groups taking on the language, laws, religions, norms, and behaviors of the dominant group (Berry, 1998; Castro, Coe, Gutierres, & Saenz, 1996; Chun, Organista, & Marin, 2002). Under the stress of assimilation, particularly monolingualism pressure and discrimination experiences, immigrants are bullied into giving up their culture of origin identities. This process is especially intense for immigrant youth (Smokowski & Bacallao, 2010). The individual perceives the dominant culture as more desirable whereas the culture of origin is seen as inferior.

Ethnic and racial discrimination play an important role in acculturation. The atmosphere upon arrival, that is, the extent to which the host culture supports or stigmatizes new immigrants, is a crucial element in determining how stressful post-immigration adjustment will be (de Anda, 1984; Berry, 1998).

In the earliest days of the US, colonists saw the new republic as the beginning of a utopian society where immigrants from different nationalities, cultures, and races blended into an idealized American "new man."

> [W]hence came all these people? They are a mixture of English, Scotch, Irish, French, Dutch, Germans, and Swedes .... What, then, is the American, this new man? He is neither a European nor the descendant of a European; hence that strange mixture of blood, which you will find in no other country ... He is an American, who, leaving behind him all his ancient prejudices and manners, receives new ones from the new mode of life he has embraced, the new government he obeys, and the new rank he holds .... The Americans were once scattered all over Europe; here they are incorporated into one of the finest systems of population which has ever appeared. (J. Hector St. John de Crevecoeur, *Letters from an American Farmer*, 1782)

In this quote from the earliest days of colonization, there are the seeds of assimilation of disparate Western European immigrants into a "new man" which is deemed "the finest population which has ever appeared." This aspirational shared identity (i.e., "Americans") was an important theme to catalyze colonization and group identity for a newly independent country; however, it also fed nativism and discrimination.

It is not difficult to see the seeds of visualizing a "master race" or chosen people in this ideology. Indeed, Eugenics, the beliefs and practices suggesting that the genetic quality of the human population should be maximized with some races superior to others, and nativism, the belief that established groups have priority over newcomers have deep roots in North America. Eugenics programs in Nazi Germany were inspired by prior work in the US and other countries. The history of Eugenics spans much of human history and cultures around the globe. In ancient Greece, Plato believed human reproduction should be controlled and monitored by the state, perhaps using a rigged lottery system where high value females were matched to high value males. This idea resurfaced in German experiments at Lebensborn where men and women with the most valued Aryan traits reproduced to further the master race. At the other extreme, early civilizations in Rome, Athens, and Sparta practiced infanticide where elders tested infants' strength and fitness; only the strong were allowed to survive while others deemed weak were left to die in the mountains. Roman law allowed patriarchs to kill deformed children at their discretion, often drowning or discarding them to die. As the philosopher Seneca (1995) wrote,

> We put down mad dogs; we kill the wild, untamed ox; we use the knife on sick sheep to stop their infecting the flock; we destroy abnormal offspring at birth; children, too, if they are born weak or deformed, we drown. Yet this is not the work of anger, but of reason—to separate the sound from the worthless

The enduring idea that some humans were sound and some worthless can be seen as underpinning the history of human discrimination, imperialism, and intergroup conflict and hate. These sentiments can be traced back thousands of years.

As a fledgling nation of immigrants who overran and exploited native people to create the country, the US has struggled with what would now be considered racist and nativist attitudes and policies for much of its history. The 1798 Alien and Sedition Acts restricted the ability of immigrants, especially radicals from *France* and *Ireland*, to gain complete political rights. In the 1830s to the 1850s Nativist parties formed to oppose *Catholic* immigrants from Ireland. In western states, throughout the 1870s, Irish American immigrants attacked *Chinese* immigrants, forcing them out of smaller towns. In 1882, the Chinese Exclusion Act limited immigration from Asian countries. From the 1840s to 1920 *German* Americans were distrusted and shunned due to their separatist social structure, their love of beer, their German-language schools, their preference for the German language over English, and their neutrality in World War I. In the 1920s people feared low-skilled immigrants (mainly from *Italy* and *Poland* flooding the labor market and today in the 2000s this same fear extends to *Mexicans*.

Figure 11.3 provides an example illustration of how political cartoons captured the nativist discriminatory views during the nineteenth century. These cartoons

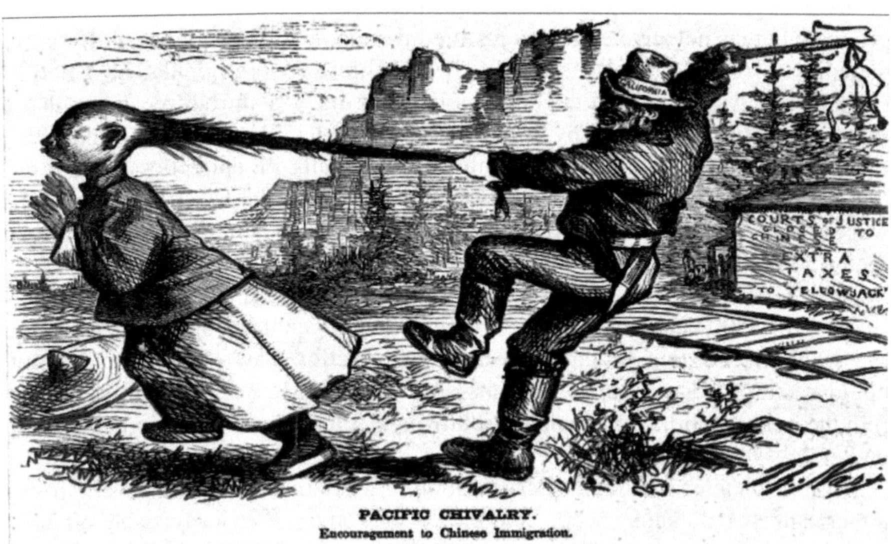

Fig. 11.3 Pacific Chivalry: encouragement to Chinese immigration, August 7, 1869 by Thomas Nast

clearly capture how intergroup bullying fuels assimilation pressure on minority groups. A simple Google search on "political cartoons and race, 1800s" provides many shocking examples of historical mistreatment of minority groups.

Charles Darwin (1809–1882), the English biologist and one of the most famous scientists in human history, popularized the concepts of natural selection, selective breeding, and evolution of species. In his seminal book *On the Origins of Species* (1859), Darwin writes in the introduction,

> As many more individuals of each species are born than can possibly survive; and as, consequently, there is a frequently recurring struggle for existence, it follows that any being, if it vary however slightly in any manner profitable to itself, under the complex and sometimes varying conditions of life, will have a better chance of surviving, and thus be naturally selected. From the strong principle of inheritance, any selected variety will tend to propagate its new and modified form (p. 5).

While Darwin was awed at the great diversity within species of plants, animals, and humans, he did not emphasize the application of his theory of natural selection to humans. He opposed slavery, but favored colonization as spreading the favorable aspects of European civilization. Unfortunately, savage peoples would become civilized or face extinction, reflecting the natural order of events even if it went against Darwin's humanitarian beliefs. Other scientists of the time were less cautious in generalizing the ideas of natural selection and evolution to humans. Francis Galton, Darwin's half cousin, vigorously promoted the idea of eugenics as a utopian plan to improve the human race. Survival of the fittest was developed as a sociological idea to justify free market economics. Colonialism, imperialism, and dog-eat-dog capitalism were all justified under the label Darwinism when Darwin never promoted his work in this way.

Applications of eugenics to social policy were stark and often devastating; positive eugenics promoted the further status and power of privileged social groups whereas negative eugenics justified the eradication of the weak. Negative eugenics to remove the "feebleminded" and inferior were popular in America, Canada and Australia, and eugenics policies in the US introduced compulsory sterilization laws, followed by several other countries. Between 1907 and 1963, over 64,000 individuals (the unfit, imbeciles, mentally ill, epileptics) were forcibly sterilized under eugenics legislation in the US (Lombardo, 2018). During the war crimes trials in Nuremberg after World War II, Nazi administrators described their 450,000 mass sterilizations as inspired by laws in the US (Kühl, 1994). The Sexual Sterilization Act enacted in 1928 in Alberta Canada led to the forced sterilization of 3500 "mentally deficit" women and indigenous people and lasted into the 1970s. According to Japan's Eugenic Protection Law (1948), sterilization could be forced on criminals, patients with genetic diseases such as total colorblindness, hemophilia, albinism and ichthyosis, schizophrenia, manic-depression, and epilepsy (Soshiren.org).

Positive eugenics justified discrimination, prioritizing Anglo races over African Americans or indigenous people and men over women. Policies focusing on positive eugenics propelled forced cultural assimilation of Aboriginal youth in Australia,

"Whitening Policies" in Brazil, Pure Blood Theory in Korea, and the One Child Policy in China which resulted in many more male babies than females. Of course, the Aryan "Master Race" was promoted in Nazi Germany.

Negative eugenics policies pressured victimized groups to accommodate, leave, or die. Assimilation sentiments and eugenics have underpinned cultural relations and prompted public policy throughout American history. During his presidency in 1801, Thomas Jefferson wrote,

> The American settlements will gradually circumscribe and approach the Indians, who will in time either incorporate with us as citizens of the United States, or remove beyond the Mississippi. Some tribes are advancing, and on these English seductions will have no effect. But the backward will yield, and be thrown further back into barbarism and misery ... and we shall be obliged to drive them with the beasts of the forest into the stony mountains. ("We Shall Remain", 2009 Chaps. 2 and 4)

Native Americans were enrolled in tribes and, because they did not have US citizenship until the Indian Citizenship Act of 1924, they were subjected to government policies of enforced cultural assimilation, also termed "Americanization." Native American children were taken from their families and placed in boarding schools to teach them how to interact in civilized society. African Americans were also excluded for not being white. Slave owners deliberately broke up families of African slaves so that they would be easier to control. Even after the Emancipation Proclamation banished slavery and made African Americans citizens, intermarriage between whites and African Americans was illegal in many US states under anti-miscegenation laws, which continued from 1883 until 1967. Asian immigrants such as Chinese, Japanese, Koreans, and Filipinos were ruled to be nonwhite and banned from marrying whites in several states where existing anti-miscegenation laws were expanded to include them. After a number of conflicting rulings in American courts, Punjabi people and others from British India were also deemed to be nonwhites. In the late nineteenth and early twentieth centuries, laws such as the Chinese Exclusion Act severely limited or banned immigration by Asians. The Immigration Act of 1924 severely restricted immigration from areas outside Northern and Western Europe.

Assimilation fervor peaks during times of national distress. There was a backlash against German immigrants during World War I. Many Japanese American adults who were imprisoned during World War II tried to discard their ethnic identity and assimilate after the end of the war, attempting to avoid any association, shame, or embarrassment that came from being imprisoned. Attitudes towards nonwhite immigrants and natives gradually improved after World War II in the second half of the twentieth century. Since the successes of the American civil rights movement and the enactment of the Immigration and Nationality Act of 1965, which allowed for a large increase in immigration from Latin America and Asia, intermarriage between white and nonwhite Americans has been increasing. However, after the terrorist attacks on the World Trade Center on September 11, 2001, assimilationist rhetoric enjoyed a resurgence and remains central to the immigrants' drama of adjusting to life in the US.

Nativist sentiment is particularly strong during the Trump Presidency, with his ongoing calls to build a "big beautiful wall" on the border with Mexico and his vocal opposition to immigrants from "shithole" countries coming to the US. The underlying anti-immigrant themes illustrated in Fig. 11.3 are clearly still salient 150 years later in contemporary politics; it is simply the immigrant group targeted for abuse and ostracism that changes. Blank (1997) stated this eloquently,

> Disproportionately, in an immigrant nation, the poor have always been the most recent immigrant group, which means they have always been "the other"—the strangers who dress differently, talk with strange accents, or follow strange customs. The stranger, the one who is different, has always caused fear (p. 47)

This fear triggers intergroup hatred and discrimination with "us versus them" evolutionary scripts.

Although the targeted group changes, nativist arguments are highly consistent. Nativist anti-immigration sentiment is typically justified with the following arguments about immigrants:

> 1) Government expense: Government expenses may exceed tax revenue relating to new immigrants; 2) Language: Immigrants isolate themselves in their own communities and refuse to learn the local language; 3) Employment: Immigrants acquire jobs which would have otherwise been available to native citizens, and suppress wages; 4) Patriotism: Immigrants damage a sense of community and nationality; 5) Consumption: Immigrants increase consumption of scarce resources; 6) Welfare: Immigrants make heavy use of social welfare systems; 7) Overpopulation: Immigrants overpopulate and have too many children; 8) Culture: Immigrants will swamp a native population and replace its culture with their own; and 9) Increase in housing costs: migrant families can reduce vacancies and cause rent increases. (http://www.thefullwiki.org/Nativism_(politics))

Many of these arguments are not borne out by evidence and data often makes the case that immigrants contribute more than they take from the host society. However, fear overtakes rationality in these ongoing debates.

Suarez-Orozco and Suarez-Orozco (2001) found that social mirroring had a particularly strong effect on immigrant adaptation. Social mirroring concerns the public perceptions, racial distortions, day-to-day interactions, and ascribed identities that characterize immigrants' relations with members of the dominant culture and the messages immigrants receive from the dominant culture media. For example, Suarez-Orozco and Suarez-Orozco (2001) reported that "fully 65 percent of our participants had a negative association to the sentence 'Most Americans think [people from the child's culture of origin] are ____'" (p. 97). Negative social mirroring is an important factor outside the home, while inside the home, immigrant parents try to reflect positive social mirroring and deflect negative social mirroring. Immigrant parents not only have to shelter their children from negative social mirroring but also need to deflect toxic messages from employers and coworkers (Smokowski & Bacallao, 2010; Suarez-Orozco & Suarez-Orozco, 2001). This dual process is oppressive and stressful, encapsulating the bullying dynamic of perpetration, victimization, and the toxic effects of using power differentials for discrimination between social groups.

11.6 Theoretical Explanations for Group Level Bullying

11.6.1 Social Capital Theory: A Missing Link for Victims and a Motivation for Bullying Behavior

11.6.1.1 Social Capital Theory and Bullying Victimization

Groups victimized by bullying often have low social status (Bagwell & Schmidt, 2011; Scholte et al., 2008) resulting in minimal social capital. Even when bullied groups have alliances, these alliances do not provide social capital because victimized groups are often rejected by the larger dominant group outside the alliance (Scholte et al., 2008). Although having one or a few alliances could serve to reinforce a group's self-worth, these relationships likely do not increase their access to valuable social information, improve their social credentials, or provide avenues to influence powerful social figures. Further, victims' limited social capital likely precludes them from being invited to social gatherings where they would have the opportunity to interact and perhaps bond with peers who could provide social capital.

Victimized groups lack of social capital intensifies and prolongs their victimization experiences and many victims lack relationships to protect them from being bullied. For example, victims are unlikely to receive help from bystanders given that research has shown only 10–20% of bystanders intervened to protect victims of bullying (Atlas & Pepler, 1998; Hawkins, Pepler, & Craig, 2001; Salmivalli, Lappalainen, & Lagerspetz, 1998). Thus, bullying behavior often continues uninterrupted and when detected often goes unpunished.

11.6.1.2 Social Capital Theory and Bullying Perpetration

Parallel to our earlier discussion of individual perpetrators, group-level bullies often have an easier time acquiring social capital and use bullying tactics as a means of amassing social capital in the form of social status (Pellegrini, 2002). High status social groups exert power over weaker groups, relegating those disempowered groups to a low position in the social hierarchy. Although bullies are usually disliked (Rodkin & Berger, 2008) they are often perceived as popular by their peer group (de Bruyn, Cillessen, & Wissink, 2010; Prinstein & Cillessen, 2003; Vaillancourt, Hymel, & McDougall, 2003). Perceived popularity indicates social status and is a form of social capital because it indicates that peers think of bullies as having power and social prestige. This power protects bullies from becoming victims and increases the likelihood of their peers rallying behind them. Indeed, bullies who are able to effectively use intimidation and humiliation tactics often become the leaders of their social groups (Pellegrini, Bartini, & Brooks, 1999). Having a group of devoted followers reinforces an individual's self-worth, which is one of the benefits of social capital. Further, being a group leader provides opportunities for making social connections with leaders of other groups, and thus expanding the individual's social credentials through bridging social capital. Once a group amasses social power, group members benefit from that social power and strive to maintain it, often times using bullying tactics as means to stay on top.

Bully-victim groups (i.e., groups both bullied and who bully others) might also turn to bullying perpetration as a means of acquiring social capital, improving their social status and ending their victimization. As groups scramble for social capital, bully-victim groups are likely victimized, resulting in a low social status and a lack of social capital. However, rather than withdrawing like most victims, bully-victim groups might search out weaker groups to bully in an effort to obtain social capital and improve their social status. This helps to explain instances of minority groups fighting against each other rather than against the dominant social group.

In summary, social capital refers to the resources embedded in social relationships. Both individuals and groups benefit from the resources of information, social influence, social credentials, and reinforcement of self-worth that social ties provide. Victims of bullying have few friends or social ties, and thus, have minimal social capital, which prevents them from exiting their role as a victim. Conversely, bullies use bullying tactics as a means of acquiring social capital in the form of perceived popularity. People often perceive bullies as powerful and popular, which serves as a form of social capital that protects bullies' social status. Finally, bully-victims attempt to end their victimization and gain social capital by bullying weaker peers, creating a social hierarchy of power and victimization.

11.6.1.3 Social Dominance Theory

Introduced in Chap. 2, Social Dominance Theory (SDT; Sidanius & Pratto, 1999) focuses on group-based social hierarchies, arguing that all societies consist of group-based social hierarchies that are based on gender (e.g., males have more power than females), age (e.g., adults have more power than children), and an arbitrary-set system (e.g., socially significant group differences such as ethnicity or social class that create hierarchies; Sidanius & Pratto, 1999). These group-based social hierarchies are formed through the mechanisms of oppression, discrimination, and injustice. Dominant groups oppress less-powerful groups to form a hierarchy with one or a few dominant groups at the top while subordinate groups are forced to the bottom. The dominant group possesses a disproportionate amount of "… positive social value, or all those materials and symbolic things for which people strive" (Sidanius & Pratto, 1999, p. 31), whereas the subordinate groups possess disproportionate amounts of negative social value. In group-based social hierarchies, the social status and power of individuals is gained from their group membership rather than individual characteristics. These hierarchies are then maintained through ongoing bullying and humiliation of victim groups.

The humiliation of being bullied violates the group's fundamental need for respect and recognition. Humiliation also undermines social standing, engendering the psychological pain of ostracism. Being bullied results in anger; this anger can be externalized as retaliation or internalized as depression. In contrast, other victim groups internalize the humiliation and feel deep despair, which manifests as depression.

11.6.1.4 The Oppression Model

Affiliation with social groups is a primary driver of identity development across the life span, reflecting the internalization of an individual's social context and cultural environment (Capuzzi & Staufer, 2019; Harro, 2000). The oppression model (Bell, 2007) emphasizes that some specific social identities have more power than others within a society (e.g., White individuals may have more privilege than minority group members; physicians and lawyers may accumulate wealth at a faster rate than other professions due to higher salaries). Dominant or "agent" groups have more power than "target" groups. In the discussion above on assimilation of immigrants and eugenics, dominant groups in the US were Anglo, male, physically "abled," heterosexual, Christian, legal citizens while targeted groups were each new wave of immigrants, regardless of culture of origin ancestry, and groups labeled inferior due to disabilities, age, religion, or low socioeconomic status. Agent groups have the power to define societal norms and determine what is "normal" or acceptable in social environments.

Oppression happens when agent groups systematically devalue or undermine the values, experiences, or beliefs of the targeted groups (e.g., assimilation pressure, laws withholding specific rights from certain groups, in extreme situations, genocide against devalued groups). This definition similarly captures our application of the bullying dynamic to higher level social groups. Agent groups bully or oppress targeted groups using prejudice, stereotypes, discrimination, and privilege (Blumenfeld & Raymond, 2000; Capuzzi & Staufer, 2019; Smith & Kehe, 2004; Smokowski & Bacallao, 2010). Just as in playground bullying, having less power, being victimized, and publicly humiliated in many cases dramatically impacts how individuals from oppressed groups see themselves, life, and agent groups (e.g., a process sometimes called psychological colonization). The targeted group's culture, language, and history is misrepresented, distorted, or eradicated while the dominant group's culture is imposed. The oppression model contends that social oppression is exerted through individual, institutional, and societal discriminatory attitudes and behaviors that are conscious or unconscious (Adams, Bell, & Griffin, 1997). The power imbalance, as seen in every reflection of bullying behavior, is key to the successful implementation of oppressive actions. As discussed in detail in previous chapters, prolonged exposure to oppressive environments may result in internalization of toxic cultural messages that impact individual and group self-esteem and mental health. Feeling disempowered by privileged agent groups or high-status bullies results in mistrust and anger that is a form of interpersonal trauma with concomitant long term negative consequences for members of minority target groups.

11.7 Conclusions

In this chapter, we applied our definition of the bullying dynamic—repeated aggression over time, power imbalance, and intent to harm—to macro level conflict between social groups. Major areas of historical and contemporary human conflict, such as genocide, human trafficking, war crimes, hate crimes, racism, xenophobia, misogyny, ableism, and classism among others can fit this bullying definition. At the group level, victimization and perpetration dynamics are similar to the playground politics between individuals (i.e., physical and relational aggression are main instruments of power-seeking perpetrators; victimized groups suffer humiliation and traumatic stress). However, group level bullying targets victims by indexing their group affiliation based on immutable characteristics (e.g., race, disability) or membership status (e.g., religion, identification with GLBT groups). Discrimination, prejudice, humiliation, exclusion, and isolation remain major weapons in group level bullying dynamics, wielded by bullies to devastate victim groups.

The Holocaust during World War II would be a common example of group level bullying magnified to horrific proportions. Yet we discussed historical examples going back to ancient Greece and ongoing struggles happening today that encapsulate the same dynamic. Social Dominance Theory, the Oppression Model, and the evolutionary competition and conflict for social capital among social groups helps explain this seemingly intractable human struggle for power and resources. We used an extended discussion of how host societies often force immigrants to adjust through assimilation pressure, leave after facing discrimination experiences, or die from exclusion and neglect to highlight how powerful social groups setting policy victimize powerless newcomers or lower status target groups.

The amount of group level bullying tolerated within a society is an indicator of equity, inclusion, civility, and the purposeful flattening of power differentials. While it is clear that progress has been made in providing women suffrage, banning slavery and protecting civil rights for racial minorities, legalizing access to the benefits of marriage between races and for same sex couples, this social progress is relatively recent compared to the thousands of years of inequalities among social groups. Further, this progress towards equality is fragile as political trends wax and wane. Current data shows growing inequality in the US, increases in hate related groups and crimes, heightening polarization, and decreasing tolerance. These trends make it all the more salient to understand group-level bullying and its corrosive effects on civilization.

References

Adams, M., Bell, L. E., & Griffin, P. (1997). *Teaching for diversity and social justice: A sourcebook*. New York, NY: Routledge.

Atlas, R. S., & Pepler, D. J. (1998). Observations of bullying in the classroom. *Journal of Educational Research, 92*(2), 86–99.

Bagwell, C. L., & Schmidt, M. E. (2011). *Friendships in childhood and adolescence*. New York, NY: Guilford Press.

Bell, L. (2007). Theoretical justifications for social justice education. In M. Adams, L. Bell, & P. Griffin (Eds.), *Teaching for diversity and social justice* (2nd ed., pp. 1–14). New York, NY: Routledge.

Berry, J. W. (1998). Acculturation stress. In P. B. Organista, K. M. Chun, & G. Marin (Eds.), *Readings in ethnic psychology* (pp. 117–122). New York, NY: Routledge.

Blank, R. M. (1997). *It takes a nation: A new agenda for fighting poverty*. New York, NY: Sage.

Blumenfeld, W., & Raymond, D. (2000). Prejudice and discrimination. In M. Adams, W. Blumenfeld, R. Castaneda, H. Hackman, M. Peters, & X. Zuniga (Eds.), *Readings for diversity and social justice: An anthology on racism, anti-semitism, sexism, heterosexism, ableism, and classism* (pp. 21–30). New York, NY: Routledge.

Boraas, S., & Rodgers, W. M. (2003). How does gender play a role in the earnings gap? An update. *Monthly Labor Review, 126*, 9–15.

Bronfenbrenner, U. (1989). Ecological systems theory. In R. Vasta (Ed.), *Annals of child development* (Vol. 6, pp. 187–251). Greenwich, CT: IAI Press.

Bureau of Labor Statistics. (2000). *Gender pay gap largest in sales, lowest in farm occupations*. Retrieved from https://www.bls.gov/opub/ted/2000/Jan/wk4/art01.htm

Capuzzi, D., & Staufer, M. D. (2019). *Foundations of group counseling*. New York, NY: Pearson.

Castro, F. G., Coe, K., Gutierres, S., & Saenz, D. (1996). Designing health promotion programs for Latinos. In P. M. Kato & T. Mann (Eds.), *Handbook of diversity issues in health psychology* (pp. 319–346). New York, NY: Plenum.

Central Intelligence Agency. (n.d.). *World factbook*. Retrieved from https://www.cia.gov/library/publications/the-world-factbook/rankorder/2172rank.html?countryname=United%20States&countrycode=us&regionCode=noa&rank=41#us

Chun, K. M., Organista, P. B., & Marin, G. (2002). *Acculturation: Advances in theory, measurement, and applied research*. Washington, DC: American Psychological Association.

Darwin, C. (1859). *On the origins of species*. Retrieved from https://www.gutenberg.org/files/1228/1228-h/1228-h.htm

de Anda, D. (1984). Bicultural socialization: Factors affecting the minority experience. *Social Work, 29*(2), 101–107.

de Bruyn, E. H., Cillessen, A. H. N., & Wissink, I. B. (2010). Associations of peer acceptance and perceived popularity with bullying and victimization in early adolescence. *The Journal of Early Adolescence, 3D*, 543–566.

Federal Bureau of Investigations. (2016). *Hate crime statistics 2016*. Retrieved from https://www.fbi.gov/news/pressrel/press-releases/fbi-releases-2016-hate-crime-statistics

Free Tibet. (n.d.). *Free Tibet*. Retrieved from https://freetibet.org/about

Freedom House. (2016). *Freedom in the world report*. Retrieved from https://freedomhouse.org/

Harro, B. (2000). The cycle of socialization. In M. Adams, W. Blumenfeld, R. Castaneda, H. Hackman, M. Peters, & X. Zuniga (Eds.), *Readings for diversity and social justice: An anthology on racism, anti-semitism, sexism, heterosexism, ableism, and classism* (pp. 15–20). New York, NY: Routledge.

Hawkins, D. L., Pepler, D. J., & Craig, W. M. (2001). Naturalistic observations of peer interventions in bullying. *Social Development, 10*(4), 512–527.

Hector St. John de Crevecoeur, J. (1782). *Letters from an American Farmer*. Retrieved from http://xroads.virginia.edu/~HYPER/crev/home.html

Kühl, S. (1994). *The Nazi connection: Eugenics, American racism, and German National Socialism*. New York, NY: Oxford University Press.

Lombardo, P. (2018). *Eugenic sterilization laws*. Retrieved from Eugenicsarchive.org

OSAPG. (2017). *Office of the UN Special Adviser on the Prevention of Genocide (OSAPG)*. Retrieved from http://www.un.org/en/genocideprevention/

Pellegrini, A. D. (2002). Bullying, victimization, and sexual harassment during the transitions to middle school. *Educational Psychologist, 37*, 151–163.

Pellegrini, A. D., Bartini, M., & Brooks, F. (1999). School bullies, victims, and aggressive victims: Factors relating to group affiliation and victimization in early adolescence. *Journal of Educational Psychology, 91*(2), 216–224.

Prinstein, M. J., & Cillessen, A. H. N. (2003). Forms and functions of adolescent peer aggression associated with high levels of peer status. *Merrill-Palmer Quarterly, 49*(3), 310–342.

Rodkin, P. C., & Berger, C. (2008). Who bullies whom? Social status asymmetries by victim gender. *International Journal of Behavioral Development, 32*, 473–486.

Salmivalli, C., Lappalainen, M., & Lagerspetz, K. M. J. (1998). Stability of change behavior in connection to bullying in schools: A two-year follow-up. *Aggressive Behavior, 24*, 205–218.

Scholte, R. H. J., Overbeek, G., ten Brink, G., Rommes, E., de Kemp, R. A. T., Goossens, L., & Engles, R. C. M. E. (2008). The significance of reciprocal and unilateral friendships for peer victimization in adolescence. *Journal of Youth and Adolescence, 89*, 89–100.

Seneca, L. A. (1995). *Seneca: Moral and political essays*. Cambridge, UK: Cambridge University Press.

Sidanius, J., & Pratto, F. (1999). *Social dominance: An intergroup theory of social hierarchy and oppression*. New York, NY: Cambridge University Press.

Smith, T., & Kehe, J. (2004). Glossary. In T. Smith (Ed.), *Practicing multiculturalism: Affirming diversity in counseling and psychology* (pp. 325–337). Boston, MA: Pearson Education.

Smokowski, P. R., & Bacallao, M. (2010). *Becoming bicultural: Risk, resilience, & Latino youth*. New York, NY: New York University Press.

Southern Poverty Law Center. (n.d.-a). *Hate groups*. Retrieved from https://www.splcenter.org/hate-map

Southern Poverty Law Center. (n.d.-b). Retrieved from www.splcenter.org

Suarez-Orozco, C., & Suarez-Orozco, M. M. (2001). *Children of immigrants*. Cambridge, MA: Harvard University Press.

Vaillancourt, T., Hymel, S., & McDougall, P. (2003). Bullying is power: Implications for school-based intervention strategies. *Journal of Applied School Psychology, 19*(2), 157–176.

We Shall Remain. (2009). *An American experience production*. Public Broadcasting Service. Retrieved from http://www.pbs.org/wgbh/amex/weshallremain/

Chapter 12
Playground Politics Across the Life Span as a Public Health Crisis: Summarizing Bullying Prevalence, Effects, Cost, Possible Solutions, and Prevention Suggestions

12.1 Overview of the Relationship Between Forms of Violence and Bullying

It has been our intent in this book to use the definition of bullying (including repetition, power imbalance, and intent to harm) as a means of illustrating how multiple forms of violence and victimization across the life span can and should be viewed through the definitional framework of bullying. Traditionally, rather than focusing on the similarities between forms of violence, as noted in Chap. 1, violence researchers study different forms of violence in isolated silos (Hamby & Grych, 2013; Wilkins, Tsao, Hertz, Davis, & Klevens, 2014), despite efforts by the Centers for Disease Control and others to "connect the dots" (CDC, 2019; Dong et al., 2004; Wilkins et al., 2014). In Chaps. 5–11, we have provided ample support to show that various forms of violence across the life span including school-age bullying, cyberbullying, child maltreatment, sibling bullying, teen dating violence, college hazing, intimate partner violence, workplace bullying, elder abuse, and large-scale violence are all forms of bullying that have power imbalance, intent to harm, and repetition in common. This suggests that researchers and practitioners working in these distinct but related fields of violence can and should apply the bullying framework to their work. However, we are not contending that forms of violence in this list that are not traditionally considered bullying (e.g., child maltreatment, teen dating violence, hazing, intimate partner violence) should only be considered as forms of bullying. For example, we are not asserting that teen dating violence be renamed teen dating bullying. We are saying that the bullying framework can help researchers and practitioners understand these forms of violence in a new and different way and can serve as a common thread that unites these forms of violence and help explain why there is such an overlap between them.

Indeed, it is quite common for youth to experience multiple forms of violent victimization. For example, as noted in Chap. 1, the National Survey of Children's Exposure to Violence ($N = 4549$) found that 64.5% of surveyed youth reported more

© Springer Nature Switzerland AG 2019

P. R. Smokowski, C. B. R. Evans, *Bullying and Victimization Across the Lifespan*, https://doi.org/10.1007/978-3-030-20293-4_12

than one type of direct victimization (i.e., conventional crime, child maltreatment, peer and sibling victimization, sexual victimization, witnessing victimization, and indirect victimization) and over one-tenth (10.9%) reported five or more types of victimization (Finkelhor, Turner, Hamby, & Ormrod, 2011). Further, physically assaulted youth were five times as likely to have been sexually assaulted and more than four times as likely to have been maltreated compared to their non-victimized counterparts (Finkelhor, Turner, Ormrod, Hamby, & Kracke, 2009). These findings, and many others, make clear that many of the forms of violence and bullying discussed in this book (e.g., child maltreatment, sibling bullying, traditional school-age bullying) overlap and are experienced in combination. There is also overlap between perpetration experiences and individuals who behaved violently in one context (e.g., school, work) are more likely to behave violently in other contexts (e.g., online, home; Foshee et al., 2015; Herrenkohl, Sousa, Tajima, Herrnkohl, & Moylan, 2008). Further, youth engaged in peer violence were more likely to be violent towards dating partners (Foshee et al., 2015) and adults who abused their partners were more likely to abuse their children (see Herrenkohl et al., 2008 for a review). Taken together, this research highlights that the similar risk factors for these forms of violence and bullying (discussed in Chap. 1) put victims at increased risk of enduring multiple forms of maltreatment simultaneously or sequentially. Table 12.1 provides a summary of these forms of violence and bullying including prevalence rates, definitions, and associated negative outcomes. Figure 12.1 provides a visual depiction of how these multiple forms of violence and bullying are related.

12.1.1 Bullying Is a Public Health Pandemic

12.1.1.1 Bullying Rates Are Unacceptably High

Surveying across all of the disparate categories of bullying discussed in this book (see Table 12.1), it is reasonable and well-grounded in the best knowledge we have to say that 25% of the US population is victimized at any given time during the life span. Considering that rates for middle school bullying (33–49% physical, 17–30% cyber), sibling bullying (30%), hazing (48%), teen dating, and intimate partner violence (32% and 36% respectively) are substantially higher, our life span estimate of 25% is conservative, perhaps optimistic. It is exceedingly difficult to get good estimates of child maltreatment, workplace bullying, and elder maltreatment due to the sensitivity of these victimization experiences, particularly when family members are perpetrators. Experts commonly agree that rates for these types of maltreatment are underreported. Many victims fear retaliation from parents, bosses, or nursing home staff, for example, and are unwilling to report their experiences; many believe that nothing will be done and resolve themselves to suffer in silence.

Based on one in four people experiencing victimization, we would like to proclaim that bullying is a pandemic. According to the CDC (2012), pandemic refers to

Table 12.1 Overview of violence and bullying across the life span

Bullying dynamic	Prevalence	Definition/negative outcomes
School-age bullying • *Intent to harm*: YES • *Repetition*: YES • *Power imbalance*: YES—Perpetrator more powerful than victim	• 35% for traditional bullying • Highest rates in middle school	• Unwanted behavior that occurs between a more powerful perpetrator(s) and weaker victim and usually occurs repeatedly over time; the behavior is intended to harm the victim and does cause harm to the victim, bystanders, and/or culture and climate within the environment where the bullying dynamic occurs • Victims—depression averaging 6.9 years, aggression and violent behavior lasting average of 6 years post-victimization
Cyberbullying • *Intent to harm*: YES • *Repetition*: YES • *Power imbalance*: YES—Those with online followers have visibility and more power than victim	• 16% of high school students were cybervictims in past year • Traditional bullying victims have higher rates of cybervictimization (YBRSS)	• Using electronic means (e.g., e-mail, instant messaging, chat rooms, websites, gaming sites, cellular phones) to threaten, humiliate, insult, exclude, or intimidate others. Youth who are traditionally bullied are often also cyberbullied • Cybervictimization associated with higher depression, binge drinking, marijuana use, stress, suicidal ideation, depression, anxiety, loneliness, low life satisfaction
Child maltreatment • *Intent to harm*: YES • *Repetition*: YES • *Power imbalance*: YES—Children have less power than parents/guardians	• 25% lifetime child maltreatment • In 2014, 3.2 million CPS reports—75% neglect, 17% physical abuse, 8% sexual abuse • About five children die of abuse each day in the US	• Abuse and/or neglect inflicted upon youth under the age of 18; includes all forms of physical and emotional mistreatment including sexual abuse, neglect, negligence, and exploitation • Maltreatment changes hippocampus and amygdala in childhood and adulthood; increases risk of violence, teenage pregnancy, mental illness
Sibling bullying • *Intent to harm*: YES • *Repetition*: YES • *Power imbalance*: YES—Age (older sibling more powerful), gender, physical size	• 30% reported being commonly bullied by their siblings • 32% physical assault, 4% physical assault with weapon or injury • 80% simple assault (no weapon no injury), 15% aggravated assaults (weapon and injury); 5% intimidation	• A repeated pattern of verbal and physical aggression where the aggressor intends to inflict harm and is motivated by the desire for power and control • Sibling bullying increases the risk of substance use, delinquency, aggression, poor mental health, low self-esteem

(continued)

Table 12.1 (continued)

Bullying dynamic	Prevalence	Definition/negative outcomes
Teen dating violence • *Intent to harm*: YES • *Repetition*: YES • *Power imbalance*: YES—Victim less powerful	• 32% experience any form TDV • 9.6% physical TDV, 10.6% sexual TDV • 27% reported dating partner "checked" on them by text 10 times per hour; 9% reported 50 times per hour	• Repeated, abusive behavior used to control a dating partner • TDV increased substance use, poor mental health, poor grades, decreased close social relationships, increased antisocial behavior, and an increased risk for future intimate partner victimization
Hazing • *Intent to harm*: YES, to initiate new recruits • *Repetition*: YES • *Power imbalance*: YES—Newcomers less powerful than veterans	• 48% of students belonging to a group reported being hazed • 43% hazed by humiliation, 23% by substance abuse, 22% in a dangerous way • 48% of high school juniors and seniors are involved in hazing • 55% of college student members reported being hazed	• An initiation process involving abuse, embarrassment, harassment, ridicule and risks emotional and/or physical harm • Hazing has resulted in injury, PTSD, poor self-esteem, sometimes death
Intimate partner violence • *Intent to harm*: YES • *Repetition*: YES • *Power imbalance*: YES—Victim less powerful, often stays out of fear, previous intimacy creates power	• 22.3% women and 14.0% men experienced lifetime physical IPV • 1.3 million women 835,000 men each year in the USA	• IPV is physical violence, sexual violence, stalking, or psychological aggression (e.g., coercive acts) by a current or former intimate partner • IPV associated with headaches, traumatic brain injury, stroke, hypertension, cardiovascular disease, stomach ulcers, diarrhea, chronic pain, inflammation, diabetes, broken bones, depression, suicidality, PTSD, heavy drinking, smoking, asthma
Workplace bullying • *Intent to Harm*: YES • *Repetition*: YES • *Power imbalance*: YES—Bully bosses have power and status	• 19% report abuse at work (9% currently, 10% past) • 15% witnessed abuse, 4% knew about it • US labor force of 161,616,000 indicating there are 30 million bullied workers and 30 million witnesses • 75% of harassment incidents go unreported due to fear of disbelief, inaction, blame, or retaliation	• Repeated, hurtful negative act or acts (physical, verbal, or psychological intimidation) that use humiliation to cause fear, distress, or harm to the individual in the workplace • Depression, PTSD, chronic stress response, poor health

(continued)

Table 12.1 (continued)

Bullying dynamic	Prevalence	Definition/negative outcomes
Elder Maltreatment • *Intent to harm*: YES • *Repetition*: YES • *Power imbalance*: YES—Older adults less powerful physically and/or mentally. Community-living, abuse by adult children. Nursing homes, abuse by caretakers and other residents	• 1 in 10 older adults in US are abused, neglected, or financially exploited each year • 11.4% of older adults living in the community reported emotional, physical, or sexual maltreatment in past year • It is estimated that 9.8% of those elders in nursing homes reported neglect and 17.4% reported abuse	• Exploitation of adults over 60; physical, sexual, and emotional abuse, neglect, abandonment, financial exploitation • Negative outcomes: trouble sleeping; depression; confusion; weight loss; signs of trauma; agitation; violent behavior; withdrawal; unexplained bruises, burns, or scars; messy appearance, unwashed hair or dirty clothes; premature death
Bullying between social groups • *Intent to harm*: YES • *Repetition*: YES • *Power imbalance*: YES—Groups with power, influence, resources disempower others	• 954 hate groups currently operating in the US in 2017, up from 457 in 1999 (52% increase) • 6063 single-bias incidents of hate speech	• Inequality and violence based on gender, race, disability, religion such as hate crimes, genocide, treatment of immigrants were examples • Trauma, fear

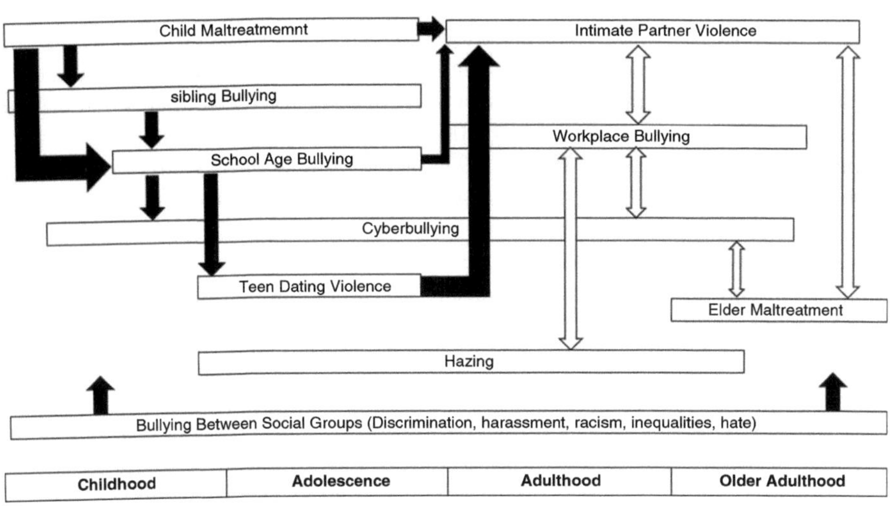

Fig. 12.1 The relationship between multiple forms of violence and bullying. Note: Black arrows indicate a causal relationship or association supported by ample research evidence; white arrows indicate a possible causal relationship or association that needs additional research

an epidemic that has spread over several countries or continents, usually affecting a large number of people. Epidemic refers to an increase, often sudden, in the number of cases of a disease above what is normally expected in that population in that area. The problem with our proclamation is the "normally expected" criterion. To some critics, bullying may be brushed off as a rite of passage, "boys being boys," "don't mess with the queen bee or you get stung," or Internet trolls using their freedom of speech. Consequently, there has been no worldwide conversation to come to any consensus concerning what is a normally expected level of victimization in social groups. Sadly, we can state with certainty that approximately one fourth of our population reports being victimized and may experience stress, trauma, and health problems as a result. We hope that the discussion in this book presents clear evidence that this level of bullying across the life span should not be normally expected or tolerated.

Some simplistic epidemiology may place the prevalence of victimization in context. In 2019, there were 7,714,576,923 people on Earth. Bullying has been identified as a global problem with rates across countries varying from 15% to 70%. Taking our 25% approximate prevalence rate, we can estimate 1.93 billion victims across the world (19,286 per 100,000 or 1928.6 per million). In contrast, the World Health Organization's estimates, in millions, for major diseases worldwide in 2004 were: hearing loss 124.2, refractive errors in vision 121.9, depression 98.7, cataracts 53.8, unintentional injuries 45, alcohol dependence and problem use 40.5, infertility 33, macular degeneration 31.9, heart disease 23.2, bipolar disorder 22.2, drug dependence and problematic use 11.8, panic disorder 13.8, Schizophrenia 16.7, and Alzheimer's and other dementias 14.9. Table 12.2 clearly shows that no major public health problem, except iron deficiency, comes close to the prevalence of bullying victimization. Indeed, if we took an exceptionally low estimate of bullying victimization, such as 10% (no survey has shown rates that low), this problem would still overshadow all other public health issues, except iron deficiency anemia, in worldwide scope. Take hearing loss as an example. In 2004, WHO estimates that mild to moderate hearing loss impacted 636,500,000 people worldwide out of 6.4 billion humans living at that time. That is 9.9% of the population, signaling a profound public health problem yet smaller in scope than bullying. Take another example; health providers and governments have invested enormous resources in finding a cure for cancer. In 2004, WHO estimated 11,474,000 cases of all cancers (excluding non-melanoma skin cancer) worldwide. That is a population rate of 0.00179, making bullying victimization at 25% 168 times more common than cancer. Based on all of these data based calculations, we can only conclude that bullying is an exceptionally high prevalence problem that should be a public health priority. To be clear, we are not saying it should be a higher priority than other major problems such as HIV, malnutrition, low vision, arthritis, or heart disease. We are saying that, based on prevalence, cost, and impact on human suffering, bullying absolutely should be considered alongside major public health priorities.

Table 12.2 Bullying victimization rates compared to other public health concerns

Disease	Rate (millions)
Bullying victimization	1928.6
Iron deficiency anemia	1159.3
Migraine headaches	324.1
Malnutrition (stunting and wasting)	238.9
Diabetes mellitus	220.5
Asthma	234.9
Hearing loss (mild/moderate)	636.5
Low vision	272.4
Unipolar depression	151.2
Osteoarthritis	151.4
Intestinal infection	150.9
Cataracts	53.8
Unintentional injuries	45
Alcohol use disorders	125
Angina pectoris	54
Infertility	33
HIV	31.4
Heart disease	23.2
Stroke	30.7
Bipolar disorder	29.5
Drug dependence	11.8
Schizophrenia	16.7
Panic disorder	13.8
Alzheimer's/dementia	24.2

12.1.1.2 Bullying Should Be Considered One of the Key Adverse Childhood Experiences

According to the CDC's National Center for Injury Prevention and Control, Adverse Child Experiences (ACEs) are traumatic events that occur during the first 18 years of life. Investigators from Kaiser Permanente conducted the seminal research on ACEs in the 1990s (Felitti et al., 1998). The original ACEs included emotional, physical and sexual abuse, neglect, exposure to intimate partner violence, mental illness, separation/divorce, substance abuse, and parental incarceration. However, subsequent research has shown that additional adversities, such as bullying, peer and community violence, and economic hardship, should be considered as ACEs because they display similar impacts on health and life outcomes (e.g., Cronholm et al., 2015; Finkelhor, Shattuck, Turner, & Hamby, 2013).

Two-thirds of adults experienced at least one ACE and nearly one quarter experience three or more ACEs (Merrick, Ford, Ports, & Guinn, 2018). In the original ACE surveys of adults in California, 61% reported at least one ACE and 16.7%

experienced four or more ACEs (34.9% emotional or verbal abuse, 26.7% parental separation or divorce, 26.1% substance abuse by household member, 19.9% physical abuse, 17.5% witnessed domestic violence, 15% had a household member with mental illness, 11.4% experienced sexual abuse, 9.3% were neglected in childhood, and 6.6% had an incarcerated family member). As discussed previously, ACEs cluster and are interrelated, making the accumulation of traumatic experiences profoundly detrimental to health and well-being across the life span. Indeed, ACEs have been associated with over 40 negative health and life outcomes, including toxic stress; physiological changes of the nervous, endocrine, and immune systems; risky health behaviors; chronic health conditions; infectious diseases; suicidal behavior; low life potential, and early death (Felitti et al., 1998; Gilbert et al., 2015; Metzler, Merrick, Klevens, Ports, & Ford, 2017; Shonkoff, 2016). Indeed, exposure to four or more ACEs has been linked to dramatically higher risk for health problems in adulthood, as shown in Table 12.3 (based on Felitti et al., 1998). It is hypothesized that exposure to ACEs in childhood leads to disrupted neurodevelopment, which causes social, emotional, and cognitive impairment. This stress and impairment raises the risk for adopting health risk behaviors (smoking, drinking) as coping mechanisms, which in turn increases disease, disability, and social problems in adulthood, ultimately increasing the chances of premature mortality. Table 12.3 shows that individuals who experienced 4 or more ACEs in childhood were 7x more likely to display alcoholism in adulthood, 10x more likely to have drug abuse problems, and 12x more likely to attempt suicide, among other problems, relative to peers without ACE exposure. This underscores a dramatic increase in health risk. Based on this research showing parallel precursors and similar consequences, we strongly assert that bullying should be considered an Adverse Childhood Experience and victimization across the life span should be a pressing public health priority based on high prevalence, cost to society, and deleterious consequences for health across the life span.

Table 12.3 Adverse Child Experiences increase the probability for other health risk behaviors

Health risk behavior	Odds—4 or more ACEs
Alcoholism	7.4
Drug abuse	10.3
Depression	4.6
Suicide attempts	12.2
Smoking	2.2
Lung disease	3.9
Liver disease	2.4
STDs	2.5
>50 sexual partners	3.2
Heart disease	2.2
Cancer	1.9
Severe obesity	1.6

Felitti et al. (1998)

12.1.1.3 Bullying Has Profound Negative Consequences on Health Across The Life Span

Bullying in childhood and adolescence can increase risk for later violent experiences, such as intimate partner violence, sexual violence, and suicide, which can have a cumulative and compounding impact on health and well-being across the life span. Violence erodes the sense of safety and security that is critical for family and community well-being. Examining the negative outcomes associated with these forms of violence and bullying in Table 12.1, it is clear that the impact on the victim is similar regardless of the form of bullying and regardless of when the bullying occurs. Thus, an older adult bullied in a nursing home will likely have a similar reaction and similar symptoms as a sixth grader bullied on the playground. The negative consequences are similar regardless of when, where, and how you get bullied or experience violent victimization. This is an exceptionally important point that warrants raising public awareness. Victims of school bullying, cyberbullying, child maltreatment, sibling bullying, teen dating violence, hazing, intimate partner violence, workplace bullying, elder maltreatment, and larger level bullying (such as discrimination and hate crimes) commonly suffer from a similar constellation of outcomes including: poor mental health (e.g., anxiety, depression, stress, post traumatic stress disorder), decreased self-esteem, heightened isolation and loneliness, difficulty sleeping, physical injuries (e.g., cuts, bruises, broken bones), increased substance use, and feelings of humiliation. Physiological reactions include stimulation of the hypothalamus-pituitary-adrenal axis, "fight, flight, or freeze" reactions to stress, dysregulation of stress hormones such as cortisol and adrenaline, and hyperarousal due to chronic stress reactivity. These biological reactions influence coping, emotional regulation, and long-term decision-making (i.e., sometimes victims "learn" never to trust others or avoid joining social groups). Social and emotional functioning is profoundly impacted because of the embarrassment, shame, humiliation, and interpersonal rejection that victims feel from the highly public aspect of bullying dynamics. One of the most important takeaways from this book is the fact that each of these forms of bullying engender severe humiliation for victims. It is this humiliation that makes the impact of victimization endure for years, if not indefinitely. The highly emotional experience of bullying victimization encodes vividly as adverse memories that are held over time due to their salience and threat to well-being. Social rejection and humiliation are particularly toxic due to human needs for interpersonal relationships and support at every point across the life span. Indeed, social rejection messages received during bullying episodes activate the same receptors in the brain as physical pain and are easy for the victim's brain to generalize. When no one helps—no bystanders, no teachers, no parents, and arguably most importantly no friends—it is tempting for the victim to begin to believe that the bully's hurtful words were correct, leading to messages of worthlessness and inadequacy that erode self-esteem and may guide negative future choices. The cognitive template that results (e.g., "people will just reject me," "I can't fit in") is carried across contexts, heightening the expectation of continuing rejection and victimization. Thus, the victimization trajectory can become a long-term self-fulfilling prophecy in which current rejections are magnified due to their triggering memories of past victimizations. The accumulation of this negativity is increasingly toxic, leading to negative coping and adoption of health risk behaviors (e.g., smoking, drinking, aggression). When severe, reactions to rejection can foster the thirst for revenge on others, leading to tragedy such as school shootings or homicide, or may be internalized into hatred against the self, also leading to tragedy in suicide.

Interestingly, perpetrators of these forms of bullying also experience similar outcomes including chronic stress, increased aggression and violence, higher risk for substance use, increased suicidality, and increased involvement in the criminal justice system. Adverse childhood experiences early in life (such as child maltreatment, witnessing domestic or community violence, neglect, divorce, having a family member incarcerated) provide role modeling for violent behavior and show children that the world is a ruthless place to survive in. Survivors of maltreatment commonly cope by suppressing their feelings of hurt and vulnerability. This underlying pain and outward learned aggression may partially define subsequent relationships with siblings, classmates, dating and intimate partners, coworkers, and others. Bullies who are successful (i.e., realize social or peer group benefits from their dominating behavior) quickly learn to generalize their use of aggression across social contexts. Having few models for positive social relationships, these bullies may prefer to be feared than to be liked. The experience of dominating and humiliating others may be a balm for their own vulnerabilities, and, in a more simplistic sense, it may be enjoyable due to the feelings of power, the dopamine and adrenaline they feel during the bullying event. Once hooked, displays of aggression may be both what bullies know through social learning and their most reliable coping strategy for reaching their goals across different life span contexts. When paired with related problems, such as alcohol and substance use, depression, and anxiety, this tendency to cope through hostility and aggression clearly raises the risks for law enforcement involvement and suicide to end this painful cycle.

12.2 The Ultimate Escalation of Power Imbalance

We have written an entire book on bullying perpetration and victimization across the life span without mentioning the one factor that encapsulates the power imbalance beyond any other—guns. The culture of bullying victimization, particularly in the US, includes the influence of guns, lots and lots of guns. Exact estimates are hard to obtain because gun research was not allowed by government agencies in the US until recently; however, the best estimates we have suggest that there are far more guns than people in the US.

In a country of 260 million people, there are approximately 393 million guns in the US. As of 2017, Gallup found that 42% of American households reported owning guns. With an estimated 118 million households in the US, per the US Census, that would mean that the country's 393 million guns are distributed among 50 million households. Considering the victimization rates in Table 12.1, it is extremely likely that guns are present in many of the households where child maltreatment, intimate partner violence, sibling bullying, teen dating violence, school bullying, and elder maltreatment are happening. The presence of a gun dramatically escalates both the power imbalance and the negative outcomes that can result from violence and bullying across the life span. Introducing a gun into the bullying dynamic produces a number of tragic scenarios:

1. A bully with a gun and intent to harm becomes lethal, no longer needing repetition to torture his/her victim(s). This intense escalation of aggression and power embodied by guns leads bullies to become murderers.
2. A victim filled with humiliation and anger seeks to nullify the power imbalance with the bully and claim revenge by carrying a gun for safety. The victim-murders-bully scenario has resulted in cases of teenagers killing abusive parents, rejected boyfriends murdering ex-lovers, siblings shooting each other, domestic violence homicides, and workers shooting up abusive workplaces, among others.

Guns complicate the bullying dynamic because whoever has the weapon takes over the power imbalance. At the same time, the situation becomes so intense the repetition criterion becomes irrelevant. Guns may be sought at the end of the bullying trajectory and tragically end the sequence in one way or another. Group-level bullying that includes hate crimes, war, and genocide are also commonly escalated by the introduction of guns. Statistics concerning gun violence in the US are shocking (see Every Town for Gun Safety website).

- Approximately 3,000,000 American children witness gun violence each year.
- Every day, 100 Americans are killed with guns.
- Firearms are the second leading cause of death for American children and teens.
- The US has the highest gun homicide rate in the world (3.6 per 100,000), a rate that is more than 7 times the rate for the second place country (Canada at 0.5 per 100,000).
- Nearly one million US women have been shot or shot at by an intimate partner.
- Black males are 16 times more likely than White males to be shot and injured in assaults involving guns.
- Access to a gun triples the risk of death by suicide.

Examining gun-related deaths leads to some important conclusions. In 2016, there were 33,594 gun deaths in the US, consisting of 14,415 homicides and 22,938 suicides. Crime and gang-related homicides in urban areas usually garner the most media publicity, and are certainly worthy of attention. At the same time, guns facilitate many more suicides than homicides. In the CDC's 2017 Youth Risk Behavior Surveillance System (YRBSS) national data, 33.9% of high school students reported being bullied (traditional or cyberbullying), 31.5% endorsed persistent sadness and hopelessness, and 17% considered suicide. In the CDC's 2015 Behavioral Risk Factor Surveillance System (BRFSS) for adults, the national suicide rate was 13.3 per 100,000 with the rate for males (21.1) nearly 4 times the rate for females (6.0). Suicide death rates are much higher for American Indians (20.0) and non-Hispanic

Whites (17.0) relative to African Americans (5.8), Hispanics (6.2) and Asian-Pacific Islanders (6.5). Suicide death rates are highest in rural areas: Wyoming (28.0), Alaska (26.9), Montana (25.3), New Mexico (23.7), Utah (22.4), Idaho (22.1), and South Dakota (20.4). Access to guns makes suicidal ideation much more dangerous, especially for males who may make an impetuous decision during a despondent period.

In contrast, homicide death rates in 2015 were 5.7 per 100,000 nationally, also 4 times higher in males (9.1) compared to females (2.2), and highest in African Americans (20.9), American Indians (9.8), Hispanics (4.9), non-Hispanic Whites (2.6), and Asian-Pacific Islanders (1.5). Homicide death rates are highest in low socioeconomic areas with high disadvantage: District of Columbia (17.5), Louisiana (12.4), Mississippi (11.3), Maryland (10.3, due to Baltimore), and Alabama (10.2; CDC, n.d.). Homicides are a function of crime, especially in urban areas, and may intensify group-level conflicts (e.g., gang disputes, hate crimes).

While only accounting for a tiny proportion of gun-related deaths (1305 out of 33,594 gun deaths in 2016), we would be remiss to not discuss mass shootings. On 20 April 1999, Eric Harris, 18, and Dylan Klebold, 17, killed 13 people and wounded more than 20 others before committing suicide at Columbine High School in Colorado. Harris and Klebold chose their victims randomly, originally intending to bomb their school in an attempt to kill hundreds of people. The attack was planned in journals for a year and a half before the attempt; 188 rounds of ammunition were fired, but the pipe bombs never detonated. Although the boys' motives remain unclear, speculation has centered on bullying victimization. The pair were gifted children who endured bullying for 4 years (an extreme accumulation of stress, see Chap. 3). Classmates reported Harris and Klebold were regularly called "faggots" and "queers," had a cup of fecal matter thrown at them, and were badgered by "jocks" at the school. Harris was born with mild chest indent, making him reluctant to take his shirt off in gym class where other students would laugh at him. According to Brooks Brown, a classmate, "People surrounded them in the commons (i.e., cafeteria) and squirted ketchup packets all over them, laughing at them, calling them faggots…That happened while teachers watched. They couldn't fight back. They wore the ketchup all day and went home covered with it." Brown described Harris and Klebold as the school's worst outcasts, "the losers of the losers" and journals kept by the killers described intense depression over lack of success with women, rage, and social isolation (Boodman, 2006).

The Columbine massacre was not the first mass shooting in the US, but it ushered in an era of intense concerns over school safety, large increases in the number of School Resource Officers, zero-tolerance policies, metal detectors, and heightened concerns over bullying policies. Unfortunately, Harris and Klebold became Internet celebrities among alienated youth, sparking copycat incidents (see Fig. 12.2). An analysis by officials at the US Secret Service of 37 premeditated school shootings found that bullying, which some of the shooters described "in terms that approached torment," played the major role in more than two-thirds of the attacks. Three hallmarks of school shooters are: (1) suicidal ideation; (2) perceived victimization; and (3) a desire for attention or fame. The humiliation and social rejection resulting

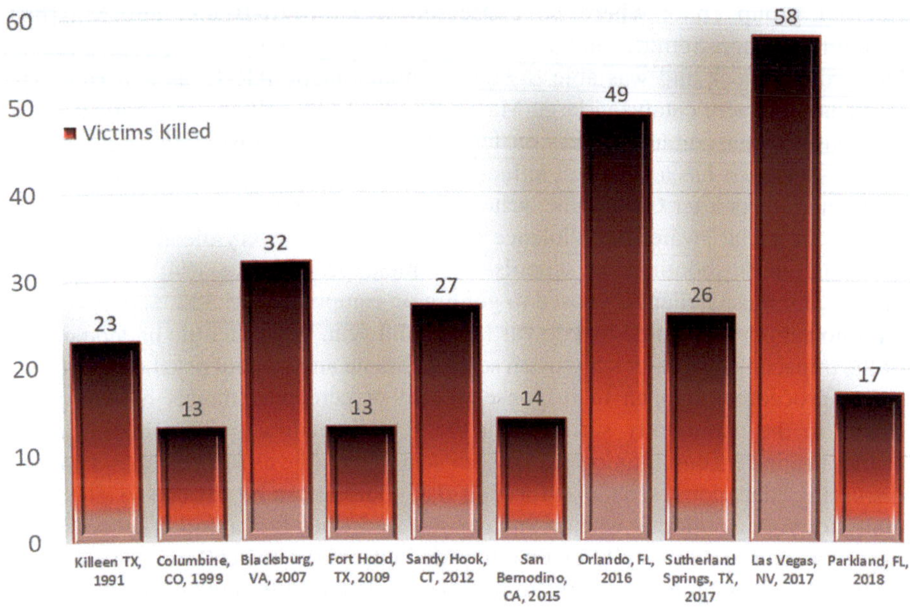

Fig. 12.2 Worst mass shootings in U.S. since 1991 by VICTIMS KILLED

from victimization may feed a lust for revenge before ending the suffering through suicide. Killing as many people as possible on your way out may bring Internet stardom and martyr status. This psychodrama is facilitated by easy access to guns.

The Columbine tragedy influenced subsequent copycat threats and plots. "Columbine" has since become a euphemism for a school shooting, rather like "going postal" is a term for seeking revenge on an employer. This has profoundly impacted the cultural consciousness and life experience of the generations of students who have followed. In 2005, Jeff Weise, an American Indian who wore a trench coat (a symbol of Columbine), killed his grandfather, who was a police officer, and his girlfriend. He took his grandfather's weapon and his squad car, and drove to his former high school in Red Lake and murdered several students before killing himself. The Virginia Tech shooter, Seung-Hui Cho, viewed Harris and Klebold as martyrs and referred to the Columbine massacre as his motivation. Adam Lanza became so obsessed with mass murder ideology, and Columbine in particular, that he killed 27 children and teachers at Sandy Hook Elementary School. Some potential shooters seek fame by planning to outdo the Columbine killers. Nikolas Cruz opened fire at Marjory Stoneman Douglas High School in Parkland, Florida, killing 17 students and staff members and injuring 17 others in February 2018. Cruz had been adopted from birth by an older couple who both died 3 months before the shooting. He had behavioral issues and was transferred between six different schools in 3 years, making it extremely difficult to fit in even with good behavior. He was purportedly diagnosed with depression, autism, and ADHD, but was not receiving any treatment. Despite repeated tips to law enforcement and a large volume of

Internet group chats where he expressed racist (anti-Black, anti-Muslim), homophobic, anti-Semitic, and anti-immigrant (xenophobic) views, Cruz passed a background check and was able to buy a semiautomatic AR-15 assault rifle. The Parkland massacre catalyzed large March for Our Lives rallies and political activism, but no measurable progress on federal gun control legislation. The National Rifle Association has a powerful influence, and Americans love their guns.

Twenty years after Columbine, school shootings, albeit rare, are deeply embedded in our social awareness. Violence in 2018 shattered every meaningful record, including most shootings at schools—25; most people shot—94; most people killed—33; most students exposed to gunfire on campuses—25,332; and more than 4 million children endured lockdowns last school year. We have little understanding of the impact of school lockdowns on school climate and student psychology. These safety procedures happen in response to real or perceived threats or dangerous events in the community surrounding the school. In low socioeconomic areas, crimes in adjacent communities can trigger school lockdowns several times a month, disrupting educational schedules for high-risk youth. It can be difficult to tell, especially for young children, when a threat is real and when it is a drill. The lockdown procedure can convince children that they are in danger; some children have written their wills, others good-bye notes to parents, while trying to remain silent during a lockdown that can last for hours. A Washington Post analyses noted that, 9 days after the Parkland shooting (Friday February 23, 2018), an Internet series of threats infectiously moved from the east to west coasts; 33 incidents caused 67 school lockdowns affecting 50,427 students across the US in 1 day! Despite being rare events, that example shows how widespread and profound the impact of guns and school shootings have had on our educational system and youth development.

12.2.1 Bullying Costs Pose an Unreasonable Burden on Society

As we continue to hire more and more School Resource Officers, buy metal detectors, cameras, and debate whether arming teachers with guns is a good idea, it is important to discuss the societal costs of bullying. As discussed in Chap. 1, the cost of bullying to individuals and families is incalculable in terms of human suffering. At the same time, the cost to society can be estimated. Bullying and violence significantly impact communities by reducing productivity, decreasing property values, and disrupting social services. There is loss of federal funding to schools when numerous students are absent because of safety concerns or drop out of school altogether. School budgets are impacted by the need to hire more School Resource Officers, social workers, counselors, and install metal detectors and surveillance cameras. Health and mental health services are needed to address physical and emotional traumas. As we previously discussed, bullies are over three times as likely to have multiple criminal convictions by their early 20s and higher self-reports of drug and alcohol use, creating law enforcement and rehabilitation service needs that are expensive. In 2016, nearly 65,000 people in the US died as a result of violence and more than 2.2 million people were treated in emergency departments for a violence-related injury. Violence can lead to other significant mental and physical health consequences such as depression and anxiety, substance abuse, pregnancy complications, chronic diseases (such as diabetes and heart disease), and even reductions in life opportunities, including educational attainment and employment (Arseneault et al., 2006; Felitti et al., 1998; Fowler, Tompsett, Braciszewski, Jacques-Tiura, & Baltes, 2009; Gilbert et al., 2015; Hillis, Mercy, & Saul, 2016; Jennings, Piquero, & Reingle, 2012; Menard, 2002; Metzler et al., 2017; Shonkoff, 2016; Wilkins et al., 2014).

Child maltreatment and intimate partner violence break up families, creating lost income, financial instability, foster care needs that are often subsidized by taxpayers. The government-financed juvenile justice system, criminal courts, and prisons are filled with individuals with past histories of perpetration, victimization, or both.

All of these costs, and others, sum to an enormous cost to society. In one of the few assessments of the labor market, income, social, health, civic, incarceration, and fiscal consequences of bullying, Sum, Khatiwada, and McLaughlin (2008) found the annual cost of bullying to be $951,327 per perpetrator and $461,668 per victim for being bullied. Here is a simple application of these costs to the US population of youth under age 18 in 2018:

- 49.7 million youth in the USA—20% victimized (9,940,000) and 15% bullies (7,455,000).
- Estimated annual perpetration cost of $7 trillion (7,455,000 × $951,327 = $7,09 2,142,785,000).
- Estimated annual victimization cost is $4.5 trillion (9,940,000 × $461,668 = $4, 588,979,920,000). Bullying costs society approximately $11.5 trillion each year.
- All US government revenue = $3.3 trillion in 2017.

A conservative estimate runs into the trillions of dollars annually. Indeed, if we cut the estimate of annual cost of $11.5 trillion in half, we would still far exceed the entire yearly revenue of the US government. Saving money is a powerful argument to convince policy makers and practitioners to implement intervention programs (Highmark Foundation, n.d.). With an astronomical cost associated with doing nothing, or doing what we currently are doing, what alternatives do we have? The next discussion outlines different ways for society to cope with the bullying dynamic, focusing on prevention to decrease the high cost of remediation.

12.3 How to Combat Playground Politics Across the Life Span

The most common question we are asked as bullying researchers is how can we stop the bullying dynamic? Concerned parents want to know how to protect their children and prevent bullying from occurring and other parents want to know how to stop bullying that is already in full swing. Teachers and school administrators inquire how they can best foster a culture of kindness and caring in their schools. Practitioners want to know how they can most effectively help their clients navigate bullying experiences at school. The conundrum of prevention extends to each and every form of violence and bullying discussed in this book. How can we put a stop to these egregious forms of violence and bullying? In the following discussion, we highlight some programs that have been found to be especially useful in ending violence and bullying. Our goal is to use the public health model for addressing social issues using this sequence:

Defining the Problem → Identify Risk and Protective Factors → Develop and Test Prevention Strategies → Assure Widespread Adoption.

Problems related to bullying across the life span are clearly articulated throughout this book, as are risk and protective factors identified by different silos of research. In this section, we describe prevention programs that have been tested for each of the reflections of bullying across the life span. Our goal is to spur widespread adoption, but also to inspire communities to use a multilevel integrative approach so that an effective package or network of prevention programs work together to eradicate bullying dynamics at key developmental stages.

12.3.1 Preventing Child Maltreatment

Results of meta-analyses indicate that, in general, parent training interventions have moderate to strong effects (Kaminski, Valle, Filene, & Boyle, 2008; Lundahl, Risser, & Lovejoy, 2006; Sandler, Schoenfelder, Wolchik, & MacKinnon, 2011). A meta-analysis by Lundahl et al. (2006) suggested that many of the positive effects of parent training interventions found at post-test were maintained at follow-up, although the follow-up effect sizes were smaller than at post-test. Major weaknesses of parent training evaluation studies include a lack of longer-term follow-up assessments beyond immediate post-test (Kaminski et al., 2008), as well as a lack of comparison groups at follow-up (Lundahl et al., 2006).

We support the use of parent-training interventions; however, it is crucial to review program implementation and evaluation details when planning a prevention initiative. Of particular importance is an intervention's effect size. Effect size is a simple statistic that measures the size or strength of an intervention's influence (Statistics Solutions, 2019). Without being overly technical, an effect size between 0 and 0.3 is considered small, 0.31–0.6 is medium, and over 0.6 would be large. Considering the expense of running a program, we would want to see medium to large effects.

Blue Prints for Healthy Youth Development (2012–2019a) provides a list of the most rigorously tested evidence-based youth violence prevention programs Searching the Blueprints for Healthy Youth Development website (blueprintsprograms.org) for child maltreatment programs renders four results; one "model" program called Nurse Family Partnership and three "promising" programs (Child First, Parent-Child Interaction Therapy [PCIT], and the Triple P System). Child First targets selected and indicated populations (parents and children 0–5) to reduce chronic stress and trauma with psychotherapeutic home visitation and care coordination (Lowell, Carter, Godoy, Paulicin, & Briggs-Gowan, 2011). The lone study evaluating Child First was a small sample that demonstrated small to medium effects with an average cost of $8000 per family served. PCIT is also a selected/indicated parent-training program for improving the parent–child relationship from preschool through elementary school. Parents are taught play therapy skills, communication, and behavior management by therapist coaches. Numerous studies have shown medium to large effects on outcomes with modest start up costs of $1210 per family. Because these are selected/indicated programs, we will spend more time highlighting the two primary prevention programs below.

12.3.1.1 Nurse Family Partnership (NFP)

NFP is a nurse home visiting program for first-time pregnant mothers that sends nurses to work one-on-one with the pregnant women to improve prenatal and child rearing practices through the child's second birthday. According to the Blueprints for Healthy Child Development archive (2012–2019b), NFP is a model program that targets multiple child outcomes, including: child maltreatment, delinquency and criminal behavior, cognitive development, physical health and well-being, preschool communication/language development, and reciprocal parent–child warmth. Specific objectives include improving women's diets; helping women monitor their weight gain and eliminate the use of cigarettes, alcohol, and drugs; teaching parents to identify the signs of pregnancy complication; encouraging regular rest, appropriate exercise, and good personal hygiene related to obstetrical health; and preparing parents for labor, delivery, and early care of the newborn.

Three NFP evaluation studies of pregnant women and their children conducted in Elmira, Memphis, and Denver found intervention-group improvements relative to the control group in the following areas: decreased domestic violence among married or cohabiting women, fewer health-care visits and hospitalization for injuries and illnesses, less emotional vulnerability in children, enhanced language and mental development in children, less child abuse and neglect, and behavioral problems caused by use of alcohol or drugs (seen in mothers at 15- and 19-year follow-up in Elmira). At 6-to-12-year follow-up in the Memphis study, NFP children displayed fewer behavioral problems at age 6, mothers reported better relationship quality with current partners, and there was less child use of substances and internalizing mental health problems at age 12. In the Elmira 15-year and 19-year follow-up, there were fewer arrests and convictions for children whose mothers received NFP. The program model suggests these outcomes are achieved by increasing prenatal health, reducing maternal hypertension and use of cigarettes, increasing responsive interactions between mothers and their children, and heightening parental social support. It is critical for potential implementation agencies to note that, while NFP is a widely disseminated program, the effect sizes for the program are small, ranging from near 0 to 0.33. Despite disappointing effects on outcomes after 1.7 years of intervention (i.e., from prenatal care to age 2), NFP is the only "model" program listed when Blueprints is searched for child maltreatment programs (Blueprints 2012–2019a). We recommend a thorough review of research findings before making the investment. Getting the label "Model" means the research evaluations of the program are strong; it does not mean that the program is highly effective.

Blueprints estimates that the total year 1 cost for launching the NFP program would be $1,014,800 to hire eight registered nurses to serve 25 families each. Two hundred families would be served at a cost of $5074 per family for 1 year of services. The program lasts approximately 1.7 years for each family with weekly or biweekly visits from pregnancy until their child turns 2. There are important long-term benefits on multiple violence and delinquency outcomes; however, it is expensive and may be difficult to recruit and retain registered nurses who are in high demand. Programs should focus NFP services on families at greater risk and use nurses (not paraprofessionals) who visit frequently, beginning during pregnancy (Olds & Kitzman, 1990, 1993).

12.3.1.2 Positive Parenting Program (Triple P)

The Triple P-Positive Parenting Program is a comprehensive, community-wide system of parenting and family support. Five intervention levels were designed to enhance parental competence and prevent or alter dysfunctional parenting practices, thereby reducing an important set of family risk factors both for child maltreatment and for children's behavioral and emotional problems (Prinz, Sanders, Shapiro, Whitaker, & Lutzker, 2009). The existing community workforce crossing several disciplines and settings (such as family and social support services, preschool and childcare settings, elementary schools and other community entities with direct contact with families) is trained to deliver the Triple P system of interventions. This workforce is then responsible for delivering the program to parents.

The Triple P Positive Parenting Program works with families who have a child birth to age 12. Using systematic training including videos, workbooks, and tip sheets, the Triple P program aims to enhance parental competence and prevent or change dysfunctional parenting practices and thereby reduce child maltreatment. The program provider works with the family in the context of multiple systems including childcare settings, elementary school, community entities, and family and social support services. Five core principles are used to support parents: (1) establishing and maintaining a safe, engaging environment, (2) establishing and maintaining a positive learning environment, (3) helping parents use assertive discipline, (4) helping parents maintain reasonable expectations, and (5) helping parents take care of themselves. These basic principles translate into 35 specific strategies and skills that parents can utilize to improve parent–child relationship, encourage desirable behavior, teach new skills and behaviors, manage misbehaviors, prevent problems in high-risk situations, improve self-regulation skills, enhance parental mood management and coping skills, and enhance partner support and communication skills. In a US study, compared to control counties, those counties that used Triple P had significantly lower rates of substantiated child maltreatment, child out-of-home placements, and hospitalizations or emergency-room visits for child maltreatment injuries (Blue Prints for Healthy Youth Development, 2012–2019c).

Triple P is a multilevel system of parenting and family support strategies for families with children from birth to age 12, with extensions to families with teenagers ages 13–16. The program has five intervention levels of increasing intensity (Blue Prints for Healthy Youth Development, 2012–2019c):

- *Level 1 (Universal Triple P)* is a media-based information strategy designed to increase community awareness of parenting resources, encourage parents to participate in programs, and communicate solutions to common behavioral and developmental concerns. The goals for this level are to (a) destigmatize parenting and family support; (b) make effective parenting strategies available to all parents; and (c) facilitate help seeking.
- *Level 2 (Selected Triple P)* provides specific advice on how to solve common child developmental issues (e.g., toilet training) and minor child behavior problems (e.g., bedtime problems). Included are parenting tip sheets and videotapes that demonstrate specific parenting strategies. Level 2 is delivered mainly through one or two brief face-to-face 20-min consultations or parenting seminars with large groups of parents.
- *Level 3 (Primary Care Triple P)* targets children with mild to moderate behavior difficulties (e.g., tantrums, fighting with siblings) and includes skills training to teach parents how to manage these behaviors. Level 3 is delivered in four 20-min sessions.
- *Level 4 (Standard Triple P and Group Triple P)*, an intensive strategy for parents of children with more severe behavior difficulties (e.g., aggressive or oppositional behavior), is designed to teach parenting skills and their application to a range of target behaviors. Level 4 is delivered in ten individual or eight group sessions totaling about 10 h.
- *Level 5 (Enhanced Triple P)* is an enhanced behavioral family strategy for families in which parenting difficulties are complicated by other sources of family distress (e.g., relationship conflict, parental depression or high levels of stress). Program modules include practice sessions to enhance parenting skills, mood management strategies, stress coping skills, and partner support skills. Enhanced Triple P extends Standard Triple P by adding three to five sessions tailored to the needs of the family.

More than 40,000 service providers around the world have received professional training in Triple P. There is a great deal of empirical evidence that Triple P is effective among culturally diverse populations parenting children with various mental health conditions, including children with attention deficit hyperactivity disorder (ADHD; Aghebati, Gharraee, Hakim Shoshtari, & Gohari, 2014), childhood anxiety disorders (Ozyurt, Gencer, Ozturk, & Ozbek, 2014), intellectual disability (Ashori, Afrooz, Arjmandnia, Pourmohamadreza-Tajrishi, & Ghobbi-Bonab, 2015), and behavioral problems (de Graaf, Speetjens, Smit, de Wolff, & Tavecchio, 2008). All forms of Triple P had moderate to large effects when outcomes were parent-reported child behaviors and parenting, with the exception of Media Triple P, which had small effects (Thomas & Zimmer-Gembeck, 2007).

According to Blueprints, it would cost communities approximately $2,367,393 for Year 1 Triple P start-up costs, mostly covering training of program staff ($1,323,795) and implementation materials ($723,598) to serve 100,000 families at a cost of $23.67 each. Once initial training and technical assistance costs are met, maintaining the program is less expensive. Based on impact, cost, quality of evaluations, and capacity for widespread adoption for large communities, we recommend Triple P as the strongest option for child maltreatment prevention.

12.3.2 Preventing Sibling Violence

Despite the fact that sibling bullying is the most widespread form of family violence, there is a glaring lack of interventions focused on this form of bullying. In 2015, researchers conducted a systematic review on interventions for sibling conflict and aggression (Tucker & Finkelhor, 2017). Of over 5330 identified studies, only five studies of four interventions were included: one study discussed the Fun with Brothers and Sisters program (ages 4–6; Kramer & Radey, 1997), one study discussed the More Fun with Brothers and Sisters Program (ages 4–8; Kennedy & Kramer, 2008), two studies discussed training parents in mediation as a means of decreasing sibling conflict (Siddiquei & Ross, 2004; Smith & Ross, 2007), and one study discussed training siblings in verbal reasoning, assertiveness, and acceptance skills over five sessions (Thomas & Roberts, 2009). The sample sizes of these studies were small, ranging from 20 to 95, and only one study had a 1-month follow-up. Overall, findings indicated that these interventions had the potential to increase emotional regulation, warmth, positivity, apologies, social skills, and conflict management and decrease conflict (Tucker & Finkelhor, 2017). It is important to note that these programs were generally for younger children or to train parents and did not specifically target sibling conflict that would be severe enough to be categorized as bullying. It is clear that research is needed to create and test family-based interventions to help with the problem of sibling bullying.

The More Fun with Sisters and Brothers program (MFWSB) targets emotional competencies and prosocial behaviors in youth ages 4–8 years of age. The program targets seven competencies: (1) initiating play with a sibling, (2) methods for accepting an invitation to play, (3) methods for declining an invitation to play, (4) perspective taking, (5) identifying and discriminating between emotions, (6) regulating emotions, and (7) problem solving/conflict management. The program teaches children how to identify, monitor, evaluate, and modify emotional reactions. Modeling, role-playing, performance feedback, and coaching were used as teaching methods. In one study 95 children were randomly assigned to participate in MFWSB (n = 55) or to a wait list control group (n = 40), parents of MFWSB participants reported that their children engaged in increased levels of warmth (effect size = 0.39) and decreased levels of agonism (e.g., conflict, aggression; effect size = 0.48) and rivalry/competition (effect size = 0.30; these effect sizes are moderate), while youth in the other group remained stable on these behaviors. However, there were no significant changes in negative sibling interactions (Kennedy & Kramer, 2008).

It is clear that research is needed in order to develop additional interventions that target sibling bullying by providing support and training for both parents and children. We recommend public health messaging and curricula development focusing on toxic sibling interactions. Currently, this bullying is brushed off too easily by parents who "choose their battles." Both parents and children need to be educated and aware of the presence of sibling bullying. Parents hold the power in a family and must intervene to protect their children if bullying is occurring in the home. This can be a tricky situation to navigate and seeking professional support from a social worker or therapist might be helpful.

In severe cases, Functional Family Therapy (FFT) would be helpful for selected/indicated families at high risk. FFT, a Blueprints model program, is a short-term family therapy intervention and juvenile diversion program helping at-risk children and delinquent youth to overcome adolescent behavior problems, conduct disorder, substance abuse and delinquency. By the time a sibling is engaged in the juvenile justice system, it may be far too late to prevent sibling bullying, but FFT may lower the risk of siblings going down the same path. With 38 years of research behind it, FFT is designed to improve family communication and supportiveness while decreasing negativity and dysfunctional patterns of behavior. A meta-analysis of effect size for eight evaluations of FFT (Aos et al., 2011) reported a mean unadjusted effect size of −0.59 (medium) and an adjusted mean effect size of −0.32 (small). The average cost per family is $2800, mostly spent on hiring therapists. While this is helpful in working on toxic family patterns, we hope to see more unique emphasis on sibling bullying directly.

12.3.3 Preventing Traditional School-Age Bullying

There are a number of interventions that exist to target bullying and various researchers have conducted systematic reviews and meta-analyses in an attempt to understand if and how these interventions are effective (e.g., Evans, Fraser, & Cotter, 2014; Farrington & Ttofi, 2009). Bullying interventions vary in their success and overall seem to be more effective when implemented outside of the US with homogeneous samples (Evans et al., 2014). Blueprints notes that Positive Action is a model program for preventing bullying, while the KiVa Antibullying program, the Olweus Bullying Prevention Program, and Steps to Respect are noted as promising (the designation of "model program" is reserved for those programs that have the highest level of evidence supporting their effectiveness, and the results have been replicated across communities; "promising programs" also have good results but require additional replication in other communities or more time to show sustainability).

KiVa. We will mention the promising programs first. KiVa includes both universal actions to prevent the occurrence of bullying and indicated actions to intervene in individual bullying cases. The program has three different developmentally appropriate versions for Grades 1–3 (Unit 1), 4–6 (Unit 2), and 7–9 (Unit 3). Blueprints has certified the evaluation evidence for grades 2–6 only, as there was no consistent pattern of results in grades 8–9 with more nonsignificant findings than significant findings and bystander behavior was in the wrong direction. This is problematic because school bullying is at its height in middle school in the US and KiVa has little support for effects at this age. With program designers in Europe, dissemination is problematic for US settings. Instead of recommending KiVa as a whole, we will consider key conceptual components from the program theory that could be translated.

The Olweus Bullying Prevention Program (OBPP). OBPP is arguably the most famous anti-bullying program. It is a universal, multilevel, multicomponent program that is appropriate for all grade levels. Reductions in bullying and victimization are generally positive in evaluation studies, but many results are mixed. The original studies in Norway produced positive results, but US replications have been disappointing with a modest effect size (0.31) for reductions in third graders reporting of bullying others (Blueprints, 2012–2019a; Olweus & Limber, 2010). Fortunately, the program costs are also modest, about $24.56 per student, mostly for training teachers.

Steps to Respect. Steps to Respect is a universal bullying prevention program for elementary school students. The program was designed to reduce bullying and destructive bystander behaviors, increase prosocial beliefs related to bullying, and increase social-emotional skills through a grade appropriate literature unit and other educational materials and lessons. The average effect size for Steps to Respect in an initial study across five social-ecological school context variables was 0.296 (range = 0.212 for staff climate to 0.382 for anti-bullying policies and strategies, indicating small to medium effects; Frey et al., 2005). However, a second study showed small effects and no significant changes in student-reported bullying perpetration and victimization (Brown, Low, Smith, & Haggerty, 2011) with $24 cost per student for curricula materials.

Positive Action (PA). PA is a universal, school-based intervention designed for elementary, middle, and high school students that aims to decrease risk factors (e.g., bullying, violence, substance use, family conflict) and increase protective factors (e.g., academic achievement, school attendance, parent–child bonding; National Registry of Evidence-Based Programs and Practices, 2014). PA is administered throughout the school year 2–3 times per week in brief 15–20 min lessons. The lessons address six main units: (1) Self-Concept—intended to improve student's self-understanding and identity; (2) Positive Actions for Your Body and Mind—designed to foster good hygiene, exercise, and creative thinking skills; (3) Managing Yourself Responsibly—teaches students time and resource management skills; (4) Treating Others the Way You Like to be Treated—teaches positive social skills; (5) Telling Yourself the Truth—teaches self-honesty; and (6) Improving Yourself Continually—teaches students to apply Positive Action skills in all areas of their life and highlights the ongoing and continual process of self-improvement (Positive Action, n.d.). Although PA does not focus solely on decreasing bullying, the lesson content increases skills that help youth engage in positive social interactions and make positive and prosocial decisions. One randomized controlled trial of 14 elementary schools found that students in schools that implemented PA had 37% fewer violence-related behaviors and 41% fewer bullying behaviors compared to control schools (Li et al., 2011). There is substantial PA research studies done in Hawaii (Washburn et al., 2011), Chicago (Li et al., 2011), and rural North Carolina (Guo et al., 2015; Smokowski et al., 2016; Stalker, Qu, Evans, & Smokowski, 2018). Effect sizes are generally medium to large, with clearinghouses considering the program a "model" or "effective." The cost per student is $27.39, which is among the lowest cost for the largest effects in this category. In the rural North Carolina studies of PA that we conducted we found some significant drawbacks to PA implementation. It was exceptionally difficult to have teachers implement a program with over 100 lessons meant to be delivered for 20 min 4 or 5 days a week. Indeed, if students liked a lesson, length often mushroomed to 40 min (i.e., unacceptable to many teachers preparing for testing). Our team streamlined and tailored the standard lessons. Even so, implementation fidelity is a serious concern for consideration. Research has also found that effects do not phase in until about 3 years of intervention. That is a very high dosage of lessons needed to achieve these medium to large effect sizes.

Considering all of these programs, we recommend an eclectic approach that integrates the best ideas and emphasizes highly consistent implementation. In our opinion, the best ideas are:

1. Form an anti-bullying committee consisting of school leaders (shows administrative buy-in), teachers, representatives from student government, and self-nominated students from each grade level. Student government reps are often popular students who may not understand bullying concerns; that is why self-nominated students should be equally represented. The popular students have social influence that should be leveraged for them to speak out against bullying in ways that will be valued by other students. This is similar to getting celebrity endorsements. This committee should try to influence school climate, like in OBPP, but should also mediate restorative resolutions to bullying incidents. Restorative resolutions would emphasize the bully repairing the harm done with apology letters or service to the school community while the victim leaves feeling supported and valued by peers.
2. Provide meaningful roles, beginning as early in school as possible. The meaningful role intervention (Ellis, Gonzalez, Volk, & Embry, 2015) is intriguing and has no start-up cost. School children at the fringes of the social network (i.e., those struggling to fit in and at risk for becoming bullies or victims) are purposely given valued roles in the classroom and school environment (e.g., tending to the class turtle, organizing art supplies). Roles must be meaningful to the student and have some social capital from the class. Problems with bullying are less likely to happen when youth feel like valued contributors to the class and school, are accepted by others, and feel that they have a place and purpose.

3. Promote inclusive sociometry and build valuable team memberships. Sociometry refers to relationships between group members (e.g., some members often are considered popular or highly chosen, some rejected, some ignored). Arguably the most powerful risk factor related to bullying is peer rejection. Teachers and counselors should actively try to counter rejection and isolation, and promote inclusion, by crafting team-building activities that value children for a variety of different traits. In many settings, sports are overvalued and academics, artistic skills, and diverse life experiences are undervalued which creates a "jocks rule" and "nerds hide" dynamic ripe for bullying. The academic environment could be reengineered so that a variety of events make a spectrum of kids feel valued. A team competition could easily consist of kickball, chess, singing or skits, drawing posters, and a science challenge all tallied up with points to show the best multi-skill team. Having multiple categories for selecting team members avoids peer rejections and heightens inclusion. Find ways to value every child's contribution.
4. Teach bystanders to be upstanders. Students provide a very large contribution to school climate. If they decide to not allow bullying behaviors, it is much more powerful than any zero-tolerance administrative policy. Bystanders need to alert adults, teachers, staff, student government reps of bullying threats, and in so doing take control of the creation of positive school atmosphere.
5. Interactive Theater can be very powerful for working with support groups for victims or the overall school population of students. Interactive Theater brings groups of victims (or all students) together to view actors portraying a bullying story of a victim. Seeing a character that shares the victimization experience with some audience members is often easier than talking about one's own personal trauma. Audience members share the common experience of the enactment without having to voice their own traumatic material. After seeing the critical scene once (e.g., a bullying episode), the group facilitator has it played a second time. At critical times, the scene is then stopped and audience members are empowered to change the narrative. They can take the roles onstage and modify the action. The group provides support and coping strategies to build resilience. Changing the scene gives students in the audience a chance for emotional release (catharsis) and an opportunity to plan new behavior that is carried out in the real world. This can teach students to be upstanders, victims how to cope, and bullies can see the consequences of their actions. Interactive theater and sociodrama has been used around the world for more than 100 years (Sternberg & Garcia, 2000).
6. Empathy is vital for preventing bullying. Empathetic children are less likely to bully others because they are able to understand the pain being victimized would cause. Further, empathetic youth are more inclined to intervene as prosocial bystanders when they witness bullying because they are able to put themselves in the victim's shoes and understand how painful it must be to be bullied. Parents can play an active role in enhancing empathy in their children by helping children express their emotional needs and addressing those needs. Helping kids verbalize how they are feeling and then addressing those feelings models empathetic behavior. Parents should help their children think about how other people

are impacted by their actions and words, for example, if Annie hits her little brother, her mother could say: "Annie, how do you think Michael feels when you hit him? How might you feel if you got hit?" Parents should also verbalize how their children's words and behaviors make them feel. For example, "James, it really hurt my feelings when you yelled that you didn't like me, it made me feel sad." In this example, it would be important to help James figure out a way to make his parent feel better, by saying sorry and then thinking about alternative ways to express his feelings. "Next time you are feeling upset James, instead of saying you don't like me, maybe you could say 'I'm feeling really frustrated right now.'" Parents can also use storybooks as a means of talking about and teaching empathy. For example, parents can ask kids: "How do you think this character feels right now?" And then help children figure out based on facial expression how the characters are feeling and how they might feel if they were in the character's position. A school social worker who understands how types of bullying are interconnected may push discussions with perpetrators to new levels by investigating adverse childhood experiences for bullies. Rather than asking the bully, "How do you think Jock felt when you called him terrible names in the cafeteria," the discussion can turn to, "Jock felt humiliated and threatened when you called him terrible names. Was there a time when someone humiliated you and it hurt your feelings? When did that happen to you and who did it?" Bullies often want the impression of power and invulnerability. Asking them about an experience when they were vulnerable is much more powerful than asking them to reverse roles with their victim, providing more insight. The onus for preventing bullying falls on all of us. Collectively, we need to maintain an open dialogue with children about bullying and fostering empathy in children is an important step that parents can make to help prevent bullying.

To summarize, school bullying has had more program development and research activity than other areas of bullying. Even so, currently available programs have small to moderate effects. More advanced prevention initiatives are needed with widely available strategies such as creating bullying committees, giving vulnerable children meaningful roles, creating inclusive group roles, encouraging upstanders, and teaching empathy early on and constantly.

12.3.4 Preventing Cyberbullying

Cyberbullying interventions are relatively new and according to a recent systematic review of cyberbullying interventions, date back to only 2011 or 2012 (Gaffney, Farrington, Espelage, & Ttofi, 2019; Hutson, Kelly, & Militello, 2018). This short duration leaves little time to extensively test the efficacy of such interventions and there is no consensus among researchers about how best to combat cyberbullying (Espelage & Hong, 2017). Further, the majority of existing interventions that target cyberbullying have been implemented in other countries (e.g., Greece, Germany,

Australia, Spain). Of the 24 programs Gaffney et al. (2019) reviewed, only three were implemented in the US (Second Step, i-SAFE internet safety curriculum, Social Networking Safety Promotion, and Cyberbullying Prevention Promotion).

Second Step is a well-known and highly tested social-emotional learning program (SEL) for middle school students that targets risk and protective factors connected to aggression, violence, and substance use. Lesson content focuses on empathy and communication, bullying, cyberbullying, sexual harassment, emotion regulation, problem-solving, and substance abuse prevention (Espelage, Low, van Ryzin, & Polanin, 2015). Although this program does not focus solely on cyberbullying, it teaches many skills that help youth become more empathetic and better decisions makers. Indeed, Second Step was found to reduce delinquent behavior, which in turn resulted in decreased cyberbullying (Espelage et al., 2015).

One simple yet common strategy to prevent cyberbullying is providing educational information to youth, parents, and school personnel on what cyberbullying is and how to avoid being a victim (Espelage & Hong, 2017). Tip sheets and websites (e.g., https://www.stopbullying.gov/cyberbullying/what-is-it/index.html; http://www.cyberbullying.ca/; https://www.prevnet.ca/) are often helpful resources, and Alfors (2010) provides a good overview of cyberbullying websites (Espelage & Hong, 2017). Espelage and Hong (2017), experts in the field of cyberbullying, provide an overview of tips for addressing cyberbulling such as the following: victims should avoid reading messages, parents must be educated about cyberbullying, schools should create and enforce internet policies for students, school faculty should be extensively trained on cyberbullying, and a whole-school prevention effort should be adopted. Cyberbullying interventions are in their nascence, and the majority have not been tested in the US; thus, it is paramount that parents and educators learn about cyberbullying and educate youth about it as well. Given the relatively new phenomenon of cyberbullying it may take a few years for research to catch up with the growing pandemic of cyberbullying. In the meantime, it is vital for parents, teachers, and practitioners to keep an open dialogue with youth about cyberbullying and to remain up to date on cyberbullying research.

12.3.5 Preventing Teen Dating Violence

Blueprints notes one promising program, Safe Dates, that can be implemented to decrease dating violence. Safe Dates is a 10-session dating abuse prevention program for middle and high school students that aims to increase participant knowledge about the differences between healthy and abusive dating in addition to the causes and consequence of dating abuse. Topics of the sessions include defining caring relationships, defining dating abuse, why people abuse, helping friends, overcoming gender stereotypes, equal power through communication, how we feel or how we deal, and preventing sexual assault. In addition to these educational sessions, which are usually conducted in school, there is a community component that provides support groups and activities for youth. Findings indicated that one month after participating in Safe Dates, participants reported 25% less psychological perpetration, 60% less sexual violence perpetration, and 60% less violence perpetrated against a current dating partner compared to the control group. The cost per student is approximately $17.40 (Blue Prints for Healthy Youth Development, 2012–2019d).

Similar to the other forms of violence and bullying previously discussed, parents should take an active role in opening up a dialogue with their children about dating violence. Making sure that youth are aware of what dating violence is and how it presents is an important step in combatting this problem. As much as possible, parents should try to meet and get to know their children's dating partners and should check in periodically with their children about their dating partners. Teenagers are often incredibly private and can bristle at parental questions; however, asking questions shows children that their parents are interested about their lives and care about what is going on. This monitoring is particularly critical when teenagers are meeting potential partners over the Internet with little background information.

12.3.6 *Preventing Hazing*

Blueprints does not review any hazing interventions as few interventions targeting hazing exist. However, the University of Arizona Life Skills Program and the National Collegiate Athletic Association created a program called Step Up! Be a leader, Make a Difference. This program is a prosocial behavior and bystander intervention program that aims to educate students about how to proactively help others. Step Up! focuses on increasing awareness of helping behaviors, increasing student motivation to help, and on developing skills and confidence to help in a variety of situations students might encounter including academics, alcohol, anger, depression, discrimination, disordered eating, gambling, relationship abuse, sexual assault, and hazing. The content on hazing defines what hazing is and provides example scenarios with questions to prompt discussion and learning, considerations to keep in mind when reading the scenarios, action steps to take if faced with hazing, and a list of resources (Step Up!, n.d.).

In addition, there are some helpful websites that provide hazing resources and education. For example, Hazingprevention.org is a national, nonprofit organization that aims to help prevent hazing through education, advocacy, and community engagement and includes online hazing prevention training (hazingprevention.org, 2018). In addition, Stop Hazing (Stophazing.org, 2019) is another educational website that provides hazing prevention resources including a hazing prevention toolkit for school campus professionals, access to state anti-hazing laws, webinars, infographics (information about hazing with pictures that could be printed and posted around a school campus), and interactive data. Although these websites are helpful, a need clearly exists for additional interventions focused on hazing. These interventions should be evaluated and added to evidenced-based archives.

12.3.7 *Preventing Intimate Partner Violence*

Domestic violence is a difficult problem to resolve. A woman in a domestic violence situation will leave an average of seven times before permanently terminating the relationship. In that time, she and her children are at risk for serious physical, psychological, and emotional trauma. There are supports available. For example, the National Domestic Violence Hotline (1-800-799-7233) is available for anonymous help and support. Further, there are multiple trauma-focused interventions for survivors of domestic violence (see Warshaw, Sullivan, & Rivera, 2013 for a review). There are also a number of batterer intervention programs; however, the research on their results is quite mixed. Some studies show that participation resulted in reduced official reports of rearrest, victim reports of reduced rearrests, self-reported improvement in women's lives, and decreased future violence. However, other studies showed high recidivism rates for domestic violence even after attending batterer intervention programs (Ferraro, 2017). Helping victims of intimate partner violence connect with a social worker or therapist is an important step to help protect victims. Mental health workers are trained in safety assessment and can help victims seek safety and/or create a safety plan.

Domestic violence is an example of bullying across the life span that requires strong laws and policies that protect victims. Unlike school-age bullying, there is not a dominant institution for launching prevention programs. Programs in shelters and mental health agencies, while helpful, are simply too late to prevent victimization trauma. Public health leaders need to work with lawmakers to put effective safeguards in place while concurrently raise awareness about victimization through information dissemination and media messaging.

12.3.8 *Preventing Workplace Bullying*

Few interventions exist that address workplace bullying. Indeed, a recent systematic review uncovered only five studies of four workplace bullying interventions. Two studies examined the Civility, Respect, and Engagement in the Workforce (CREW) intervention, an organizational/employer level intervention, the goal of which is to assist work units in identifying their strengths and areas for improvement in regard to civility. There are weekly workgroup conversations about civility and a comprehensive educational toolkit. Results indicated a 5% increase in civility from baseline to 6- and 12-month follow-up and a decrease in number of days absent the previous month at 6-month follow-up. A multilevel intervention looked at the effectiveness of a combination of policy communication, stress management training, and negative behavior awareness training; however, this did not result in decreased bullying victimization, in fact, bullying victimization was 13.6% prior to the intervention and 14.3% after the intervention. In terms of individual–job interface level interventions, one cognitive behavioral intervention resulted in no differences in rates of perpetration or victimization before or after the intervention. And another study used expressive writing as an intervention, which resulted in decreased incivility perpetration, but there was not change in incivility victimization (see Gillen, Sinclair, Kernohan, Begley, & Luyben, 2017 for a review).

Taken together, few workplace bullying interventions exist and those that exist have minimal impact on decreasing workplace bullying. Given the tremendously negative impact workplace bullying has on individual physical and mental health, work productivity, work attendance, and work atmosphere it is imperative that researchers and practitioners focus efforts on creating and testing additional workplace bullying interventions. Programs should target organization leaders because these executives set the tone for workplace interactions, create and enforce (or ignore) relevant policies, and are in control of the power to change culture and climate. Federal policies primarily protect against sexual harassment, leaving 80% of workplace bullying legal and little recourse for other types of victims. Indeed, most victims and witnesses never report offenses for fear of retaliation and lack of responsiveness. Responsive leaders who do not protect bullies, even when perpetrators are superstars in the office, can make an enormous difference in workplace bullying. Employers must set the tone for workplace climate and model civility.

12.3.9 Preventing Elder Maltreatment

One key way to prevent elder maltreatment is by identifying it. Many maltreated elders suffer in silence, thus, screening by healthcare providers by interviewing the elderly could be helpful. However, difficulty arises due to a lack of valid and reliable screening tools, the fact that the abuser often accompanies the elder person to appointments, and the victim might be too frail or confused to answer questions accurately. Therefore, clinicians should be well educated on elder maltreatment (through workplace training on elder abuse) and should be aware and sensitive to the signs and symptoms; clinicians should rely on their knowledge as opposed to screening instruments for elder abuse identification (see Pillemer, Mueller-Johnson, Mock, Suitor, & Lachs, 2007 for a review). In addition, all states have adult protective services that can be called for help and support in abusive situations; this service serves as tertiary prevention and could help extricate the elderly from an already abusive situation. Caregiver support interventions to lower stress are also a potential means of preventing elder abuse. Some services help by offering respite care, caregiver support groups, housekeeping, meal preparations, and day care to give the caregiver a break and relieve stress. It is also important to educate potential victims about elder abuse (see Pillemer et al., 2007 for a review). Taken together, preventing elder abuse is a difficult task that requires health care education as well as educating the elderly.

12.3.10 Preventing Large-Scale Bullying

Large-scale bullying is difficult to eradicate, as is abundantly evidenced by the inequalities, social conflicts, and genocidal wars happening around the world. Reducing bullying of all kinds is challenging for two primary reasons: the joy of power and the power of prejudice. Both of these reasons can be linked to inherent, perhaps primal, drives and evolutionary psychology. The joy of power comes when a person or group feels dominant and in control of the environment. There is a deep-seated survival need to control resources such as land, territory, food sources, and mating resources that is encoded in our Neanderthal brain regions (i.e., the amygdala and autonomic nervous system). Successfully seizing food, mates, and safe territory protects the tribe and floods human brains with endorphins that make you feel good, thus creating the joy of power. Indeed, the history of human civilization is largely a chronicle of conflict and war with competitive sports for leisure time. The oldest cave paintings reflect competition in battle, wrestling, hunting, swimming, and fighting. The joy of power comes from winning, which is a biological impulse that is difficult to temper.

The power of prejudice can be seen as the flip side of the joy of power. If our biology wants our team or tribe ("us") to win, our impulse is equally as strong to have others (i.e., foreigners, visitors, strangers, the "not us") to lose. Social science shows that people tend to choose friends and mates who are similar to themselves; this is called propinquity (e.g., proximity and similarity, sameness, "birds of a feather"). Our primal brains also judge others who are different as threat, generating prejudice. These others might stand in our way or threaten our joy of power, triggering competitive individual and group impulses. Indeed, emerging neuroscience suggests that some people have stronger brain responses around threatening stimuli and these individuals tend to also hold conservative political and group-based ideologies. Feeling threatened from outsiders breeds strong group affiliations for protection. Others who have less sensitive responses to threat tend to hold liberal beliefs and display more empathy. Interestingly, this research has been extended to examine brain responses to disgust (appropriately labeled the science of "disgustology"). When shown photos of disgusting stimuli, such as garbage, vomit, and feces, some people have stronger reactions of disgust or revulsion. The emerging science shows individuals who experience disgust more strongly tend to hold more conservative beliefs, feel threatened perhaps in unconscious fear of contamination (i.e., germs or disease), and make harsher moral judgments. Their reaction to cope is to stay within the similarity of their social circle and minimize potential threats from foreigners or outsiders who may carry disease. High disgust sensitivity is relevant to bullying because individuals with these strong gut reactions see strangers, outsiders, foreigners, and others not like them as threats and this revulsion response prompts them to exercise their power to isolate and eradicate the threat (i.e., victim). This line of reasoning is interesting because so much of bullying interactions are based on the victim being different (e.g., too short, too tall, too skinny, too fat, too smart, too dumb) and difference attributes are framed with disgust (e.g., "you stink," "your pimples are disgusting"). These revulsion reactions become group-based (e.g., immigrants are criminals who will take our jobs. Let's build a wall!). That creates the power of prejudice.

Preventing group-based bullying requires reducing both the joy of power and the power of prejudice. This happens through social action and legislation; individuals speaking out and banding together in advocacy against social inequalities. For humiliated victims whose inclination is to hide, it is extremely difficult to raise their voices against powerful bullies. Most of the time speaking up can be an exercise in frustration, when there is no response and a strong risk for further degradation, when there is active retaliation. However, personal health and social justice is only made possible by shining light on disparities, reducing feelings of threat, and increasing empathy. Bullies lose when victims reject the power differential and toxic messages, standing up with conviction and courage. Aggregate these courageous individuals into a community and further up into a social movement and change, albeit sometimes incremental and slow, can happen. Women won the right to vote, own property, and attend college after a century and a half of fighting for these rights. Minorities won civil rights. The gay and lesbian community won the right to marry. All of these are examples of successes, but also each is a work in progress, tenuous victories with much more to address. The only group-level bullying prevention program we know of is education, which is modestly effective in the short run but has large effects over long periods of time.

12.4 Conclusion

We strongly assert that bullying across the life span should be viewed as a public health priority, if not a pandemic. With a conservative estimate of 25%, the prevalence of bullying is far too high, eclipsing many other social problems. The annual costs to society are equally shocking and unacceptable. Without effective prevention programs widely disseminated, bullying victimization and perpetration are antecedents to short- and long-term health problems, including increased stress, trauma, anxiety, depression, aggression, violence, substance use, obesity, smoking, heart and lung disease, criminality and suicidal behavior. We recommend a multicomponent package of anti-bullying prevention programs, such as the Positive Parenting Program (Triple P), Positive Action, and Safe Dates; however, these programs tend to have modest effects. New initiatives integrating an array of creative ideas are greatly needed.

References

Aghebati, A., Gharraee, B., Hakim Shoshtari, M., & Gohari, M. R. (2014). Triple P-Positive Parenting Program for mothers of ADHD children. *Iranian Journal of Psychiatry Behavioral Sciences, 8*(1), 59–65.

Alfors, R. (2010). Many sources, one theme: Analysis of cyberbullying prevention and intervention websites. *Journal of Social Sciences, 6*(4), 515–522.

Aos, S., Lee, S., Drake, E., Pennucci, A., Klima, T., Miller, M., … Burley, M. (2011, July). *Return on investment: Evidence-based options to improve statewide outcomes* (Document No. 11-07-1201A). Olympia, WA: Washington State Institute for Public Policy.

Arseneault, L., Walsh, E., Trzeniewski, K., Newcombe, R., Caspi, A., & Moffitt, T. E. (2006). Bullying victimization uniquely contributes to adjustment problems in young children: A nationally representative cohort study. *Pediatrics, 118*(1), 130–138.

Ashori, M., Afrooz, G., Arjmandnia, A., Pourmohamadreza-Tajrishi, M., & Ghobbi-Bonab, B. (2015). The effectiveness of group positive parenting Program (Triple P) on the mother-child relationships with intellectual disability. *Iranian Journal of Public Health, 44*(2), 290–291.

Blue Prints for Healthy Youth Development. (2012–2019a). *Blueprints*. Retrieved from https://www.blueprintsprograms.org/

Blue Prints for Healthy Youth Development. (2012–2019b). *Nurse-family partnership*. Retrieved from https://www.blueprintsprograms.org/factsheet/nurse-family-partnership

Blue Prints for Healthy Youth Development. (2012–2019c). *Triple P system*. Retrieved from https://www.blueprintsprograms.org/factsheet/triple-p-system

Blue Prints for Healthy Youth Development. (2012–2019d). *Safe dates*. Retrieved from https://www.blueprintsprograms.org/factsheet/safe-dates

Boodman, S. G. (2006, May 16). Gifted and tormented. *The Washington Post*. Retrieved October 15, 2018.

Brown, E. C., Low, S., Smith, B. H., & Haggerty, K. P. (2011). Outcomes from a school-randomized control trial of Steps to Respect. *School Psychology Review, 40*(3), 423–443.

Centers for Disease Control and Prevention. (2012). *Introduction to epidemiology*. Retrieved from https://www.cdc.gov/ophss/csels/dsepd/ss1978/lesson1/section11.html

Centers for Disease Control and Prevention. (2019). *Preventing multiple forms of violence: A strategic vision for connecting the dots*. Atlanta, GA: Division of Violence Prevention, National Center for Injury Prevention and Control. Retrieved from https://www.cdc.gov/violenceprevention/overview/strategicvision.html

Centers for Disease Control and Prevention. (n.d.). *Sortable risk factors and health indicators*. Retrieved from https://sortablestats.cdc.gov/#/summary

Cronholm, P. F., Forke, C. M., Wade, R., Bair-Merrit, M. H., Davis, M., Harkins-Schwarz, M., & Fein, J. A. (2015). Adverse childhood experiences: Expanding the concept of adversity. *American Journal of Preventive Medicine, 49*(3), 354–361.

de Graaf, I., Speetjens, P., Smit, F., de Wolff, M., & Tavecchio, L. (2008). Effectiveness of the Triple P Positive Parenting Program on behavioral problems in children. *Behavior Modifications, 32*(5), 714–735.

Dong, M., Anda, R. F., Felitti, V. J., Dube, S. R., Williamson, D. F., Thompson, T. J., & Giles, H. (2004). The interrelatedness of multiple forms of childhood abuse, neglect, and household dysfunction. *Child Abuse Neglect, 28*(7), 771–784.

Ellis, B. J., Gonzalez, J., Volk, A. A., & Embry, D. D. (2015). The meaningful roles intervention: An evolutionary approach to reducing bullying and increasing prosocial behavior. *Journal of Research on Adolescence, 26*, 622–637.

Espelage, D. L., & Hong, J. S. (2017). Cyberbullying prevention and intervention efforts: Current knowledge and future directions. *Canadian Journal of Psychiatry, 62*(6), 374–380.

Espelage, D. L., Low, S., van Ryzin, M. J., & Polanin, J. R. (2015). Clinical trial of second step middle school program: Impact on bullying, cyberbullying, homophobic teasing, and sexual harassment perpetration. *School Psychology Review, 44*(4), 464–479.

Evans, C. B. R., Fraser, M. L., & Cotter, K. L. (2014). The effectiveness of school-based bullying prevention programs: A systematic review. *Aggression and Violent Behavior, 19*, 532–544.

Farrington, D. P., & Ttofi, M. M. (2009). School-based programs to reduce bullying and victimization. *Campbell Systematic Reviews*. https://doi.org/10.4073/csr.2009.6

Felitti, V. J., Anda, R. F., Nordenberg, D., Williamson, D. F., Spitz, A. M., Edwards, V., & Marks, J. S. (1998). Relationship of childhood abuse and household dysfunction to many of the leading causes of death in adults: The adverse childhood experiences (ACE) study. *American Journal of Preventive Medicine, 14*, 245–258.

Ferraro, K. J. (2017). *Current research on batterer intervention programs and implications for policy*. Battered Women's Justice Project. Retrieved from https://www.bwjp.org/assets/batterer-intervention-paper-final-2018.pdf

Finkelhor, D., Shattuck, A., Turner, H., & Hamby, S. (2013). Improving the Adverse Childhood Experiences Study Scale. *JAMA Pediatrics, 167*(1), 70–75.

Finkelhor, D., Turner, H., Hamby, S., & Ormrod, R. (2011). *Polyvictimization: Children's exposure to multiple types of violence, crime, and abuse*. Washington, DC: U.S. Department of Justice, Office of Justice Programs, Office of Juvenile Justice and Delinquency Prevention.

Finkelhor, D., Turner, H. A., Ormrod, R., Hamby, S. L., & Kracke, K. (2009). *Children's exposure to violence: A comprehensive national survey*. Washington, DC: U.S. Department of Justice, Office of Justice Programs, Office of Juvenile Justice and Delinquency Prevention.

Foshee, V. A., Reyes, L. M., Tharp, A. T., Chang, L., Ennett, S. T., Simon, S. T., … Suchindran, C. (2015). Shared longitudinal predictors of physical peer and dating violence. *Journal of Adolescent Health, 56*(1), 106–112.

Fowler, P. J., Tompsett, C. J., Braciszewski, J. M., Jacques-Tiura, A. J., & Baltes, B. B. (2009). Community violence: A meta-analysis on the effect of exposure and mental health outcomes of children and adolescents. *Developmental Psychopathology, 21*(1), 227–259.

Frey, K. S., Hirschstein, J. L., Snell, J. L., Van Schoiack Edstrom, L., MacKenzie, E. P., & Broderick, C. J. (2005). Reducing playground bullying and supporting beliefs: An experimental trial of the Steps to Respect program. *Developmental Psychology, 41*(3), 479–491.

Gaffney, H., Farrington, D. P., Espelage, D. L., & Ttofi, M. M. (2019). Are cyberbullying intervention and prevention programs effective? A systematic and meta-analytical review. *Aggression and Violent Behavior, 45*, 134–153.

Gilbert, L. K., Breiding, M. J., Merrick, M. T., Thompson, W. W., Ford, D. C., Dhingra, S. S., & Parks, S. E. (2015). Childhood adversity and adult chronic disease: An update from ten states and the District of Columbia, 2010. *American Journal of Preventive Medicine, 48*(3), 345–349.

Gillen, P. A., Sinclair, M., Kernohan, W. G., Begley, C. M., & Luyben, A. G. (2017). Interventions for prevention of bullying in the workplace (review). *Cochrane Database of Systematic Reviews*, (1), CD009778.

Guo, S., Wu, Q., Smokowski, P. R., Bacallao, M., Evans, C. B. R., & Cotter, K. L. (2015). A longitudinal evaluation of the Positive Action program in a low-income, racially diverse, rural county: Effects on self-esteem, school hassles, aggression, and internalizing symptoms. *Journal of Youth and Adolescence, 44*, 2337–2358.

Hamby, S., & Grych, J. (2013). *The web of violence: Exploring connections among different forms of interpersonal violence and abuse*. New York, NY: Springer Briefs in Sociology.

Hazingprevention.org. (2018). *Who we are*. Retrieved from https://hazingprevention.org/home/about/who-we-are/

Herrenkohl, T. I., Sousa, C., Tajima, E. A., Herrnkohl, R. C., & Moylan, C. A. (2008). Intersection of child abuse and children's exposure to domestic violence. *Trauma, Violence, & Abuse, 9*(2), 84–99.

Highmark Foundation. (n.d.). *The cost benefit of bullying prevention: A first-time analysis of savings*. Retrieved from https://www.highmarkfoundation.org/pdf/publications/HMK_Bullying%20Report_final.pdf

Hillis, S., Mercy, J. A., & Saul, J. R. (2016). The enduring impact of violence against children. *Psychology, Health & Medicine, 22*(4), 393–405.

Hutson, E., Kelly, S., & Militello, L. K. (2018). Systematic review of cyberbullying interventions for youth and parents with implications for evidence-based practice. *Worldviews on Evidence-Based Nursing, 15*(1), 72–79.

Jennings, W. G., Piquero, A. R., & Reingle, J. M. (2012). On the overlap between victimization and offending: A review of the literature. *Aggressive and Violent Behavior, 17*(1), 16–26.

Kaminski, J. W., Valle, L. A., Filene, J. H., & Boyle, C. L. (2008). A meta-analytic review of components associated with parent training program effectiveness. *Journal of Abnormal Child Psychology, 36*(4), 567–589. https://doi.org/10.1007/s10802-007-9201-9

Kennedy, D. K., & Kramer, L. (2008). Improving emotion regulation and sibling relationship quality: The More Fun with Sisters and Brothers Program. *Family Relations, 57*, 567–578.

Kramer, L., & Radey, C. (1997). Improving sibling relationships among young children: A social skills training model. *Family Relations, 46*, 237–246.

Li, K. K., Washburn, I., DuBois, D. L., Vuchinich, S., Ji, P., Brechling, V., … Flay, B. R. (2011). Effects of the Positive Action programme on problem behaviors in elementary school students: A match-pair randomised control trial in Chicago. *Psychology and Health, 26*(2), 187–204.

Lowell, D. I., Carter, A. S., Godoy, L., Paulicin, B., & Briggs-Gowan, M. J. (2011). A randomized controlled trial of Child FIRST: A comprehensive home-based intervention translating research into early childhood practice. *Child Development, 82*(1), 193–208.

Lundahl, B. I., Risser, H. J., & Lovejoy, M. C. (2006). A meta-analysis of parent training: Moderators and follow-up effects. *Clinical Psychology Review, 26*(1), 86–104.

Menard, S. (2002). *Short- and long-term consequences of adolescent victimization. Youth Violence Research Bulletin*. Washington, DC: U.S. Department of Justice, Office of Justice Programs, Office of Juvenile Justice and Delinquency Prevention. Retrieved from https://www.ncjrs.gov/pdffiles1/ojjdp/191210.pdf

Merrick, M. T., Ford, D. C., Ports, K. A., & Guinn, A. S. (2018). Prevalence of adverse childhood experiences from the 2011–2014 behavioral risk factor surveillance system in 23 states. *JAMA Pediatrics*. Retrieved from https://jamanetwork.com/journals/jamapediatrics/fullarticle/2702204

Metzler, M., Merrick, M. T., Klevens, J., Ports, K. A., & Ford, D. C. (2017). Adverse childhood experiences and life opportunities: Shifting the narrative. *Children and Youth Services Review, 72*, 141–149.

National Registry of Evidence-Based Programs and Practices. (2014). *Positive action*. Retrieved from http://www.nrepp.samhsa.gov/ViewIntervention.aspx?id=400

Olds, D. L., & Kitzman, H. (1990). Can home visitation improve the health of women and children at environmental risk? *Pediatrics, 86*, 108–116.

Olds, D. L., & Kitzman, H. (1993). Review of research on home visiting for pregnant women and parents of young children. *The Future of Children: Home Visiting, 3*, 53–92.

Olweus, D., & Limber, S. P. (2010). Bullying in school: Evaluation and dissemination of the Olweus Bullying Prevention Program. *American Journal of Orthopsychiatry, 80*(1), 124–134. https://doi.org/10.1111/j.1939-0025.2010.01015.x

Ozyurt, G., Gencer, O., Ozturk, Y., & Ozbek, A. (2014). Long term effectiveness of Triple P Positive Parenting Program on childhood anxiety disorders: A randomized controlled trial. *European Neuropsychopharmacology, 24*, S613.

Pillemer, K. A., Mueller-Johnson, K. U., Mock, S. E., Suitor, J. J., & Lachs, M. S. (2007). Interventions to prevent elder mistreatment. In L. S. Doll, S. E. Bonzo, J. A. Mercy, D. A. Sleet, & E. N. Hass (Eds.), *Handbook of injury and violence prevention* (pp. 241–254). New York, NY: Springer.

Positive Action. (n.d.) *Positive Action overview*. Retrieved from https://www.positiveaction.net/

Prinz, R. J., Sanders, M. R., Shapiro, C. J., Whitaker, D. J., & Lutzker, J. R. (2009). Population-based prevention of child maltreatment: The U.S. Triple P System Population Trial. *Prevention Science, 10*, 1–12.

Sandler, I. N., Schoenfelder, E. N., Wolchik, S. A., & MacKinnon, D. P. (2011). Long-term impact of prevention programs to promote effective parenting: Lasting effects but uncertain processes. *Annual Review of Psychology, 62*, 299–329. https://doi.org/10.1146/annurev.psych.121208.131619

Shonkoff, J. P. (2016). Capitalizing on advances in science to reduce the health consequences of early childhood adversity. *JAMA Pediatrics, 170*(10), 1003–1007.

Siddiquei, A., & Ross, H. (2004). Mediation as a method of parent intervention in children's disputes. *Journal of Family Psychology, 18*, 147–159.

Smith, J., & Ross, H. (2007). Training parents to mediate sibling disputes affects children's negotiation and conflict understanding. *Child Development, 78*, 790–805.

Smokowski, P. R., Guo, S., Wu, Q., Evans, C. B. R., Cotter, K. L., & Bacallao, M. (2016). Evaluating dosage effects for the Positive Action program: How implementation impacts internalizing symptoms, aggression, school hassles, and self-esteem. *American Journal of Orthopsychiatry*. https://doi.org/10.1037/ort0000167

Stalker, K. C., Qu, Q., Evans, C. B. R., & Smokowski, P. R. (2018). The impact of the positive action program on substance use, aggression, and psychological functioning: Is school climate a mechanism of change? *Children and Youth Services Review, 84*, 143–151.

Statistics Solutions. (2019). *Effect size*. Retrieved from https://www.statisticssolutions.com/statistical-analyses-effect-size/

Step Up! (n.d.). *Hazing*. Retrieved from http://stepupprogram.org/topics/hazing/

Sternberg, P., & Garcia, A. (2000). *Sociodrama: Who's in your shoes?* (2nd ed.). West Port, CT: Praeger.

Stop Hazing. (2019). *Stop hazing: Prevention through education*. Retrieved from https://www.stophazing.org/hazing-prevention-resources/

Sum, A., Khatiwada, I., & McLaughlin, J. (2008). An assessment of the labor market, income, social, health, civic, incarceration, and fiscal consequences of dropping out of high school: Findings for Michigan adults in the 21st century. Unpublished report. C.S. Mott Foundation: Flint, MI. Online, available: http://www.gongwer.com/public/Mottreportentire.pdf.

Thomas, B. W., & Roberts, M. W. (2009). Sibling conflict resolution skills: Assessment and training. *Journal of Child & Family Studies, 18*, 447–453.

Thomas, R., & Zimmer-Gembeck, M. J. (2007). Behavioral outcomes of Parent-Child Interaction Therapy and Triple P-Positive Parenting Program: A review and meta-analysis. *Journal of Abnormal Child Psychology, 35*, 475–495.

Tucker, C. J., & Finkelhor, D. (2017). The state of interventions for sibling conflict and aggression: A systematic review. *Trauma, Violence, & Abuse, 18*, 396–406.

Warshaw, C., Sullivan, C. M., & Rivera, E. A. (2013). *A systematic review of trauma-focused interventions for domestic violence*. National Center on Domestic Violence, Trauma, & Mental Health. Retrieved from http://www.nationalcenterdvtraumamh.org/wp-content/uploads/2013/03/NCDVTMH_EBPLitReview2013.pdf

Washburn, I. J., Acock, A., Vuchinich, S., Snyder, F., Li, K. K., Ji, P., … Flay, B. R. (2011). Effects of a social-emotional and character development program on the trajectory of behaviors associated with social-emotional and character development: Findings from three randomized trials. *Prevention Science, 12*(3), 314–323.

Wilkins, N., Tsao, B., Hertz, M., Davis, R., & Klevens, J. (2014). *Connecting the dots: An overview of the links among multiple forms of violence*. Atlanta, GA: National Center for Injury Prevention and Control, Centers for Disease Control and Prevention Oakland, CA: Prevention Institute.

Index

© Springer Nature Switzerland AG 2019

P. R. Smokowski, C. B. R. Evans, *Bullying and Victimization Across the Lifespan*, https://doi.org/10.1007/978-3-030-20293-4

MIX
Papier aus verantwortungsvollen Quellen
Paper from responsible sources
FSC® C105338

If you have any concerns about our products,
you can contact us on
ProductSafety@springernature.com

In case Publisher is established outside the EU,
the EU authorized representative is:
Springer Nature Customer Service Center GmbH
Europaplatz 3, 69115 Heidelberg, Germany

Printed by Libri Plureos GmbH
in Hamburg, Germany